ADULT SEVERE
MENTAL ILLNESS

To

Annie-Louise, Rosalind, Laurie and Wendy

ADULT SEVERE
MENTAL ILLNESS

Edited by

Dr Alain Gregoire MB, BS, DRCOG, MRCPsych

Consultant and Honorary Senior Lecturer in
Psychiatry

GMM

© 2000

Greenwich Medical Media Ltd.
137 Euston Road
London
NW1 2AA

ISBN 1 900 151 52 9

First Published 2000

A catalogue record for this book is available from the British Library

Production and Design by
Saxon Graphics Limited, Derby

Printed in the UK by
the Alden Group

**Visit our website at
www.greenwich-medical.co.uk**

CONTENTS

FOREWORDS vii

PREFACE xi

CONTRIBUTORS xiii

1   DEFINING SEVERE MENTAL ILLNESS 1
Andrew Barker and Alain Gregoire

2   SCHIZOPHRENIA 11
Robin McCreadie

3   AFFECTIVE DISORDERS 33
David S. Baldwin

4   ANXIETY DISORDERS 53
Caroline Bell, Hugh Middleton, Pam Jezzard-Clark and David Nutt

5   EATING DISORDERS 85
Janet Treasure and Simone Fox

6   SOMATOFORM DISORDERS 109
Christopher Bass

7   SEVERE MENTAL ILLNESS IN OLD AGE 123
Sarah Craig and Alistair Burns

8   PERSONALITY DISORDERS – WHAT ROLE
FOR THE MENTAL HEALTH SERVICES? 155
Connor Duggan

9   UNDERSTANDING THE NEED 177
Graham Thornicroft, Sonia Johnson, Michael Phelan and Mike Slade

10   MODELS OF CARE FOR SEVERE MENTAL
ILLNESS 201
Richard Ford and Matt Muijen

11   POLICY DEVELOPMENT FOR SEVERE
MENTAL ILLNESS: THE UK EXPERIENCE 231
Amanda Reynolds, John Bindman and Graham Thornicroft

12 MODELS OF MENTAL HEALTHCARE FOR THE ELDERLY 243
Sube Banerjee

13 FORENSIC PSYCHIATRY SERVICES 257
Huw Stone and Amanda Taylor

14 SERVICES FOR SEVERE SOMATOFORM DISORDERS 283
Eleanor J. Feldman

15 PSYCHOLOGICAL APPROACHES TO PSYCHOTIC ILLNESS 293
Zaffer Iqbal and Max Birchwood

16 SUICIDE PREVENTION 321
Louis Appleby and Tim Amos

17 MENTALLY ILL PARENTS 343
Alain Gregoire

18 MONITORING EFFECTIVENESS AND INCREASING KNOWLEDGE: EDUCATION, AUDIT AND RESEARCH 367
Jed Boardman

FOREWORD

This is not a textbook; or perhaps it is more accurate to say that it is a novel kind of textbook. Despite the aspirations of their authors, traditional textbooks are read mainly by candidates for examinations, and their content is often geared more or less explicitly to the syllabus of an examination. This multi-author volume is written not for examination candidates but for those who are responsible either for providing or for commissioning services for people with 'severe mental illness'.

The roles of commissioners and providers are complementary, and both need to understand the other's priorities and assumptions, and the constraints under which they are acting. At times providers need to stand back from immediate service pressures to consider whether there might be more effective or cost effective ways of meeting the demands upon them, and to consider how analogous services in other part of the country, or abroad, are organised and delivered. Commissioners, on the other hand, need to understand the perspective of the psychiatrists and other mental health professionals responsible for existing services. The latter will have a clear view, based on their own clinical experience and the wider literature, of current needs and demands, which aspects of these needs and demands are being met and which are not, what constraints are imposed by a shortage of trained staff or equipment and what views are not always the same as those of patients and carers, or indeed those of ministers and departmental officials, but they are generally firmly grounded in clinical realities, and so need to be understood and taken seriously.

Psychiatric symptoms of various kinds are extremely common. The survey of the adult population in Britain conducted by the Office of Population Censuses and Surveys (OPCS) in 1993–93 established that, in any given week, 14% of the population had clinically significant symptoms, and surveys in other countries have generated similar findings. Although these symptoms are often short-lived, and never brought to the attention even of primary medical services, they are, almost by definition, troublesome enough to justify clinical attention, and therefore constitute a huge potential demand for mental health services. It was against this background that the term 'severe mental illness' was coined – to embrace all the most severe and handicapping forms of psychiatric morbidity on which the attention of specialised mental health services ought to be focused. It is, of course, easier to see the need for such a term than to provide it with a precise definition; Dr Barker and Dr Gregoire discuss the problem in the first chapter of this book and conclude that, in the absence of an agreed definition, it is probably best to accept a variety of local definitions, provided they are based on the general principles set out by the Department of Health in 1995. The next six chapters of the book describe the main kinds of 'severe mental illness' from a practical rather than a theoretical perspective. The final ten chapters describe the ways in which services for people suffering from these disorders, and their carers, are, or could be, planned, organised, delivered and audited. All of them are written by experts who are thoroughly familiar with the realities of the contemporary National Health Service as well as with service needs and the aspirations of patients and carers.

This book was conceived shortly after the UK Health Departments designated mental health as a priority topic for the NHS, along with cancer and heart disease. More recently the Secretary of State has committed an additional £700 million over three years to the development of mental health services for adults of working age, and also published a National Service Framework for Mental Health setting comprehensive and ambitious standards against which the performance of the NHS and social services in England are to be measured. The book is therefore appearing at a time of unique importance and opportunity both to the commissioners and providers of services. It should be invaluable to both of them.

Robert Kendell

Formerly President of the Royal College of Psychiatrists
and Chief Medical Officer for Scotland

FOREWORD

Most countries in the world are undergoing mental health reform to a greater or lesser extent; reform from old style custodial and institutional care and/or community neglect to care which is local, needs-led, in as least restrictive an environment as is compatible with the health and safety of the affected individual, their family and the public. Many countries are also contemplating reform of the legislative framework so that it supports appropriate care in the community, enabling professionals to deliver care in flexible settings with appropriate attention to human rights. Both these movements require reform of other areas – reform of training for mental health professionals and primary care workers so that they are adequately equipped to tackle mental health needs in their country; and formation or reform of the intersectoral links that are needed to deliver mental health care (primary and secondary health care, social care, housing, welfare benefits, criminal justice system, education and industry).

This book addresses the need for training of mental health professionals, managers and planners of specialist services.

Even the richest of countries cannot afford anything like sufficient specialists to tackle the whole range of mental disorders. It therefore makes sense to target specialists on those with greatest needs, and to support and resource primary care to tackle those with less severe needs.

This book is a highly readable account of the role of specialist services in tackling those with severe mental illness – not of course just psychosis, although that is a major element, but also severe neurotic disorders, suicidality, dementia and personality disorders. Of interest throughout the book is an holistic approach to assessment and treatment, and the importance of disability, duration and distress in assessment and treatment, as well as of diagnosis itself.

Professor Rachel Jenkins
Director, WHO Collaborating Centre
Institute of Psychiatry
London

PREFACE

Delivering the best possible mental healthcare is an extraordinarily complex challenge. Not only are we dealing with disorders of the human brain, the most complex structure in the universe, but also we are treating dysfunction of the mind, an entity with no concrete form yet which is the essence of our being, arising from the interaction between the brain and every aspect of its environment. Our understanding of the normal brain and mind is at best patchy and probably in its infancy: we cannot be sure of how developed our knowledge is as we do not even know how much there is to know. Yet there are further levels of complexity to the task as clinical, research, organisational, philosophical, social, economic and political issues abound in this field of healthcare, possibly more than any other. Severe mental illness not only affects the sufferers with symptoms and disability but also has effects on all the people around them and on the rest of society. These are not simple one-way effects but rather interactive ones which are fluid over time. Thus, the individual's reaction to their suffering, the disabilities they develop and the reactions of others have feedback effects on the course and nature of the mental illness. This is a challenge for all those involved in the provision of services aimed at alleviating or preventing mental illness to which we cannot claim to have found the best solutions. However, it is not just our rudimentary knowledge which limits the effectiveness of mental healthcare: even in countries with relatively well-developed mental health services the application of what we do know is restricted by deficiencies in expertise, vision and the allocation of resources.

My intention in producing this book has been to draw together some of the very considerable expertise which the authors have developed while facing the academic and clinical challenges presented to them during the recent intense period of modernisation of mental health care in the UK National Health Service. In doing so, I have been guided by a number of principles which I hope are reflected in the final product. Firstly, I believe that the aims of health provision should always be firmly clinical rather than administrative, but at the same time high-quality, well-informed management of services and resource distribution is essential to the delivery of high-quality care by clinicians. Indeed, in the field of mental health possibly more than any other, clinical and service management are so interdependent that one cannot function well unless the other does so, as has become evident in the UK where mental health is unique amongst the specialties in requiring specialist health trusts to optimise quality of provision. It follows that managers and planners at every level need to be well informed about clinical issues and, although it has been a difficult balance, this book is aimed at them as well as clinicians. The chapters in the first part of the book deal principally with aspects of disorders which have practical rather than purely academic relevance. Although the second half of the book focuses on service delivery, the emphasis throughout is on the clinical issues rather than administrative ones.

Secondly, I hope to dispel the frequent dysfunctional automatic thought which equates 'severe mental illness' with 'dramatic, acute, disturbed and risky symptoms'. Professionals should not be misled or collude with the journalistic and popular conception of the severely mentally ill as the crazy, psychotic and homicidal youths of the headlines. Public services are right to prioritise scarce specialist provision to those who are most in need, or who will benefit most from it, but in defining this group we must consider severity of symptoms, disability, duration, economic and psychosocial costs to others and the benefit to be gained from specialist secondary care input. Bearing this in mind, the reader should not be surprised to see a chapter on anxiety disorders which have global economic implications and one on eating disorders, such as anorexia nervosa with its high mortality.

Thirdly, I make no apology for including a chapter on personality disorder. It is included because, whatever the current emotional, political or organisational response to people with personality disorders, the reality is that mental health workers are inevitably involved in their care or management. Furthermore, we should not hide behind imperfect classificatory systems to justify the neglect of a group who has severe needs, some of whom may be helped by mental health services. Without wishing to advocate a medical model for such disorders, I think one should nevertheless acknowledge that, as we develop our understanding of the bio-psychosocial nature of these disorders and more importantly if we lose our therapeutic nihilism about them, we may become more prepared to see them as a form of mental 'ill-health' or even illness rather than a form of mental deviance. An eventual shift of this kind would not be surprising if one considers that this has been the usual historical pattern in the development of our understanding of mental illnesses.

Finally, this is not designed to be a comprehensive textbook of psychiatry: it concentrates on clinical and service-based issues with the greatest impact and does not consider areas such as sexual dysfunction, dissociative disorders or acute organic disorders. Substance abuse is only discussed in the context of its interaction with severe mental illness.

I would like to express my gratitude to the authors who have contributed their expertise and effort to this project, to the teachers and colleagues who have inspired me, to the staff of Greenwich Medical Media for their help and patience, to my secretary, Sue Wallis, and, last but not least, to my family for their support and tolerance.

CONTRIBUTORS

Dr Tim Amos
University Department of Psychiatry
Withington Hospital
Manchester

Professor Louis Appleby
University Department of Psychiatry
Withington Hospital
Manchester

Dr David Baldwin
Mental Health Group
Faculty of Medicine, Health and Biological
 Sciences
University of Southampton

Dr Sube Banerjee
Senior Lecturer in Old Age Psychiatry
Institute of Psychiatry
London

Dr Andrew Barker
Consultant in Old Age Psychiatry
Thornhill Research Unit
Moorgreen Hospital
Southampton

Dr Christopher Bass
Department of Psychological Medicine
John Radcliffe Hospital
Oxford

Dr Caroline Bell
Psychopharmacology Unit
University of Bristol
Bristol

Dr Richard Ford
Head of Service Evaluation
Sainsbury Centre for Mental Health
London

Dr Simone Fox
Eating Disorder Unit
Institute of Psychiatry
London

Dr Alain Gregoire
University Department of Psychiatry
Southampton

Dr Zaffer Iqbal
Institute of Psychiatry
London

Dr Pam Jezzard-Clark
Psychopharmacology Unit
University of Bristol
Bristol

Sonia Johnson
Department of Psychiatry and Behavioural
    Sciences
University College London Medical School
London

Dr Robin McCreadie
Department of Clinical Research
Crichton Royal Hospital
Dumfries

Dr Hugh Middleton
Psychopharmacology Unit
University of Bristol
Bristol

Dr Matt Muijen
Sainsbury Centre for Mental Health
London

Professor David Nutt
Psychopharmacology Unit
University of Bristol
Bristol

Dr Michael Phelan
Charing Cross Hospital
London

Dr Amanda Reynolds
Section of Community Psychiatry
Institute of Psychiatry
London

Dr Mike Slade
Charing Cross Hospital
London

Dr Huw Stone
Consultant Forensic Psychiatrist
Ravenswood House
Medium Secure Unit
Southampton

Dr Amanda Taylor
Consultant Forensic Psychiatrist
Ravenswood House
Medium Secure Unit
Southampton

Professor Graham Thornicroft
Section of Community Psychiatry
Institute of Psychiatry
London

Dr Janet Treasure
The Eating Disorders Unit
Institute of Psychiatry
London

1

DEFINING SEVERE MENTAL ILLNESS

Andrew Barker and Alain Gregoire

> The broad area of severe mental illness has suffered, in our view, from the lack of a clear working definition and it is time that one was agreed among those working in this field. This is necessary at national level for assessing overall needs and resources and at local level for responding sensitively but explicitly to those persons in need of most help. An accepted definition is not an academic nicety, but is essential for identifying those people who are most vulnerable and ensuring that appropriate resources are available to meet their needs.
>
> (Mental Health Foundation 1994)

The requirement for a precise yet workable definition of severe mental illness arises principally from two sources: the need to prioritize in cash-limited health services, and the need to aid the coordination of multiple agencies in planning, delivering and monitoring services targeted towards particularly vulnerable people. A survey in the USA suggested that 28% of the population fulfils criteria for a psychiatric diagnosis (Regier et al. 1998). Clearly no service could cope with providing mental healthcare to all of these, nor do all people so identified necessarily need such care. The challenge is to find a way of defining and identifying those who do. Explicit prioritizing of limited and expensive specialist mental health services and the continued development of community care has made the need for a suitable definition of severe mental illness increasingly evident. Highly publicized incidents of failure of community care of psychiatric patients have undoubtedly increased the political incentive to make explicit the group of psychiatric patients for whose care health and social services staff should be accountable. Despite this, no widely accepted criteria for severe mental illness exist, perhaps because of the variety of national and local purposes such a definition is required to fulfil. The purpose of this chapter is to examine the need for a definition of severe mental illness and to present progress in moving towards such a definition.

THE NEED FOR PRIORITIZATION AND THE DIFFICULTIES OF IMPLEMENTATION

Following the Second World War, the UK, in keeping with other Western countries, experienced economic growth that allowed the development of the post-war liberal attitude towards the provision of health and social care. Unfortunately, economic performance and demand for services did not match expectations, and declines in growth occurred over a period which also saw increasing costs of healthcare due to developments in health technology, the demographic shift towards the elderly and increasingly exacting demands of consumers. The expectation of more state provision of healthcare has been difficult to restrain; this is seen in the gradually increasing proportion of public funding in healthcare expenditure in most western countries over the past 20 years (OECD 1993). Indefinite growth is unsustainable and governments have been re-examining the role of the State in the provision of healthcare and exploring methods of containing expenditure.

The primary policy of the governments of most Western countries (OECD 1994) is adequacy and equity in access to some minimum of healthcare for all citizens, closely followed by the objective of containing costs to an acceptable share of national resources. The NHS reforms in the late 1980s and early 1990s implemented economic theories of the 'market' as the best way to maximize efficiency and consumer satisfaction while maintaining quality. However, it became increasingly evident that the market alone could not address issues of adequacy of services and equity of access, which are essential components of a national organization in which a social welfare function is an essential part. A second widely used method to contain costs internationally is by defining the types and level of healthcare which are the responsibility of the State.

Part of the original attraction of introducing market principles into the NHS was as a means to push through long overdue changes in organization while allowing government to distance itself from the unpopular decisions that were necessary. As time has passed since the initiation of the reforms, the language of competition has moved towards collaboration. Fragmentation and decentralized purchasing decisions over the types and levels of services to be provided locally by primary and secondary care have been overtaken by more explicit centralized descriptions of core services to be provided. The 1996 Department of Health publication 'The Spectrum of Care' details the components that should make up a comprehensive local service for people with mental health problems. It indicates that people with less severe disorders should be exclusively managed in primary care. Government policy required that 'the specialist mental health services target their resources and efforts first and foremost on severely mentally ill people' (DoH 1995).

The fact that this had previously not been the case in the UK was demonstrated in the influential Audit Commission report 'Finding a Place: A Review of Mental Health Services for Adults' (1994). It reported on the way that services were targeted for people with severe mental illness. The researchers divided mental illness into three categories by criteria of diagnosis and record of hospital admission and examined the caseloads of community psychiatric teams using these criteria. Markedly differing case mixes were found with the implication that some teams were not sufficiently targeted at those with more severe mental illnesses. No strong relationship was found between the numbers of people with severe mental illness and the total caseload size, the frequency with which clients were seen or the length of time patients stayed on caseloads. The report indicated that nationally the work of community psychiatric nurses (CPN) had shifted away from severe mental illness, and quoted one study where one-quarter of CPNs' caseloads had been found to not include any people with schizophrenia (Wooff et al. 1986, White 1990). Similar findings arose in the USA from studies of community mental health centres established without explicit prioritization of client group (Mechanic 1991).

The proportion of occupied bed days accounted for by people with severe mental illness also differed widely between districts. This is very relevant when examining the differing roles of primary and secondary care. Nearly ten times as much is spent on inpatient psychiatric care for a given district population than for general practitioner (GP) consultations with people with neurotic illness (Wing et al. 1992), despite the vastly greater numbers of people accounted for by the latter. This, of course, reinforces the argument for carefully targeting such very expensive forms of care.

One of the great strengths of the UK system in terms of cost containment has been the strong primary care function in gatekeeping access to resource intensive specialist services. In an organization that aims to be led by patients' needs rather than being service led and one that aims to give equity of access, it is only rational to have a centrally determined indication of what level or type of mental illness requires specialist input. The difficulty is partly in the definition of severity of illness, but also in addressing funding and operational issues across the primary/secondary interface.

In a document giving guidance for GPs on the management of people with severe mental illness in the community, the British Medical Association's General Medical Services Committee (1996) highlighted the Government's dilemma:

> The GMSC supports the need for a care programme approach as a means of ensuring the safety of patients and the general public. The committee, however, is concerned that implementation of the care programme approach without additional resources for mental health services diverts mental healthcare from less seriously disturbed people. The committee believes that any diversion of resources from the much larger group of patients with lower grade anxiety and depression, from whom the next generation of severely ill patients will be drawn, is misguided. The care programme approach should not be delivered at the expense of other mental health services, which, in some areas, are already severely limited. The care programme approach is a new, and desirable, activity which requires separate and new funding.

The guidance also stated that a GP's responsibility towards someone with severe mental illness, beyond that for general medical services, was discharged once assessment and referral to secondary care had been carried out. This aspect of the guidance seems retrogressive and goes against the view that GPs should be more closely involved in the care of people with severe mental illness (Nazareth et al. 1995).

Close working between primary and secondary care is recommended in 'Building Bridges: A Guide to Inter-Agency Working for the Care and Protection of Severely Mentally Ill People' (DoH 1995). This document was produced in response to the report of the Clunis Inquiry (Ritchie et al. 1994) into a much publicized incident, which involved Christopher Clunis, a man known to be suffering from schizophrenia who stabbed to death Jonathan Zito, a complete stranger. The report was extremely critical of most of the agencies that had been involved in the care of Clunis, and many instances of lack of coordination of services were identified. The document was, therefore, designed to promote close and effective collaborative inter-agency work. It brought together existing guidance for the care of the mentally ill, primarily based around the Care Programme Approach, a scheme introduced in 1991 to provide a framework by which health authorities, social service departments and other parties agree arrangements for care and treatment of mentally ill people in the community.

THE SEARCH FOR A DEFINITION

During the 1980s a number of definitions of severe mental illness were proposed. These tended to be principally based on diagnostic categories and reflected a very medical view of the concept of severity and by implication the need for services (Goldman 1981, Tyrer et al. 1985, McLean and Liebowitz 1989). Falloon (1988) tried to move away from this rather narrow view by devising a framework designed to provide a health/social services interagency definition of severe mental illness based on concepts of impairment, disability and handicap. However, the definition does not encompass important issues such as duration and risk of harm to self or others. The House of Commons Health Committee, frustrated by this lack of clarity, had recommended that the Department of Health should assist in formulating a definition of severe mental illness (House of Commons 1994). It was in the 'Building Bridges' document that such help was forthcoming. The definition offered in 'Building Bridges' improved on those previous:

In referring to 'people suffering from severe mental illness' we mean individuals who:

1. are diagnosed as suffering from some sort of mental illness (typically people suffering from schizophrenia or a severe affective disorder, but including dementia);

2. suffer substantial disability as a result of their illness, such as an inability to care for themselves independently, sustain relationships or work;

3. a) are currently displaying florid symptoms; or
   b) are suffering from a chronic enduring condition;

4. have suffered recurring crises leading to frequent admissions/interventions;

5. occasion significant risk to their own safety or that of others.

The report also presented dimensions of severe mental illness that Powell and Slade (1995) had found common to definitions used by twenty NHS and social care providers. The '3 Ds' of diagnosis, duration and disability had previously been described by Schinnar et al. (1990), who found them common to 17 published definitions of severe and persistent mental illness. To these were added the two dimensions of safety to self and others, and presence of formal or informal care. How relative weightings should be applied to these five dimensions was not stated, but clearly service use alone would not suffice for any national definition since this is so heavily influenced by service provision.

Even a definition with five dimensions is likely to prove inadequate. Any definition used to inform allocation of major financial and clinical resources should logically take into account a much broader view of the consequences of severe mental illness. Our knowledge of such consequences now extends far beyond distress and disability for the individual and danger of physical harm to others. We are now well able to predict the likely future course for most disorders and evidence is also available which allows us to predict other important consequences including burden on carers (e.g. Fadden et al. 1987), impact on dependent children (see Chapter 17), and costs to services (McCrone et al. 1994, Salize and Rossler 1996). Furthermore, although more difficult to define and identify, there is no doubt that severe mental illnesses also have important consequences for society as a whole. These include both abstract effects such as the societal reactions to mental illness and disabilities and the effects of these on social behaviour and policy (Wing 1993). More concrete effects such as the costs to nations are now increasingly understood. The Global Burden of Disease study, initiated by the World Bank, measured the burden of disease for 107 disorders using Disability Adjusted Life Years (DALY), a measure derived from life years lost due to premature mortality and years lived with disability, adjusted for severity. This estimated that in 1990 mental disorders accounted for 9.1% of the burden of disease across the world and 22.4% of the burden of disease in established market economies. About half of the burden of disease is attributable to unipolar depression and anxiety disorders (other non-psychotic disorders were not examined) (Andrews 1998). Unipolar depression was the fourth leading cause of DALY in the world in 1990 and is projected as being the second most important cause of global DALY, very closely second only to ischaemic heart disease, by 2020 (Murray and Lopez 1996).

ARRIVING AT A LOCAL OPERATIONAL DEFINITION

Powell and Slade (1995) advised that top-down and bottom-up approaches should be used to negotiate local criteria, and certainly local ownership would enhance the benefit of guidelines. They also suggested that no definition of severe mental illness could be imposed nationally. This is no doubt true, but it is inevitable that any significant disparity in definitions will compromise equity of access in different areas. Perhaps a universally adopted definition that unambiguously defines a core priority group but incorporates flexibility of interpretations in some areas would satisfy the need for local ownership and appropriateness to specific local characteristics.

The operational definition described in Table 1.1 is one that we developed locally for general adult mental health services and agreed with the health authority and social services, with targets for contacting sufferers during any single year. It describes mental illness which, due to its chronic nature or current effects, is severe

---

One of A or B

A. One of the following:

    i.   Symptomatic psychotic illnesses: schizophrenia, persistent delusional disorder, schizo-affective disorder or psychotic symptoms that have lasted more than 1 week

    ii. Symptomatic Bipolar Affective Disorder

    iii. Receiving antipsychotic or mood stabilizing medication for diagnosis in (i) or (ii)

B. Unipolar depression; neurotic, stress-related and somatoform disorders; behavioural syndromes; organic disorders; **and** one of 1 or 2

    1. Functional impact – the mental disorder is causing a severe disability in maintaining usual or expected roles and behaviours for at least 3 months. This may be seen in the following areas:

- maintaining accommodation by paying bills or maintaining basic living conditions
- caring for dependants
- applying for or holding down a job in open employment
- pursuing usual recreational activities
- maintaining socially acceptable personal hygiene
- maintaining a diet adequate for physical health
- recognizing and responding appropriately to household risks
- forming and/or sustaining interpersonal relationships

    2. Significant risk of suicide or of serious harm to others.

Table 1.1 – Example of a locally determined definition of severe mental illness for general adult psychiatry.

enough to require the involvement of general adult mental health services. It does not include people with a sole diagnosis of personality disorder or those with a brief but recurrent neurotic disorder.

It was argued that people with a psychotic illness or bipolar affective disorder, even if currently stable on medication, have such vulnerability to relapse and potential side effects from medication to warrant being followed up by psychiatric services. A definition based on presence of psychosis alone would not be sufficient though, since non-psychotic illness can be extremely disabling and prolonged, and in many cases more so than well-controlled psychotic illnesses. Any workable definition must also encompass the need for a psychiatric service to be involved in the care of people at serious risk to themselves or others even if only for a short while.

Conversely, with a strong primary care function and financially stretched public funding, it is not necessary to have resource-intensive secondary care involved in the care of people suffering from disorders with mild symptoms that will be self-limiting or remediable by simple interventions. For these disorders, therefore, some measure of disability in addition is required. Here we start entering a difficult area. How can the severity of two disorders be compared when one is of mild degree but suffered for decades, and one severely disabling, but of a duration of weeks or even days? Milder degrees of disability should qualify after a period that would allow most self-limiting disorder to resolve or be appropriately treated by primary care services. As an essentially arbitrary though clinically reasonable period, we would suggest 3 months for this.

An operational definition of severe mental illness is obviously only useful and indeed valid if the context for its use is clear. This depends on locally agreed operational policies being developed which should, for example, define the proportion of clients in a service who would be expected to meet the agreed definition for severe mental illness.

SUMMARY

The concept of mental illness encompasses a number of medical and social parameters, which are further complicated by attempting to define a severe mental illness subgroup. A definition of severe mental illness is essential to enable limited specialist mental health services to target those most in need. A number of definitions have been described. Because the concept of severe mental illness is not absolute and depends on its intended purpose, no universally applicable definition exists. However, there are core parameters or axes that should be considered when attempting to derive a local operational definition.

References

Andrews G. The burden of anxiety and depressive disorders. Current Opinion in Psychiatry 1998; 11: 121–123.

Audit Commission. Finding a Place: A Review of Mental Health Services for Adults. London: HMSO, 1994.

Department of Health. Building Bridges: A Guide to Inter-Agency Working for the Care and Protection of Severely Mentally Ill People. London: HMSO, 1995.

Department of Health. The Spectrum of Care: Local Services for People with Mental Health Problems. London: HMSO, 1996.

Fadden G, Bebbington P, Kuipers L. The impact of functional psychiatric illness on the patient's family. British Journal of Psychiatry 1987; 150: 285–292.

Falloon I. The prevention of morbidity in schizophrenia. In Falloon I (ed.), Handbook of Behavioural Family Therapy. London: Hutchinson, 1988.

General Medical Services Committee. Mentally Disordered People: Continuing Care in the Community: Guidance for GPs. London: British Medical Association, 1996.

Goldman H, Gattozzi A, Taube C. Defining and counting the chronically mentally ill. Community Psychiatry 1981; 31: 21.

House of Commons. First Report of the Health Committee: Better Off in the Community? The Care of People who are Seriously Mentally Ill. London: HMSO, 1994.

McLean E, Liebowitz J. Towards a working definition of the long-term mentally ill. Psychiatric Bulletin 1989; 13: 251–252.

McCrone P, Beecham J, Knapp M. Community Psychiatric Nurse Teams: cost-effectiveness of intensive support versus generic care. British Journal of Psychiatry 1994; 165: 218–221.

Mechanic D. Strategies for integrating public mental health services. Hospital and Community Psychiatry 1991; 42: 797–801.

Mental Health Foundation. Creating Community Care: Report of the Mental Health Foundation Inquiry into Community Care for People with Severe Mental Illness. London: Mental Health Foundation, 1994.

Murray CJL, Lopez AD. Evidence-based health policy – lessons from the Global Burden of Disease Study. Science 1996; 274: 740–743.

Nazareth I, King M, Davies S. Care of schizophrenia in general practice: the general practitioner and the patient. British Journal of General Practice 1995; 45: 343–347.

OECD. The Reform of Health Care Systems: A Review of Seventeen OECD Countries. Paris: OECD, 1994.

OECD. OECD Health Systems: Facts and Trends 1960–1991, vol. 1. Health Policy Studies no. 3. Paris: OECD, 1993.

Powell R, Slade M. Defining severe mental illness. In Thornicroft G, Strathdee G (eds), Commissioning Mental Health Services. London: HMSO, 1995.

Regier DA, Kaelber CT, Rae DS et al. Limitations of diagnostic criteria and assessment instruments for mental disorders. Archives of General Psychiatry 1998; 55: 109–115.

Ritchie J, Dick D, Lingham R. The Report of the Inquiry into the Care and Treatment of Christopher Clunis. London: HMSO, 1994.

Salize HJ, Rossler W. The cost of comprehensive care of people with schizophrenia living in the community – a cost evaluation from a German catchment area. British Journal of Psychiatry 1996; 169: 42–48.

Schinnar AP, Rothbard AB, Kanter R et al. An empirical literature review of definitions of severe and persistent mental illness. American Journal of Psychiatry 1990; 147: 1602–1608.

Tyrer P. The 'Hive' system: a model for a psychiatric services. British Journal of Psychiatry 1985; 146: 571–575.

White E. Surveying CPNs. Nursing Times 1990; 86: 62–64.

Wing J. Social consequences of severe and persistent psychiatric disorders. In Bhugra D, Leff J (eds), Principles of Social Psychiatry. Oxford: Blackwell, 1993.

Wing J, Brewin CG, Thornicroft G. Defining mental health needs. In Thornicroft G, Brewin CR, Wing J (eds), Measuring Mental Health Needs. London: Gaskell, 1992.

Wooff K, Goldberg D, Fryers T. Patients in receipt of community psychiatric nursing care in Salford 1976–1982. Psychological Medicine 1986; 16: 407–414.

2

SCHIZOPHRENIA

Robin McCreadie

INTRODUCTION

Schizophrenia and affective disorders are the two principal major mental illnesses affecting the young and middle-aged adult today. A measure of the severity of the illness is the cost in treating schizophrenia. It has been estimated (Davies and Drummond 1994) that 1.6% of the total UK healthcare budget is used to treat patients with schizophrenia and that hospital- and community-based residential care accounts for nearly three-quarters of these costs. Less than 50% of the patients account for 97% of the costs. This chapter can only hope to touch on some of the important growth points in the understanding of schizophrenia. There are two international journals dealing solely with schizophrenia, and the psychiatric journals with the highest impact factors devote much of their space to schizophrenia research.

DEFINITION

The term 'schizophrenia' was coined by Bleuler (1911) and is derived from the Greek, a literal translation being 'a splitting of the mind'. The term has crept into everyday use, but unfortunately when used by the layman, it is taken as 'a split mind', that is, a Jekyll and Hyde personality. This, of course, is not schizophrenia, but if it exists at all it is part of the dissociative disorders, namely dissociative identity disorder (APA 1994). By using 'splitting of the mind', Bleuler intended it to mean the disintegration of many aspects, including mood, thinking and behaviour.

INCIDENCE AND PREVALENCE

The lifetime incidence is about 9 per 1000 of the general population (Jablensky 1994). The incidence is much the same in different cultures and different countries (Sartorius et al. 1986). 'Pockets' of increased incidence such as in African-

Caribbeans born in England (Wesseley et al. 1991) are of obvious interest and warrant further exploration as they may throw light on possible aetiological factors. Controversy continues about whether the incidence of schizophrenia has been falling in recent decades (Der et al. 1990).

The point prevalence of schizophrenia is probably between 3 and 5 per 1000 general population (Leach and Scherer 1992). Thus, in the UK a group general practice of, say, 10 000 at any given time will have 30–50 schizophrenic patients 'on their books'. As of today the vast majority of people with schizophrenia live outside hospital (McCreadie et al. 1997). This will amount to a considerable caseload for each practice.

AETIOLOGY

Both genetic and environmental factors are probably important in the aetiology of schizophrenia. The relative importance of each remains controversial with some authors maintaining that genetic factors alone can explain almost all cases of schizophrenia (McGuffin et al. 1994). Others take a more cautious line (Eagles 1994).

GENETIC FACTORS

The lifetime incidence of schizophrenia in the general population is about 1% but is 6–10% in first-degree relatives of schizophrenic patients (Gottesman and Shields 1982). Thus, schizophrenia is a familial disorder. There are two principal ways in which genetic and environmental factors can be examined in familial disorders, namely through twin and adoption studies.

Twin studies

The relative importance of genetic factors can be examined by comparing the concordance for an illness between members of monozygotic (MZ) and dizygotic (DZ) twin pairs. Since MZ twins have exactly the same genetic make-up, while DZ twins share on average 50% of their genes, then if the concordance among MZ twins is greater than among DZ twins, this will reflect a genetic influence. It is assumed that MZ and DZ twins share their environment to the same extent.

The concordance rate for schizophrenia in MZ twins has been estimated to be between 35 and 58% and for DZ twins between 9 and 27% (Gottesman and Shields 1982); that is, MZ concordance rates are about three times higher than DZ rates. This suggests that genetic factors are probably important. The concordance rate, however, in MZ twins is not 100%. This suggests that environmental factors may also be a contributory aetiological factor. It has recently been shown, however (Gottesman and Bertelsen 1989), that the incidence of schizophrenia in the offspring of non-affected MZ twins is as high as it is in the offspring of the twins that do develop a schizophrenic illness. This suggests that individuals may carry the genes for the illness but not themselves develop it.

Adoption studies

The classic studies in this area come from the USA (Heston 1966) and Denmark (Kety et al. 1976). In the US study the incidence of schizophrenia was compared in children born to 47 schizophrenic mothers and who were adopted away at birth with the incidence in children also adopted but born to psychiatrically well mothers. Five of the children born to schizophrenic mothers developed schizophrenia, but none of the children of non-schizophrenic mothers did so.

In the Danish study the research workers started with individuals who had been adopted and who had developed schizophrenia. They found that 20% of 118 biological parents also had schizophrenia, compared with only 6% of 224 adoptive parents of schizophrenic patients which was the same rate as in parents of control adoptees.

These studies argue very persuasively for genetic factors in the aetiology of schizophrenia.

The mode of inheritance may be through a single gene, a small number of genes or many genes having a small but additive effect. It is certain there are some families with multiply affected members and it is more than likely that within these families there may be a single gene responsible for the illness. However, what that gene might be has not been elucidated. One study has suggested a gene (Sherrington et al. 1988) only for that finding not to be replicated (Kennedy et al. 1988).

With most patients with schizophrenia there is in fact no family history of the disorder; multiply affected families are rare. It is probable that schizophrenia is genetically heterogeneous; it may be transmitted by a few genes, each of only moderate effect, or by many genes, each of only small effect.

ENVIRONMENTAL FACTORS

Both physical and emotional aspects of the environment appear to be important in the aetiology of schizophrenia.

Physical environment

One of the few consistent findings in schizophrenia research is the small excess of late winter births in those who eventually develop schizophrenia; this is the case both north and south of the Equator (Bradbury and Miller 1985, McGrath et al. 1985). It is not clear what it is about the winter that predisposes to schizophrenia, but much work has suggested that exposure of the foetus to the influenza virus, possibly in the second trimester, predisposes to the later development of schizophrenia (Adams et al. 1993). Influenza, of course, is more common during the winter months.

It is also now widely accepted that there is an association between obstetric complications and the later development of schizophrenia (Geddes and Lawrie 1995). Association, of course, does not imply causality. It may be that the difficult birth is the result of some foetal dysfunction and not that the obstetric complication causes minimal brain damage which predisposes that individual to develop schizophrenia in later life. A recent study (McCreadie 1997) suggested that a lack of breast milk might also be a further environmental risk factor. Breast milk contains the fatty acid docosahexaenoic acid, which is essential to the developing brain (O'Brien et al. 1964). Cow's milk does not contain it, and neither do most formula feeds (Carlson et al. 1986).

Schizophrenia is more common in lower socio-economic classes (Freeman 1994). This cannot be explained simply by the drift of schizophrenic patients into lower classes as the association holds well when class is defined by the occupation of the patient's father. Overcrowding, exposure to infection, bottle rather than breast feeding, and harsh economic circumstances are likely to be more common in individuals born into lower social classes. These environmental factors may have something to do with the increased incidence of schizophrenia in these lower social groups.

It is also noteworthy that in some western countries the incidence of schizophrenia is higher in urban areas (Takei et al. 1992) where the physical environment is likely to be harsher than in rural areas. Also, the increased incidence in urban areas is especially found among the non-white population (Wesseley et al. 1991) and indeed this may be the principal factor explaining the rural-urban difference in some areas (McCreadie et al 1997).

Emotional environment

A 30-year-old study found that schizophrenic patients have experienced more life events than expected in the 3 weeks before the onset or relapse of the illness (Brown and Birley 1968). This finding was more recently confirmed in the Camberwell Collaborative Psychosis Study (Bebbington et al. 1993); when 51 patients were compared with a psychiatrically healthy group, there was a significant excess particularly in the 3 months before relapse.

The course of the illness after the first episode is closely associated with the patient's home environment (Bebbington and Kuipers 1994). An environment where there is criticism or over-involvement is more likely to lead to relapse than an atmosphere that is warm and supportive. Once again, association does not imply causality. It may indeed be that critical and over-involved relatives (usually parents) promote a further relapse. It may be, however, that a patient who is more seriously ill is likely to affect the home environment and produce criticism and over-involvement. Probably there is a two-way interaction between patient and relatives; the result is a poorer prognosis.

BRAIN CHANGES

Brain structure

When groups of schizophrenic patients are compared with non-schizophrenic individuals, there are small but significant differences in brain structure (Lewis 1990). The brains of schizophrenic patients are smaller and the ventricles, especially the lateral ventricle, are larger. Structural abnormalities have been most frequently found in the temporal cortex (Suddath et al. 1989). Post-mortem studies (Roberts et al. 1986) suggest that it is a failure of the brain to develop properly rather than a degenerative process that underlies the structural abnormality.

Brain function

Studies of brain function using neuro-imaging techniques, such as single photon-emission computerized tomography (SPECT) and positive-emission tomography (PET), show that there is diminished blood flow in the frontal regions of the brain (Buchsbaum et al. 1982, Rubin et al. 1991). Blood flow reflects metabolism and, therefore, there is likely to be hypometabolism in frontal areas.

It must be emphasized that these changes in structure and function are very subtle and that there is no way a person can be 'diagnosed' as suffering from schizophrenia simply by examining brain scans.

THE DOPAMINE HYPOTHESIS

At a neuronal and synaptic level in the brain, it has been postulated that an abnormality of the system mediated by the neurotransmitter dopamine may be aetiologically important. This hypothesis arose out of the finding that there was a close relationship in standard antipsychotic drugs between the dose required to produce a clinical effect and the degree of blockade of dopamine receptors (Carlsson 1978).

It is, of course, too simple to implicate a single neuro-transmitter system as the only pathway for the mediation of schizophrenia. Recently introduced and effective antipsychotic drugs such as clozapine and risperidone (see below) have a more profound effect on neurotransmitter systems other than the dopamine system. Clozapine, for example, acts also on 5-HT_2, muscarinic and α-receptors. The excitatory amino acid glutamate and the inhibitory transmitter GABA (γ-amino butyric acid) have also been implicated. It is more than likely that there is interplay between different systems leading to schizophrenic illness.

SIGNS AND SYMPTOMS OF SCHIZOPHRENIA

The signs and symptoms of schizophrenia can be broadly divided into positive and negative symptoms (Crow 1980). Positive symptoms are the presence of phenomena that are not present in a normal individual; negative symptoms are the absence of certain functions that should be present in a normal individual.

Positive symptoms

The principal positive symptoms in schizophrenia are delusions, hallucinations, disorder in the form of thinking and inappropriate mood.

A delusion is a fixed false belief that is not held by other members of that person's social and cultural background. In schizophrenia, delusions, which are said to be typical of the disorder, are so-called 'primary' delusions. This is a false belief that arises *de novo* and is not preceded by any other psychological phenomenon. Secondary delusions are obviously false beliefs that are secondary to other psychological events.

The content of the delusions of a schizophrenic patient can vary widely, but many patients show evidence of persecutory delusions. Grandiose delusions are also common. A delusional perception is also said to be typical of schizophrenia. In this instance, a patient not only perceives something as having an ordinary meaning, but also makes a delusional interpretation of it. (For a discussion of cognitive modelling of delusions, see Chapter 15.)

Passivity phenomena are difficult to classify, but are said to be typical of schizophrenia. Examples include thought insertion where patients believe that thoughts which they are thinking are not their own but have been put into their mind by some external agency; thought withdrawal, where patients believe that thoughts have been taken out of their mind by an external force; and thought broadcasting, where patients believe that their thoughts escape into the outside world where they are experienced by others.

A hallucination is a perception in the absence of an external stimulus. Hallucinations can occur in any modality in schizophrenia, but the most common are auditory hallucinations. Three types of auditory hallucination are said to be typical of schizophrenia. They are third-person auditory hallucinations, where the patient hears imaginary voices talking about them in the third person; running commentary hallucinations, where the voices comment on the patient's actions; and thought echo, where the patient hears their thoughts spoken out loud. (For a discussion of cognitive modelling of hallucinations, see Chapter 15.)

The form of thinking may be disturbed in schizophrenia. Patients may have difficulty thinking clearly and so what they say may be difficult to follow; one idea does not logically follow on from another. There are various types of formal thought disorder and words such as 'derailment', 'loosening of association' and 'knights move thinking' have been used to describe them. In very serious formal thought disorder, a patient's speech may be almost incoherent, giving rise to a so-called 'word salad'.

The patient may show an inappropriate affect in relation to thought content. This may lead, for example, to the patient laughing and giggling inappropriately when talking of a serious event, for example the death of their mother.

Negative symptoms

The two main negative symptoms are flattening of affect and poverty of thought. In flattening of mood patients will be unresponsive to changes in their environment and there will be a narrowing of the range of emotional expression. In poverty of thought, the patient thinks little. This can show itself in speech, which is vague, hesitant and lacking in content.

Other 'negative' symptoms that the patient may have may not be primary but secondary to other symptoms, especially positive ones. For example, a patient may show social withdrawal and a lack of interest in their surroundings. This may be secondary, for example, to persecutory ideas.

Recent work (Liddle and Barnes 1990) using factor analysis suggests that rather than a simple division of schizophrenic symptoms into positive and negative ones it may be more appropriate to describe three clusters of symptoms, namely psychomotor poverty (poverty of speech, flattened affect and decreased spontaneous movement), disorganization (formal thought disorder and inappropriate affect) and reality distortion (delusions and hallucinations). PET showed that psychomotor poverty was associated with decreased left frontal activity, disorganization with increased cingulate activity on the right, and delusions and hallucinations with increased activity in the left hippocampal regions.

DIAGNOSIS

In the UK, for the purposes of collecting health statistics, the diagnosis of schizophrenia is made using the criteria outlined in the 10th edn of the International Classification of Diseases (WHO 1992). In the USA, the diagnosis is made using criteria in the Diagnostic and Statistical Manual of Mental Disorders, 4th edn (DSM-IV) (APA 1994). Tables 2.1 and 2.2 outline the diagnostic criteria.

It can be seen that in both diagnostic systems there is a 'menu' of signs and symptoms. The principal differences between the two systems are that DSM-IV requires a 6-month duration of illness and deterioration in social functioning.

A **Characteristic symptoms:** Two (or more) of the following each present for a significant portion of time during 1 month (or less if successfully treated):

- delusions
- hallucinations
- disorganized speech (e.g. frequent derailment or incoherence)
- grossly disorganized or catatonic behaviour
- negative symptoms, i.e. affective flattening, alogia or avolition

Note: Only one Criterion A symptom is required if delusions are bizarre or hallucinations consist of a voice keeping up a running commentary on the person's behaviour or thoughts, or two or more voices conversing with each other.

B **Social/occupational dysfunction:** For a significant portion of the time since the onset of the disturbance, one or more major areas of functioning such as work, interpersonal relations or self-care are markedly below the level achieved prior to the onset (or when the onset is in childhood or adolescence, failure to achieve level of interpersonal, academic or occupational achievement).

C **Duration:** Continuous signs of the disturbance persist for at least 6 months. This period must include at least 1 month of symptoms (or less if successfully treated) that meet Criterion A (i.e. active-phase symptoms) and may include periods of prodromal or residual symptoms. During these prodromal or residual periods, the signs of the disturbance may be manifested by only negative symptoms or two or more symptoms listed in Criterion A present in an attenuated form (e.g odd belief, unusual perceptual experiences).

D **Schizo-affective and mood disorder exclusion:** Schizo-affective disorder and mood disorder with psychotic features have been ruled out because either (1) no major depressive, manic or mixed episodes have occurred concurrently with their active-phase symptoms; or (2) if mood episodes have occurred during active-phase symptoms, their total duration has been brief relative to the duration of the active and residual periods.

E **Substance/general medical condition exclusion:** The disturbance is not due to the direct physiological effects of a substance (e.g. a drug of abuse, a medication) or a general medical condition.

F **Relationship to a pervasive development disorder:** If there is a history of autistic disorder or another pervasive development disorder, the additional diagnosis of schizophrenia is made only if prominent delusions or hallucinations are also present for at least 1 month (or less if successfully treated).

Table 2.1 – Diagnostic Criteria for Schizophrenia: DSM-IV.

It might seem from the plethora of signs and symptoms in both lists that the diagnosis of schizophrenia is easy. This is certainly not the case especially in the early stages of illness. A detailed history and full mental state examination is necessary. The diagnosis must not be made lightly as once made it may be difficult to remove. Also, with the continued stigma of mental illness, great care must be taken before 'labelling' someone as suffering from schizophrenia. However, caution in making the diagnosis should not lead to a delay in treating psychotic symptoms which can adversely affect outcome.

Although no strictly pathognomic symptoms can be identified, for practical purposes it is useful to divide symptoms into groups that have special importance for the diagnosis and often occur together such as;

1. Thought echo, thought insertion or withdrawal and thought broadcasting.

2. Delusions of control, influence or passivity clearly referred to body or limb or specific thoughts, action or sensations: delusional perception.

3. Hallucinatory voices giving a running commentary on the patient's behaviour, or discussing the patient among themselves or other types of hallucinatory voices coming from some part of the body.

4. Persistent delusions of other kinds that are culturally inappropriate and completely impossible, such as religious or political identity, or superhuman powers and abilities (e.g being able to control the weather or being in communication with aliens from another world).

5. Persistent hallucination in any modality, when accompanied either by fleeting or half-formed delusions without clear affective content, or by persistent over-valued ideas, or when occurring every day for weeks or months on end.

6. Breaks or interpolations in the train of thought, resulting in incoherence or irrelevant speech or neologisms.

7. Catatonic behaviour such as excitement, posturing or waxy flexibility, negativism, mutism and stupor.

8. Negative symptoms such as marked apathy, paucity of speech and blunting or incongruity of emotional responses, usually resulting in social withdrawal and lowering of social performance; it must be clear that these are not due to depression or to neuroleptic medication.

9. A significant and consistent change in the overall quality of some aspects of personal behaviour, manifest as loss of interest, aimlessness, idleness, a self-absorbed attitude and social withdrawal.

Diagnostic guidelines
The normal requirement for a diagnosis of schizophrenia is that a minimum of one very clear symptom (and usually two or more if less clear-cut) belonging to any one of the groups listed as 1 and 4 above, or symptoms from at least two of the groups referred to as 5 to 8 should have been clearly present for most of the time *during 1 month or more*. Conditions meeting such symptomatic requirements but of duration less than 1 month (whether treated or not) should be diagnosed in the first instance as acute schizophrenia-like psychotic disorder (F23.2) and re-classified as schizophrenia if the symptoms persist for longer periods.

Table 2.2 – Diagnostic Criteria for Schizophrenia: ICD–10.

TREATMENT

The first episode

Although there is currently great pressure on admission beds in psychiatric units in the UK (Marshall 1997), admission to inpatient care of someone with a first episode of schizophrenia is usually desirable as it allows a full and detailed assessment. The assessment will be made not only by the psychiatrist, but also will involve other disciplines including nurses, social workers and occupational therapists. During a patient's inpatient stay, not only will the patient's mental state be assessed, but also the importance of any social and psychological factors can be determined. Examination of the patient over a period of up to 1 week in the absence of specific antipsychotic medication should be sufficient to make a clear diagnosis.

Admission to hospital in most instances will be on a voluntary basis. However, where people are experiencing a first episode of schizophrenia they may be perplexed and bewildered, and have no clear understanding that they are mentally ill. They may refuse admission. The law in most countries, however, acknowledges the right of patients to receive treatment. In the UK admission to hospital may be necessary using the relevant sections of the different Mental Health Acts.

The initial drug treatment of the patient experiencing a first episode will depend on the level of behaviour disturbance. If there is severe behaviour disturbance and the patient needs sedation but is unwilling to take medication, then a short-acting intramuscular antipsychotic drug such as haloperidol or droperidol can be used. It may also be possible to use a longer acting intramuscular antipsychotic drug such as zuclopenthixol acetate, but as it has an action of up to 72 h it should not be used unless the diagnosis of undoubted psychosis has already been made. For more sedation a benzodiazepine can be added.

Further drug treatment will remain dependent on whether there is continuing behaviour disturbance. If there is no such disturbance then a non-sedating antipsychotic should be used. Such drugs include sulpiride, haloperidol and trifluoperazine. The two latter drugs, however, can produce marked extrapyramidal side-effects (see below), especially in patients who have never before been exposed to an antipsychotic. There are also newer 'atypical' antipsychotics such as risperidone, olanzapine, quetiapine and amisulpride. These drugs certainly cause less in the way of extrapyramidal side-effects (Peuskens et al. 1995), but because of their high costs they are not yet firmly established as first-line treatment in first episode schizophrenia. However, because compliance is associated with side-effects (see below) and as it is important to win the patient's cooperation, clinical grounds indicate that the 'atypicals' should probably be used as first-line treatment.

If there is continuing behaviour disturbance, the patient should be given a non-sedating antipsychotic plus an additional sedating drug such as a benzodiazepine (e.g. lorazepam or diazepam). When the behaviour disturbance settles, the benzodiazepine can be stopped and the same antipsychotic drug continued.

Positive versus negative symptoms

The drug treatment of schizophrenia mainly improves the positive symptoms, namely delusions, hallucinations, inappropriate affect and incoherence of thinking. The negative symptoms such as flattening of affect and poverty of thought are much more resistant to antipsychotic drugs. It has been suggested that the atypical antipsychotics may have an effect on negative symptoms (Peuskens et al. 1995). The failure of drugs to tackle negative symptoms adequately leads to the typical picture of the chronic schizophrenic patient in whom hallucinations and delusions might be causing them little serious trouble but apathy, loss of drive and isolation are much more serious problems (see below).

Antipsychotic drugs usually do not act right away. They can take up to 2–6 weeks to produce a satisfactory antipsychotic effect (Keck et al. 1989). Patients must, therefore, be encouraged to take medication for this period and on a regular basis if beneficial effects are to be seen.

Compliance is crucial in the management of the first (and, of course, subsequent) episodes if the patient's symptoms are to be brought under control. Compliance is affected not only by drug side-effects (see below), but also by lack of insight. The bewildered and distressed individual who is lacking insight will obviously be reluctant to take medication. This is a further reason for inpatient care of a first-episode patient where skilled nursing care plays an important part in helping the patient recover.

The sooner treatment with drugs is started in a first episode of schizophrenia, the better is the longer term prognosis. For example (May et al. 1976), when 228 patients were randomly allocated to receive either drugs, electroconvulsive therapy (ECT), psychotherapy, milieu therapy or drugs and psychotherapy, it was found that during treatment of the acute episode, drugs and/or ECT were better than psychotherapy. In the longer term, patients who had initially received psychotherapy but were then given drugs had a poorer outcome over the following 3–5 years compared with those who received drugs right from the very beginning of treatment. This work was confirmed by others (Loebel et al. 1993) when it was found that the longer a patient had been ill before they first received antipsychotic drugs, the longer it took for that patient to remit. Also the level of remission was poorer.

Acute side-effects of antipsychotic medication

Patients who have never received antipsychotic drugs, so-called 'drug-naive patients', are especially sensitive to such medication. Up to three-quarters of drug-naive patients given standard antipsychotic drugs develop parkinsonian side-effects such as tremor and rigidity, which are sufficiently distressing to warrant the prescription of anti-parkinsonian medication (Scottish Schizophrenia Research Group 1987). Even with an atypical antipsychotic drug such as risperidone more than half of the first-episode patients will require anti-parkinsonian medication (Emsley et al. 1999).

As these side-effects are dose-related, interest has recently focussed on low-dose treatment. Studies have consistently demonstrated that lower doses (haloperidol 2–6 mg equiv. daily) are as effective as higher doses, at least in first episode schizophrenia (Bollini et al. 1994).

Compliance with drugs is affected by side-effects, including the extrapyramidal side-effects of parkinsonism, akathisia (motor restlessness) and dystonia. The experience of akathisia, which responds little if at all to anti-cholinergics, especially affects compliance (van Putten 1974).

Recurrent episodes

After recovery from the first episode, about one third of patients will probably have no more episodes over the following 5 years (Scottish Schizophrenia Research Group 1992). The other two thirds will. Although ability to predict relapse is at present very poor, much research is currently examining prodromes in the hope of improving prediction and targeting prevention (see Chapter 15).

A possible algorithm (McCreadie 1995) for the treatment of relapses is shown in figure 2.1.

If a patient relapses but responded well to an antipsychotic drug during the first episode, then obviously that drug should be tried again and at the dose previously used. If the patient does not respond to a standard antipsychotic, then an atypical antipsychotic should be tried. If the patient does not respond to one of these drugs, then there should be a trial of an intra-muscular long-acting antipsychotic such as fluphenazine decanoate or flupenthixol decanoate; the possibility of failure to respond because of poor compliance or poor absorption will be avoided. If the patient still does not respond to medication, then they can be said to be drug-resistant and clozapine should be tried (see below).

Maintenance therapy

As two-thirds of patients are likely to relapse in the 5 years after the first episode (see above), then it is probably good practice for them to be offered maintenance therapy after recovery from the first episode. Unfortunately, it is not possible to forecast which patients will be free of further episodes, but sometimes it is only the occurrence of subsequent relapses that establishes the diagnosis. The best course of action is to err on the side of caution and offer all patients maintenance treatment. Maintenance treatment should probably continue for 1–2 years. The choice of treatment will depend on assessment of compliance. If a patient is thought to be compliant, then probably oral medication should be given. The drug should be the same as that which produced an improvement during the first episode. If compliance is thought to be poor, then consideration should be given to the use of a long-acting intramuscular antipsychotic drug such as fluphenazine decanoate,

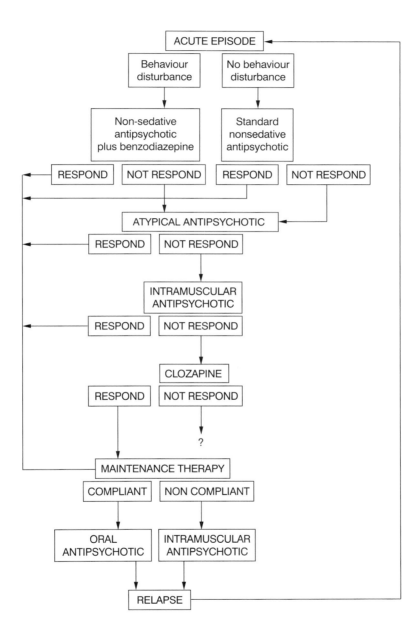

Figure 2.1 – A drug treatment algorithm

flupenthixol decanoate or haloperidol decanoate. Such drugs can be given by injection once every 2–4 weeks. However, many patients resent intramuscular drugs especially when given for lengthy periods.

If an antipsychotic drug is to be given for lengthy periods then obviously side-effects should be avoided wherever possible. This might lead to a decision to prescribe one of the atypical antipsychotics. Again, cost has to be taken into account.

Longer term side-effects

Mention has already been made of the common acute extrapyramidal side-effects. When antipsychotic drugs are given for lengthy periods, a common side-effect is tardive dyskinesia. This takes the form of abnormal movements, especially affecting the lower face, jaw, lips and tongue, but also the trunk and limbs. Patients are largely unaware of this side-effect which can be disfiguring. Estimates of the prevalence of dyskinesia vary, but probably at any given time about one-third of patients on long-term medication will show this disorder to some extent (McCreadie et al. 1992).

The 'drug-resistant' patient

A useful definition of drug resistance is where the patient has failed to respond to at least two antipsychotic drugs both given at adequate doses for an adequate period. In such a patient, the use of clozapine should be considered. Clozapine has been shown to be helpful in at least one third of so-called drug-resistant schizophrenic patients (Kane et al. 1988) and possibly may help up to two-thirds (Meltzer et al. 1990). Clozapine is used in the UK only for drug resistant patients as it can produce a serious blood disorder, i.e. agranulocytosis. As a result regular blood checks must be made, initially on a weekly basis for 18 weeks, two weekly for up to 1 year, and monthly thereafter. Up until recently in the UK it has only been possible to obtain clozapine from the hospital pharmacy, but now arrangements can be made where it can be obtained from community pharmacies.

The atypical antipsychotics

A final word about the atypicals. The scene is changing rapidly. Many psychiatrists are coming around to the idea that because atypicals undoubtedly cause less extrapyramidal side-effects and may help negative symptoms, then they should be the drugs of first choice in the treatment of the first episode and relapse, and in maintenance therapy. Studies are currently examining effectiveness of atypicals in drug-resistant schizophrenia and carrying out economic evaluations of their use.

THE COMMUNITY MANAGEMENT OF SCHIZOPHRENIA

The management of schizophrenic patients depends not only on the use of antipsychotic drugs, but also social and other measures are necessary. Assessing the level of need for such services is described in Chapter 9; service models are discussed in Chapter 10. New psychological approaches are detailed in Chapter 15. Psychosocial issues, which need to be considered, are described below.

Living arrangements

A generation ago substantial numbers of schizophrenic patients were in long-stay wards of large psychiatric hospitals. The run down and closure of many of these hospitals has meant that alternative accommodation has had to be found as there is little consistent evidence that the incidence of schizophrenia is falling (Der et al. 1990). Today, few schizophrenic patients live with their parents (Kelly et al. 1998). It seems that the parents of today are less willing to care for their sick adult offspring than those of a generation ago.

The fall in the number of patients living with parents is matched by the increasing number of those living in supported accommodation. This usually consists of patients living in small groups in houses, often in residential parts of town. The support workers, some of whom have come from a nursing background (but many have not), provide a range of support from daily visits to 24-h staffed waking cover. For the most part these are not 'half-way houses'. This is permanent accommodation for chronically ill schizophrenic patients, mainly young and usually male, who a generation ago would have been moving towards long-term care in a psychiatric hospital or creating considerable havoc in the parental home. It is a paradox that, in the community care of schizophrenic patients in the UK today, many of the most disturbed patients are now being cared for by the least-trained staff.

Patients in supported accommodation will be encouraged to do much for themselves, but they may require help with budgeting, shopping, cooking, cleaning, etc. There will be varying degrees of success.

Homelessness in rural areas is uncommon (Kelly et al. 1998). The same, however, cannot be said of inner-city areas where the prevalence of schizophrenia is higher in hostels for the homeless than among the general population (Geddes et al. 1994). Lack of permanent accommodation will inevitably be associated with a lack of almost everything else, including medication and good physical health. Assertive outreach services in the community must take a special interest in those patients.

Occupational activities

Unemployment among schizophrenic patients is high. A recent community survey (Kelly et al. 1998) found that only 8% were in open employment. Work is an integral part of most people's lives. Without it many people lack self worth and a sense of purpose. Schizophrenic patients are no exception. Providing sheltered work brings not only general benefits, but also can have a specific role to play in schizophrenia. It has long been known that an understimulating environment can exacerbate negative symptoms (Wing and Brown 1970). Attending a workplace can provide more stimulation and perhaps ameliorate some of the more severe negative symptoms. Too busy a workplace, of course, may *over*stimulate the vulnerable patient and an acute relapse may occur.

If work is not an option, and it will not be for most schizophrenic patients, what other activities could or should be provided? The most obvious are activities of daily living. Members of the rehabilitation team should have different roles. The occupational therapist can help with important areas such as budgeting, cooking, shopping, housework and personal hygiene. The clinical psychologist (few of whom in the UK, however, are involved in the care of the severely mentally ill; McCreadie et al. 1993) can provide a range of interventions to change patterns of thinking or behaviour, e.g. to improve social skills or increase assertiveness. Nursing staff often takes part in these activities and can also help to organize the patient's leisure time, including holidays. However, it must be recognized that many patients simply do not want to take part in organized activities. Their mere attendance at a unit, however, can be therapy enough for some patients (Mitchell and Birley 1983).

Support services

Patients living outside hospital need support from a wide variety of sources. Recent years have seen the development of community mental health teams. Such teams include nurses, psychiatrists, occupational therapists, psychologists and social workers. From time to time additional input will be required from clinical pharmacists, dieticians, clinical secretaries and local community workers. The team, of course, should have a leader who is often, but not necessarily, the consultant psychiatrist. The team should cover a defined sector and be responsible for delivering a specialized level of care. The functions of the team should include (Scottish Office DoH 1996): assessment and regular review of all care programme approach and community care order patients; identifying at risk patients and regularly reviewing those so identified; pro-active psychological and physical treatments; assertive outreach to support those requiring acute intervention and their carers; acute care backup with responsibility for admission and discharge; liaison on a regular basis with primary care services; and involvement with a range of day and residential settings from hospitals to domiciliary care including intensively staffed homes with NHS staff. The team should give service priority to people with severe and enduring mental health problems (see Chapter 10).

Psychosocial education and family management

There is no doubt that carers and patients, but especially the former, are thirsty for knowledge about all aspects of schizophrenia. Community psychiatric nurses are well placed to give this information. There is little evidence that 'psychosocial education' alone cuts down on the relapse rate in schizophrenia (Tarrier et al. 1989), but education of groups of patients can improve their social functioning and quality of life (Atkinson et al. 1996).

It has already been mentioned that relapse is associated with the patient returning to a critical or over involved family. Much work has been done in recent years to develop family interventions that improve the family atmosphere (Lam 1991). These usually include education, relatives' groups and family support. There is little doubt that such family interventions can cut down on subsequent relapse rates (Lam 1991) (see Chapter 15).

Current interest in drug-resistant patients has stimulated non-drug approaches to such patients. One approach is cognitive–behavioural therapy (Kingdon et al. 1994), described in Chapter 15. Recently strategies to improve treatment 'compliance' have also been developed (Sair et al. 1998). 'Adherence' or 'cooperation' are probably better words as they place responsibility on the clinicians to form a treatment alliance. Education, medication management and other strategies such as explicit written instructions have been used.

OUTCOME

As already stated, about one-third of patients will recover from their first episode of schizophrenia and have no further episodes for at least the next 5 years. The outcome for the other two-thirds of patients is not so good. A minority will not even recover from the first episode and will enter into a chronic disturbed state. The remainder will fall into two groups: the first will recover from the first episode but have subsequent relapses. However, between relapses their level of social functioning will be sufficient to allow them not only to be at home, but also perhaps to live a life approaching that of normality. The second group will also have further episodes, but between episodes they will not return to their previous level of functioning. Work and family relations will suffer and there will be a stepwise deterioration. There is evidence that this decline tends to occur early in the illness and plateaus with the deterioration in the first 2 years predicting subsequent course (Harrison et al. 1996).

CONCLUSION

The explosion of interest in biological aspects of schizophrenia in recent years has led to an improvement in the understanding of the disease process. The introduction of the novel antipsychotics has brought an improvement in treatment options. Psychosocial interventions, especially family management, are undoubtedly effective. However, schizophrenia remains for many patients a chronic and debilitating disorder.

ACKNOWLEDGEMENTS

The author thanks Dawn Hiddleston and Mary Muirhead for secretarial help.

References

Adams W, Kendell RE, Hare EA, Monk-Jorgensen P. Epidemiological evidence that maternal influenza contributes to the aetiology of schizophrenia: an analysis of Scottish, English and Danish data. British Journal of Psychiatry 1993; 163: 522–534.

American Psychiatric Association. Diagnostic and Statistical Manual of Mental Health Disorders, 4th edn. Washington, DC: APA, 1994.

Atkinson JM, Coia DA, Gilmour WH, Harper JP. The impact of education groups for people with schizophrenia on social functioning and quality of life. British Journal of Psychiatry 1996, 168: 199–204.

Bebbington P, Kuipers L. The predictive utility of expressed emotion in schizophrenia: an aggregate analysis. Psychological Medicine 1994; 24: 707–718.

Bebbington PE, Wilkins S, Jones P et al. Life events and psychosis: initial results from the Camberwell Collaborative Psychosis Study. British Journal of Psychiatry 1993; 162: 72–79.

Bleuler E. Dementia Praecox or the Group of Schizophrenias. New York: International Universities Press, 1911.

Bollini P, Pampallona S, Orza MJ et al. Antipsychotic drugs: is more worse? A meta-analysis of the published randomised control trials. Psychological Medicine 1994; 24: 307–316.

Bradbury TN, Miller GA. Season of birth in schizophrenia: a review of evidence, methodology and aetiology. Psychological Bulletin 1985; 98: 569–594.

Brown GW, Birley JLT. Crises and life changes and the onset of schizophrenia. Journal of Health and Social Behaviour 1968; 9: 203–214.

Buchsbaum MS, Ingavar DH, Kessler R, Waters RN, Cappelletti J, van Kammen DP. Cerebral glucography with positron tomography. Use in normal subjects and patients with schizophrenia. Archives of General Psychiatry 1982; 39: 251–259.

Carlson S, Rhodes PG, Ferguson MG. Docosahexaenoic acid status of pre-term infants at birth and following feeding with human milk or formula. American Journal of Clinical Nutrition 1986; 44: 798–804.

Carlsson A. Mechanism of action of neuroleptic drugs. In Lipton MA, Di Mascio A, Killam KF (eds), Psychopharmacology: A Generation of Progress. New York: Raven, 1978.

Crow TJ. Molecular pathology of schizophrenia: more than one disease process? British Medical Journal 1980; 280: 66–68.

Davies LM, Drummond, MR. Economics and schizophrenia: the real cost. British Journal of Psychiatry 1994; 165 (suppl. 25): 18–21.

Der G, Gupta S, Murray RM. Is schizophrenia disappearing? Lancet 1990; 335: 513–516.

Eagles JM. Strength of the genetic effect in schizophrenia. British Journal of Psychiatry 1994; 165: 266.

Emsley RA and the Risperidone Working Group. Risperidone in the treatment of first episode psychotic patients (in press) Schizophrenia Bulletin.

Freeman H. Schizophrenia and city residence. British Journal of Psychiatry 1994; 164 (suppl. 23): 39–50.

Geddes JR, Lawrie SM. Obstetric complications and schizophrenia: a meta-analysis. British Journal of Psychiatry 1995; 167: 786–793.

Geddes JR, Newton R, Young G, Bailey S, Freeman C, Priest R. Comparison of prevalence of schizophrenia among residents of hostels for homeless people in 1966 and 1992. British Medical Journal 1994; 308; 816–819.

Gottesman II, Bertelsen A. Confirming unexpressed genotypes for schizophrenia – risks in the offspring of Fischer's Danish identical and fraternal discordant twins. Archives of General Psychiatry 1989; 46: 867–872.

Gottesman II, Shields J. Schizophrenia: The Epigenetic Puzzle. Cambridge: Cambridge University Press, 1982.

Harrison G, Crondace T, Mason P, Glazebrook C, Medley I. Predicting the long-term outcome of schizophrenia. Psychological Medicine 1996; 26: 697–705.

Heston LL. Psychiatric disorders in foster home reared children of schizophrenic mothers. British Journal of Psychiatry 1966; 122: 819–825.

Jablensky A. The epidemiology of schizophrenia. Current Opinions in Psychiatry 1994; 6: 43–52.

Kane J, Honigfeld G, Singer J, Meltzer HY and the Clozaril Collaborative Study Group. Clozapine for treatment-resistant schizophrenia: a double blind comparison with chlorpromazine. Archives of General Psychiatry 1988; 45: 789–796.

Keck PE, Cohen BM, Baldessarini RJ, McElroy SL. Time course of antipsychotic effects of neuroleptic drugs. American Journal of Psychiatry 1989; 146: 1289–1292.

Kelly C, McCreadie RG, MacEwan T, Carey S. Nithsdale schizophrenia surveys 17. Fifteen year review. British Journal of Psychiatry 1998; 172: 513–518.

Kennedy JL, Guiffra LA, Moises HW et al. Evidence against linkage of schizophrenia to markers on chromosome 5 in a northern Swedish pedigree. Nature 1988; 336: 167–169.

Kety SS, Rosenthal D, Wender PH et al. Mental illness in the biological and adoptive families of individuals who have become schizophrenic. Behaviour Genetics 1976; 6: 219–225.

Kingdon D, Turkington D, John C. Cognitive behaviour therapy of schizophrenia. British Journal of Psychiatry 1994; 164: 581–587.

Lam D. Overview: psychological family intervention in schizophrenia: a review of empirical studies. Psychological Medicine 1991; 21: 423–441.

Leach A, Scherer S. The epidemiology of schizophrenia. Current Opinions in Psychiatry 1992; 5: 20–24.

Lewis SW. Computerised tomography in schizophrenia 15 years on. British Journal of Psychiatry 1990; 157 (suppl. 9): 16–24.

Liddle PF, Barnes TRE. Syndromes of chronic schizophrenia. British Journal of Psychiatry 1990; 157: 558–561.

Loebel AD, Liberman JA, Aluir JM, Mayerhoff DI, Geisler SH, Szymanski SR. Duration of psychosis and outcome in first episode schizophrenia. American Journal of Psychiatry 1993; 149: 1183–1188.

Marshall M. London's mental health services in crisis. British Medical Journal 1997; 314: 246.

May PRA, Tuma AH, Yale C, Potepan P, Dixon WJ. Schizophrenia. A follow-up study of results of treatment. Archives of General Psychiatry 1976; 33: 481–486.

McCreadie RG, Williamson DJ, Robertson LJ. Scottish rehabilitation services: eight year follow-up. Psychiatric Bulletin 1993; 17: 341–343.

McCreadie RG. Recent advances in the drug treatment of schizophrenia. Primary Care Psychiatry 1995; 1; 163–167.

McCreadie RG. The Nithsdale schizophrenia surveys XVI. Breast feeding and schizophrenia: preliminary results and hypotheses. British Journal of Psychiatry 1997; 170: 334–337.

McCreadie RG, Leese M, Tilak-Singh D, Loftus L, MacEwan T, Thornicroft G. Nithsdale, Nunhead and Norwood: similarities and differences in prevalence of schizophrenia and utilisation of services in rural and urban areas. British Journal of Psychiatry 1997; 170: 31–36.

McCreadie RG, Robertson LJ, Wiles D. The Nithsdale schizophrenia surveys IX. Akathisia, parkinsonism, tardive dyskinesia and plasma neuroleptic levels. British Journal of Psychiatry 1992; 161: 793–799.

McGrath J, Welham J, Pemberton M. Month of birth, hemisphere of birth and schizophrenia. British Journal of Psychiatry 1995; 167: 783–785.

McGuffin P, Asherson P, Owen M, Farmer A. The strength of the genetic effect. Is there room for an environmental influence in the aetiology of schizophrenia? British Journal of Psychiatry 1994; 164: 593–599.

Meltzer HY, Burnett S, Bastam B, Ramirez LF. Effect of six months of clozapine treatment on the quality of life of chronic schizophrenic patients. Hospital and Community Psychiatry 1990; 41: 892–897.

Mitchell SF, Birley JL. The use of ward support by psychiatric patients in the community. British Journal of Psychiatry 1983; 142: 9–15.

O'Brien JS, Fillerup DL, Mean JF. Quantification and fatty acid and fatty aldehyde composition of ethanolamine, choline and serine glycerophosphatides in human cerebral grey and white matter. Journal of Lipid Research 1964; 5: 329–338.

Peuskens J and the Risperidone Study Group. Risperidone in the treatment of patients with chronic schizophrenia. British Journal of Psychiatry 1995; 166: 712–726.

Roberts GW, Colter N, Lofthouse R, Bogerts B, Zecai M, Crow TJ. Gliosis in schizophrenia: a survey. Biological Psychiatry 1986; 21: 1043–1050.

Rubin P, Holm S, Friberg L, Videbech P, Anderson HS, Bendsen BB. Altered modulations of prefrontal and subcortical brain activity in newly diagnosed schizophrenia and schizophreniform disorder. A regional cerebral blood flow study. Archives of General Psychiatry 1991; 48: 987–995.

Sair A, Bhui S, Haq S, Strathdee G. Improving treatment adherence among patients with chronic psychoses. Psychiatry Bulletin 1998; 22: 77–81.

Sartorius N, Jablensky A, Korten A, Ernberg G, Anker M, Cooper JE, Day R. Early manifestations and first-contact incidence of schizophrenia in different cultures. Psychological Medicine 1986; 16: 909–928.

Scottish Office Department of Health. Draft Framework for Mental Health Services in Scotland. Edinburgh: Scottish Office DoH, 1996.

Scottish Schizophrenia Research Group. Scottish first episode schizophrenia study II. Treatment: pimozide versus flupenthixol. British Journal of Psychiatry 1987; 150: 334–338.

Scottish Schizophrenia Research Group. The Scottish first episode schizophrenia study VIII. Five year follow-up. British Journal of Psychiatry 1992; 161: 496–500.

Sherrington R, Brynjolffson J, Petersson H et al. Localisation of a susceptibility locus for schizophrenia on chromosome 5. Nature 1988; 336: 164–167.

Speller JC, Barnes TRE, Curson DA, Pautellis C, Alberts JL. One year, low dose neuroleptic study of inpatients with chronic schizophrenia characterized by persistent negative symptoms. British Journal of Psychiatry 1997; 171: 564–568.

Suddath RL, Casanova MF, Goldberg TE, Daniel DG, Kelsoe JR, Weinberger DR. Temporal lobe pathology in schizophrenia. American Journal of Psychiatry 1989; 146: 464–472.

Takei N, O'Callaghan E, Sham P, Glover G, Murray RM. Winter birth excess in schizophrenia: its relationship to place of birth. Schizophrenia Research 1992; 6: 102.

Tarrier N, Barrowclough C, Vaughn C, Bamrah JS, Porceddu K, Watts S, Freeman H. Community management of schizophrenia. A two year follow-up of a behavioural intervention with families. British Journal of Psychiatry 1989; 154: 625–628.

Van Putten T. Why do schizophrenic patients refuse to take their drugs? Archives of General Psychiatry 1974; 31: 67–72.

Wesseley S, Castle D, Der G, Murray R. Schizophrenia in Afro-Caribbeans. A case control study. British Journal of Psychiatry 1991; 159: 795–801.

Wing JK, Bennett DA, Denham J. The Industrial Rehabilitation of Long-stay Schizophrenic Patients. Medical Research Council Memo no. 42. London: HMSO, 1964.

Wing JK, Brown GW. Institutionalism and Schizophrenia. Cambridge: Cambridge University Press, 1970.

World Health Organisation. The ICD–10 Classification of Mental and Behavioural Disorders. Geneva: WHO, 1992.

3

AFFECTIVE DISORDERS

David S. Baldwin

INTRODUCTION

Taken together, the 'affective disorders' represent a group of related conditions, in which the primary disturbance is thought to be one of mood or **affect**. Traditionally, this group includes the depressive disorders, mania and hypomania, and the anxiety disorders; but better delineation of the latter group, together with their often selective response to treatment, has led to the anxiety disorders being considered separately from depression. Although this approach is taken in this volume it is acknowledged that this is somewhat controversial: a recent review (Piccinelli 1998) concluded that there are no clear boundaries between depression and generalized anxiety.

Unhappiness is not only part of the usual reaction to adversity, but also can occur without an obvious cause: the symptom of depressed mood is present when unhappiness lasts longer than expected, appears out of proportion to circumstances, or seems beyond control. Depressed mood occurs in certain physical illnesses (such as hepatitis or glandular fever) and as part of many different psychiatric syndromes: the characteristic features of the depressive disorders include low mood, reduced energy and loss of interest or enjoyment. Other common symptoms in depressive episodes include poor concentration, reduced self-confidence, guilty thoughts, pessimism, ideas of self-harm or suicide, disturbed sleep and altered appetite (WHO 1992). The designated severity of depressive episodes varies, being dependent on the number, type and intensity of symptoms, and the associated impairment at work and in personal or family life.

Consequences of depression

Depression causes much personal suffering and imposes a significant burden on society: the under-recognition and generally rather poor treatment of depression together constitute a major public health issue (Table 3.1). Depression is undoubtedly a common disorder and one that is often severe: it can have serious personal, inter-personal and societal consequences. For the individual, depression causes significant psychological distress, reduces quality of life and increases the mortality rate from suicide, accidents and cardiovascular disease; it can contribute to marital and family breakdown, and in depressed mothers can delay the development of their children (Thompson et al. 1996) (see Chapter 17). The economic burden on society arises not only from direct health and social care costs, but also from the costs of reduced work productivity in patients and carers (Wells et al. 1989), and the costs of premature mortality due to suicide, which is the cause of death in about 10% of patients with a severe recurrent depressive disorder (Harris and Barraclough 1997).

Despite this, the management of people with depression is often far from ideal. Stigma and discrimination together make people reluctant to present for treatment; even after presentation with psychological symptoms, recognition by doctors and other health professionals is variable and often poor; delivery of care and treatment is patchy and sometimes inadequate; and few patients are offered the range of treatments shown to have value in consolidating clinical recovery and preventing a return of illness (Brugha and Bebbington 1992).

CLINICAL DESCRIPTIONS

The brief account of depressive symptoms given in the introductory section is essentially a summary of a 'depressive episode' as described by the World Health Organisation ICD–10 classification (1992) (Table 3.2); the symptoms included within the American Psychiatric Association DSM-IV (1994) diagnostic criteria for major depression are very similar. This type of depression is common in psychiatric outpatient settings. However, psychiatrists see a rather unrepresentative sample of patients, being likely to see the most severely ill, and those with 'co-morbid' disorders (Shepherd et al. 1981). In primary care, many depressed patients do not fulfil the accepted criteria for major depression/depressive episode, either because their illness is too mild or too short, too long or without

---

- Common
- Severe
- Marked associated impairment
- Effective treatments
- Acceptable treatments
- Significant public concern

Table 3.1 – Criteria for a clinical condition to be considered a public health issue.

social consequences. The most recent classificatory schemes include a number of 'by-product' depressive disorders, in an attempt to describe important groups of patients, who otherwise could not be allocated a diagnosis. For example, both the DSM-IV classification and the ICD–10 system include dysthymia (a chronic mild depressive disorder), and the ICD–10 also incorporates recurrent brief depressive disorder (RBD) within the group of mood disorders (Baldwin and Sinclair 1997).

Recurrent unipolar depression

Depression is usually an intermittent condition, most patients experiencing multiple depressive episodes over their lifetime; individual episodes varying in length, severity and impairment, and in the response to treatment. This 'recurrent unipolar depression', may account for up to 10% of consultations in general practice (Ormel and Tiemans 1997). Many depressed patients also describe anxiety symptoms: in some these may be more prominent, the underlying depressive symptoms being found only after direct questioning. 'Biological' (in ICD–10, 'somatic') depressive symptoms (including weight loss, feeling worst earliest in the day and early morning wakening) predict a better response to antidepressant drugs. Some severely ill patients may experience psychotic symptoms, which predict a good response to electro-convulsive therapy (ECT).

- Typical symptoms
  - Depressed mood
  - Loss of interest and enjoyment
  - Reduced energy
- Other common symptoms
  - Reduced concentration and attention
  - Reduced self-esteem and self-confidence
  - Ideas of guilt and unworthiness
  - Bleak and pessimistic view of the future
  - Ideas or acts of self-harm or suicide
  - Disturbed sleep
  - Diminished appetite
- Severity graded according to symptom burden and associated impairment
- Duration of at least 2 weeks is usually required for diagnosis

Based upon ICD–10 Classification of Mental and Behavioural Disorders

---

Table 3.2 – Simplified clinical description of an ICD–10 depressive episode.

Dysthymia

Dysthymic disorder (dysthymia) was introduced into the group of affective disorders in the DSM-III classification in 1980. Although relatively little was known about dysthymia then, subsequent research has resulted in a more detailed understanding of the phenomenology, epidemiology, associated co-morbidity and treatment of this disorder. Accurate diagnosis of dysthymia is often difficult, since it is largely dependent on the recall of symptoms by patients (Baldwin et al. 1995). Simplified diagnostic criteria for dysthymia are given in Table 3.3.

Recurrent brief depression

Community studies, predominantly of young adults, indicate that many of those receiving treatment for 'depression' do not fulfil diagnostic criteria for major depression. These patients experience episodes that are rather short-lived, i.e. less than 2 weeks, but otherwise indistinguishable from major depression (Angst et al. 1990). In a large minority, these 'brief' depressions recur at least monthly and are associated with significant social and occupational impairment. The 'Zurich criteria' for recurrent brief depression are shown in Table 3.4: broadly similar descriptions are included within the ICD–10 (WHO 1992) and Appendix B of the DSM-IV (APA 1994).

A Depressed mood for most of the day, more days than not, for at least 2 years

B Presence, while depressed, of at least two of the following:

- Poor appetite or overeating
- Insomnia or hypersomnia
- Low energy or fatigue
- Low self-esteem
- Poor concentration or difficulty making decisions
- Feelings of hopelessness

C Never without symptoms in A or B for more than 2 months within 2 years

D No evidence of unequivocal major depression during the first 2 years of the disturbance

E No history of mania or an unequivocal hypomanic episode

F Not superimposed on a chronic psychotic disorder

G Not initiated or maintained by organic factors

H Causes clinically significant distress or impairment in social, occupational or other important areas of functioning

---

Table 3.3 – DSM-IV criteria for dysthymia (simplified).

1. Dysphoric mood or loss of interest or pleasure
2. Four of eight symptoms as listed for DSM-III major depression
    - Poor appetite or significant weight loss
    - Insomnia or hypersomnia
    - Psychomotor agitation or retardation
    - Loss of interest or pleasure in usual activities, or decrease in sexual drive
    - Feelings of worthlessness, self re-approach or excessive guilt
    - Diminished ability to think or concentrate; indecisiveness
    - Recurrent thoughts of death, suicidal thoughts, wishes to be dead or suicide attempts
3. Present less than 2 weeks but recurring at least monthly over 1 year
4. Reduced subjective capacity at work

Table 3.4 – Recurrent brief depression: Zurich criteria (modified) (Angst et al. 1990).

Mixed anxiety and depressive disorder

The ICD–10, but not the DSM-IV, includes a new category of mixed anxiety and depressive disorder (MADD), to be recorded when symptoms of both anxiety and depression are present, but neither set of symptoms, considered separately, is sufficiently severe to justify a diagnosis (WHO 1992). As the criteria for the condition are disputed, very little epidemiological research has been conducted. The recent UK household survey of psychiatric morbidity found a point prevalence for MADD of 7.7%, compared with a prevalence of only 2.1% for depressive episodes (Meltzer et al. 1995), as defined by ICD–10. The course of MADD is unknown, but the disorder may be of particular relevance in primary care settings.

Bipolar affective disorder

While lifting of mood is part of the usual response to good fortune, elation can also occur without an obvious cause; alternatively, it may seem unduly excessive or rather too prolonged. Elation may be a symptom or sign of several psychiatric syndromes, including manic episodes, acute schizophrenic episodes and certain drug-induced states. The abundant energy and increased activity of people experiencing manic episodes is usually accompanied by an exaggerated sense of subjective well-being, although many feel irritable and exasperated, and the euphoric mood is sometimes tinged with sadness. Typically, elation is reflected in excessive talkativeness (pressure of speech) and the quick succession of grandiose ideas and unrealistic plans: this impairment of judgement can lead to financial or sexual indiscretions that may ruin personal and family life. Insight into the changes in mood, activity and interpersonal relationships is usually impaired, contributing to the high rates of compulsory admission of manic patients to hospital.

Manic episodes rarely occur in isolation; more characteristically, episodes recur irregularly, becoming interspersed with depressive episodes, which may become relatively more frequent with time. The cyclical pattern of mania and depression was previously called 'manic-depressive psychosis'. The current term of bipolar affective disorder or bipolar illness is better as many patients with marked disturbance of affect do not experience psychotic phenomena, such as delusions or hallucinations.

ATTITUDES TOWARDS DEPRESSION

Depression seems to be a much-misunderstood condition. Repeated surveys of the UK general population, and questionnaire surveys of members of depression 'user groups', reveal widespread attitudes that may hinder optimal outcomes for people with depression. Opinion poll findings indicated a steady increase in the proportion of the population who believe depressed patients should be treated with antidepressants, although this belief is still only shared by a quarter of the population (Paykel et al. 1998); 'counselling' (which has unproven efficacy in the treatment of depression) remains a popular choice. More people appear to accept that 'biological changes in the brain' could cause depression, but the vast majority of the sampled population believes that antidepressants are addictive. Small but significant changes in attitudes towards depression have occurred over the last decade (Paykel et al. 1998): whether these changes have led to altered behaviour (e.g. a greater readiness to consult general practitioners, when troubled by psychological symptoms) is unknown.

Misunderstandings and misgivings are also widespread in the medical and other health professions. For example, many doctors believe that if a depression seems somehow 'understandable', then it should not be treated; others are unaware of the need for long-term pharmacological or psychological treatment, used to prevent early relapse or later recurrence of illness. Primary and secondary care budget holders worry about the cost of seemingly expensive new treatments for depression; policy-makers tend to focus on 'severe mental illness', overlooking the fact that depression is potentially a fatal disorder. When combined with the widespread fear of mental illness, the stigma of a psychiatric diagnosis, and the resulting discrimination in work opportunities, these misunderstandings serve to maintain suboptimal clinical outcomes (Byrne 1999).

EPIDEMIOLOGY

In Western societies, community surveys indicate that significant depressive symptoms are reported by about 15% of the population and some 10% of consultations in primary care settings are probably due to depressive disorders (Ormel and Tiemens 1997). Women are twice as often affected by depression as men, the lifetime prevalence being about 20 and 10% respectively. There is good evidence that women develop more complex and severe clinical pictures, and probably a more troublesome course (Angst 1997). Although the prevalence of depressive symptoms increases with age, major depressive illness may be no more common, or even less common in the elderly. Recent studies suggest a rising incidence of depression in younger age groups: in young men this may be linked to the rise in suicide rates (see Chapter 16). While depressive symptoms are more frequent in the socially excluded and economically disadvantaged, depressive illness can affect people from all sections of society. Major depression in childhood or adolescence is no longer considered rare, the point prevalence in children lying in the range 0.5–2.5% (Harrington 1993).

The accuracy of the reported rates of dysthymia is affected by the phenomenon of forgetting. Lifetime prevalence rates vary between 1 and 12%. All studies of the prevalence of dysthymia have found higher rates in women than in men. There is some evidence that dysthymia and minor depression are more prevalent in the elderly, at the expense of major depression, which seems to be less common in this age group (Angst 1997).

Recurrent brief depression (RBD) appears common in the general population, but there has been relatively little research into the epidemiology of the condition. One-year prevalence rates vary between 4 and 8%; 14.6% of the population in the Zurich study had fulfilled criteria for RBD by 35 years of age. The WHO primary care study found a point prevalence of 5.2% for 'pure' RBD, together with 4.8% for RBD associated with other depressive disorders (Weiller et al. 1994).

While seasonal variations in mood are well established, there is little consensus between epidemiological studies about which season shows a peak of depression. Retrospective investigations have found peak incidences of depressed mood in autumn, winter, spring and even late summer! Although the concept of 'seasonal affective disorder' has gained a degree of recognition in both the ICD–10 and DSM-IV classifications, there is little epidemiological data to support the notion that it is a separate depressive disorder (Angst 1997).

Bipolar affective disorder is not a rare condition. Community surveys in industrialized countries indicate that the lifetime risk for bipolar disorder is about 1%. Similar rates are seen in other cultures where, like unipolar depression, rates of bipolar disorder are higher in urban areas (Angst 1997). Women and men are affected as frequently; the mean age of onset is 21 years, earlier than for major depression; and there is no convincing association with any particular social class.

CO-MORBIDITY

Depression and anxiety often occur together, both in community and clinical samples (Piccinelli 1998). This 'co-morbidity' is typical: up to two-thirds of those with a lifetime history of major depression have a lifetime history of another psychiatric disorder, and an even higher proportion of those with anxiety having multiple previous disorders (Robins et al. 1991). The vast majority of people experiencing a current depressive episode or anxiety disorder also fulfil criteria for another psychiatric disorder, if hierarchical rules relating to diagnosis are relaxed (Kessler et al. 1994).

In some respects, the extensive 'co-morbidity' of anxiety and depression is artefactual, resulting from an excessively categorical approach to psychiatric diagnosis: a more 'dimensional' approach, in which the severity of individual symptoms and signs is described, rather than the current approach of counting symptoms, would reduce apparent co-morbidity, and possibly may be more relevant to clinical practice. A dimensional approach may also have more long-term stability, since categorical approaches change as more becomes known about the features of individual mental disorders. It seems clear that when patients have significant co-existing depressive and anxiety disorders, the associated impairment and use of health services resources is increased; the prognosis is less good, with greater persistence of symptoms; and the risk of suicidal behaviour may be increased (Kessler 1998).

These unfavourable associations may result from the somewhat poorer response of patients with multiple syndromes to traditional pharmacological and psychological treatment approaches. However, some recent studies with selective serotonin re-uptake inhibitors and some other antidepressant drugs suggest that the presence of marked anxiety or agitation is not an impediment to responding to treatment (Boyer and Feighner 1998).

Whether people with certain types of personality are more prone to developing depression is the subject of much controversy. Personality assessments made while an individual is depressed are unreliable, being affected by the anxiety, irritability and negative cognitions associated with depression. Furthermore, assessments performed after full recovery may also be an inaccurate reflection of true 'premorbid' personality, since personality traits may have been affected by the depressive episode. Ideally, the best way to study the interactions of personality and mood is to perform a prospective investigation in which a group of young adults are followed up over many years: this type of research is difficult to perform and is comparatively rare (Hirshfield et al. 1997).

Certain personality traits may confer a predisposition to mental disorder in general, rather than to depression alone. The trait most often associated with a predisposition to depression is undue interpersonal dependence, i.e. an excessive need for reassurance, support and attention from other people. This trait may not be predictive in young people (aged 17–30 years), but when present in older age groups it may confer some risk to developing depression. What is more clear is that the presence of clear-cut personality disorder, i.e. the presence of persisting maladaptive personality traits causing significant personal or interpersonal suffering, adversely affects clinical outcomes in depression. This may be due to the difficulty in engaging in collaborative relationships with health professionals, as much as it is due to the reduced opportunities for establishing wider patterns of psychosocial support at home and at work.

SUICIDE

There are about 4000–5000 deaths by suicide each year in England and Wales, of which 400–500 involve overdoses of antidepressant drugs. Many countries have set targets for reductions in suicide rates, enshrined within policy documents, and have embarked on professional training exercises designed to improve the detection of those at particular risk of committing suicide. The prevention of suicide is described in more detail elsewhere (see Chapter 16).

Two particular groups of patients are at significantly increased risk of suicide: those with a history of suicide attempts, and those recently discharged from psychiatric inpatient care. A recent meta-analysis estimated the standardized mortality ratio for completed suicide of those who had previously attempted suicide to be over 4000, higher than the risk attached to any particular psychiatric disorder, including major depression or alcoholism (Harris and Barraclough 1997). About 10–15% of patients in contact with health services following a suicide attempt will eventually die by suicide, this risk being greatest during the first year after an attempt (Cullberg et al. 1998). Accurate identification of persisting risk, and more assertive follow-up of those at higher risk, may be a useful strategy in reducing completed suicide rates; however, there is at present little evidence to suggest that treatments aimed against repetition of deliberate self-harm are effective (Hawton et al. 1998). Furthermore, recent research in Finland found that 62% of male suicide victims died at their first suicide attempt (Isometsa and Lonnqvist 1998), so this strategy may only be helpful in women.

Up to 41% of suicide victims have received psychiatric inpatient care in the year before death, and up to 9% of suicide victims kill themselves within one day of discharge (Pirkis and Burgess 1998). It is difficult to identify those at particular risk within the general population of psychiatric inpatients; further research is required before targeted interventions can be recommended. At present, it seems that a history of compulsory admission to hospital, suicidal thoughts being noted while in hospital, with a history of suicide attempts and of being separated, are common among those at greatest risk of suicide within 12 months of discharge.

If accurate identification of those patients at particular risk becomes possible, within the setting of standard clinical practice, then it may be possible to 'target' measures to reduce risk of death from suicide, such as the use of psychotropic drugs that are less toxic in overdose.

AETIOLOGY

Depression has many causes: in most patients, depressive episodes arise from the combination of familial, biological, psychological and social factors. Genetic influences are most marked in patients with more severe depressive disorders and 'biological' symptoms: the morbid risk in first-degree relatives is increased in all studies, this elevation being independent of environment or upbringing.

Potential genetic markers for affective disorders have been localized to chromosomes X, 4, 5, 11, 18 and 21. Some of these sites have been linked to the neurobiology of depression: for example, two of the putative markers on the long arm of chromosome 5 contain candidate genes contributing to the receptors for noradrenaline, dopamine, γ-amino butyric acid and glutamate (Souery et al. 1997). It seems increasingly clear that no single genetic abnormality could account for more than a small proportion of cases of affective disorder (Holmes and Lovestone 1997).

The response of depressed patients to antidepressant drugs, and the results of certain investigations, together suggest that abnormalities in the level or function of the neurotransmitters serotonin, noradrenaline and dopamine may be important in the pathophysiology of depression, although this evidence is not conclusive.

There is considerable evidence that aspects of serotonergic neurotransmission are altered in patients with major depression, although some of these abnormalities (such as increased numbers of platelet and brain $5\text{-}HT_2$ receptors) may be linked to suicidal behaviour, rather than to the depressive syndrome. The results of neuroendocrine studies suggest that depression is associated with decreased neurotransmission at post-synaptic $5\text{-}HT_{1a}$ receptors. Some of the changes in brain 5-HT function seen in depressed patients may themselves result from hyper-secretion of cortisol (Cowen and Smith 1997).

Abnormalities of noradrenergic and dopaminergic neurotransmission may be as important as those within the serotonergic system. Although there is no consistent change in noradrenergic receptor function in patients with depression, down-regulation of α-2 receptors by antidepressant drugs may underlie the treatment response (Anand and Charney 1997). Dopaminergic dysfunction has been reported in psychotic and bipolar depression, seasonal affective disorder and depression associated with Parkinson's disease: antidepressants may resolve anhedonia and loss of drive by increasing the sensitization of dopamine D2 and D3 receptors (Anand and Charney 1997).

Low self-esteem, the experience of adversity in childhood and maladaptive negative patterns of thinking about oneself and others, are all psychological 'risk factors' for depression (Hirschfeld and Shea 1992). Social factors include excessive undesirable recent life events, usually involving loss (such as bereavement, divorce and redundancy), and persisting major difficulties including being a lone parent, prolonged unemployment, poverty, and lack of social support or intimacy (Brown et al. 1988).

There is no single cause for bipolar affective disorder: like unipolar depression, individual episodes usually result from the combination of familial, biological, psychological and social factors. The genetic 'loading' for bipolar illness seems greater than that for unipolar depression; for example, the concordance rate for bipolar disorder among monozygotic (identical) twins is about 70%. However, attempts to identify definite genetic markers for the condition have not been successful (Holmes and Lovestone 1997). As is the case for unipolar depression, abnormalities in the level or function of the neurotransmitters serotonin and noradrenaline may be important in bipolar illness. Manic episodes may be associated with overactivity in dopamine pathways within the brain, as mania can be provoked by dopamine-releasing psychostimulants, such as cocaine and amphetamine. Depressed bipolar patients may be more likely to respond than unipolar patients to dopamine-enhancing agents such as bromocriptine or L-dopa (Anand and Charney 1997). A study of dopamine receptor sensitivity postpartum suggests that increased sensitivity precedes the onset of symptoms in affective psychotic relapse (Wieck et al. 1991).

Psychosocial factors, particularly family dynamics, are undoubtedly important in influencing the course of bipolar illness once established; however, their role in causing the condition to appear is unclear. Studies of the impact of adverse life events have produced contradictory findings, although bereavement can be a common precipitant for a manic relapse (Sclare and Creed 1990).

TREATMENT

Unfortunately, for most patients depression is a recurring and sometimes chronic condition. Epidemiological studies, and prospective investigations in clinical samples, reveal high rates of recurrence for both unipolar and bipolar depression; typically, 75% of patients will experience a second depressive episode within 10 years of their first (Paykel and Priest 1992).

Unipolar depression

The risk for future episodes increases with each episode, as if some form of psychological or cerebral 'scarring' has occurred: the length of the 'healthy' interval shortens progressively, and disability and quality of life can worsen with each new episode. Furthermore there is some evidence that 'treatment responsitivity' to antidepressants decreases over time (Kasper 1993). For these reasons, unipolar depression should be considered to be a potentially lifelong condition, and management should focus not only on acute treatment (i.e. getting ill patients well), but also on the perhaps rather harder task of long-term treatment, designed to prevent early relapse or later recurrence of illness (Kasper 1993). Because most depressive episodes result from the combination of biological and psychosocial factors, the optimal treatment of depressed patients usually involves integrating psychological and physical treatment approaches with practical and emotional social support.

'Physical' methods of treatment include the judicious use of antidepressant drugs, and occasionally ECT; light therapy may be helpful for some patients with seasonal affective disorder. Neurosurgery is used exceedingly rarely, being restricted for severely and chronically ill patients who previously derived no benefit from multiple, combined, specialist treatment approaches. Other physical treatments include transcranial magnetic stimulation, but the evidence for its efficacy is still rather limited (Reid et al. 1998).

Antidepressant drugs include the tricyclic antidepressants (TCA), mono-amine oxidase inhibitors (MAOI), selective serotonin re-uptake inhibitors (SSRI) and a disparate group of other compounds. In standard practice, about 70% of patients with moderate or severe depressive episodes will be substantially improved within 3 months of starting treatment: by continuing with antidepressants beyond symptomatic recovery, the risk of relapse can be halved, and longer term treatment can prevent the emergence of new depressive episodes. However, the antidepressant drugs are not ideal (Table 3.5), side-effects limiting their use in some patients. The older drugs (e.g. TCA) can cause drowsiness and interfere with work, and are dangerous when taken in overdose: newer drugs (e.g. SSRI) are somewhat better tolerated (Anderson and Tomenson 1994), and relatively safer, but treatment-emergent insomnia and sexual dysfunction are common problems (Baldwin et al. 1996). The place of newer antidepressants (such as venlafaxine, nefazodone, mirtazapine and reboxetine) in the therapeutics of patients with depression is still being evaluated.

- Effective across a range of depressive disorders
- Effective in short- and long-term treatment
- Rapid onset of action
- Suitable for once-daily dosage
- Effective across the range of age groups
- Well tolerated
- No behavioural toxicity
- Suitable for the physically ill
- Free from interactions with food or drugs
- Safe in overdose
- Cheap

Table 3.5 – The 'ideal' antidepressant.

Many of the mildly depressed patients seen in primary care settings can be helped by simple counselling, and instruction in cognitive, behavioural or problem-solving techniques (Mynors-Wallis et al. 1995). However, moderately or severely ill patients generally probably require more 'intensive' psychological approaches, such as cognitive therapy or interpersonal therapy (Frank et al. 1990). The psychological treatment approaches which have the best evidence of efficacy in depressed patients are those which are semi-manualized (i.e. conducted according to the treatment manual), relatively short-term and focused on particular issues or problems. These directive, problem-focused, time-limited treatments are effective in the short-term, and possibly have some value in delaying the onset of new depressive episodes (Fonagy and Roth 1996). Unfortunately, access to specialized psychological treatments is variable, and often limited. Marital or couple therapy can be a useful accompaniment to other treatment methods (Kasper 1993); and many patients describe some benefit from complementary approaches such as instruction in the Alexander technique or meditation, although 'scientific' evidence for efficacy (i.e. randomized controlled trials) is lacking.

Bipolar depression

It is usually advisable to admit patients with manic episodes to hospital; even the less severe (hypomanic) episodes are disruptive and can lead to reckless behaviour or financial destitution. Considerable nursing skill is required to settle the euphoric, often overactive and sometimes insightless manic patient. The acute treatment of mania usually involves antipsychotic drugs or lithium, often in combination: antipsychotic drugs are more quickly effective, but less well tolerated, at least in the case of traditional antipsychotics.

Lithium is more frequently used as a prophylactic treatment, designed to reduce the risk of future manic or depressive episodes. When prescribed rationally, and when taken regularly lithium can have startling effects, altering the course of illness dramatically: it may also reduce the excess mortality of bipolar illness (Fonagy and Roth 1996). However, many patients will derive little or no benefit, and experience only side-effects such as thirst, tremor and weight gain. Randomized controlled trials with lithium have found that it is effective in 60–90% of acutely ill patients with mania, and in up to 80% of patients when used in the prophylaxis of bipolar disorder. Although effective in the prophylaxis of unipolar depression, the efficacy of lithium in this indication is less good than that of antidepressant drugs (Souza and Goodwin 1991). Unfortunately, the good results seen with lithium in patients participating in treatment studies are not replicated in routine clinical practice, where lithium therapy is not always undertaken in a rigorous way: treatment can be improved through the development of protocols for care and specialized 'lithium clinics' (Schou 1993). In bipolar illness best results are seen when compliance with treatment is good, when there is a family history of bipolar illness and when the pattern of affective episodes is mania followed by depression; results are less good in the presence of rapid cycling illness, paranoid features, and co-morbid substance abuse (Abou-Saleh and Coppen 1990).

Anticonvulsant drugs, more frequently used in the treatment of epilepsy, can be effective in patients who respond only partially to treatment with lithium, or in those with particularly 'rapid-cycling' affective disorder or mixed affective episodes (Post et al. 1997). There is good evidence for the use of sodium valproate and carbamazepine in the acute treatment of mania, and in longer term treatment of rapid cycling bipolar disorder: the evidence is less strong for their use in prophylaxis in bipolar illness, although both have been found helpful as adjuvant treatment, with lithium (Post et al. 1997)

Psychological approaches to the long-term management of bipolar illness have not been studied extensively: however, 'self-management' including heightened mood awareness, the acquisition of appropriate assertiveness, and the spacing apart of activities and life events has been advocated enthusiastically (Guiness 1997).

Dysthymia

Although patients with chronic mild depression make considerable use of health service resources, and often receive prescriptions of psychotropic drugs, the treatment of dysthymia has not been investigated extensively. Furthermore, the methods used in many published studies of the treatment of dysthymia are flawed. Nevertheless, recent research supports the use of antidepressant drugs in certain groups of patients. Benefits have been described with imipramine, certain SSRI (sertraline and fluoxetine) and moclobemide – particularly in patients with so-called 'double depression', in whom depressive episodes complicate an underlying dysthymic disorder (Baldwin et al. 1995). 'Focused' psychotherapies (such as cognitive-behavioural therapy) may improve social functioning, rather than improving depressive symptoms. It seems sensible to offer a combined approach, using both antidepressant drugs and focused psychotherapy, to optimize clinical outcomes in patients with dysthymia (Fonagy and Roth 1996).

Recurrent brief depression

RBD has been formally recognized only recently, and as yet no treatment is established. It is probably misguided to attempt to manage acute episodes with psychotropic drugs, as the episode will usually have resolved before any agent has become effective. Double-blind placebo-controlled studies of fluoxetine, paroxetine, imipramine and moclobemide have not found any evidence that drug treatment reduces the frequency, severity or duration of individual episodes (Kasper et al. 1995, Baldwin and Sinclair 1997). Similarly, no forms of psychological treatment can be recommended, as no formal studies of psychotherapeutic approaches in RBD have been undertaken. Training in problem-solving skills may be of some value in preventing repetition of deliberate self-harm, and could be helpful in the overall management of RBD. It seems sensible to advise patients to limit their alcohol consumption and possibly to avoid the use of benzodiazepines (Baldwin and Sinclair 1997).

'Resistant depression'

The long-term outcome of depression is not as favourable as was previously assumed: between 20 and 35% of patients do not recover fully from a given depressive episode (Prien and Kocsis 1995), although full recovery is possible, even after 10 years of depressive illness (Mueller et al. 1996). A number of factors predict chronicity in depression, including demographic factors (elderly, female), type of illness ('double' depression, psychotic depression), co-morbid physical illness and mental disorder, positive family history and an anxiety-prone pre-morbid personality (Scott 1994). Other factors include delay in starting treatment, inappropriate or suboptimal treatment, poor compliance and therapeutic nihilism (Quitkin 1985).

Research into 'resistant' depression has been hampered by the lack of consensus as to what constitutes 'resistance' (Checkley 1998). However, a number of double-blind placebo-controlled studies have been performed, with a variety of approaches (Nolen et al. 1994). Typically, about 50% of patients improve (though do not necessarily recover) with adjuvant treatments, including lithium, carbamazepine, tryptophan and liothyronine: combining antidepressants, using drugs from different classes, can also be helpful (Berlanga and Ortega-Soto 1995). The management of resistant depression is a complex and time-consuming task, and is probably best left to specialist mental health services.

Long-term treatment in affective disorder

Increasingly, both uni- and bipolar depression are regarded as potentially lifelong, episodic conditions: as such, the focus of treatment is shifting towards long-term management, designed to minimize the risks of relapse and recurrence of affective illness. The efficacy of many antidepressants, and some psychological therapies, in continuation and prophylactic treatment has been evaluated and most have been found beneficial, although there is no good evidence to support the use of nortriptyline or mianserin in long-term treatment (Kasper 1997). When used in maintenance treatment, the dosage of antidepressant used should be the same as that which helped resolve that acute episode of illness (Kasper 1997). Steadily, consensus has been reached on the optimal duration of continuation treatment: it is clear that antidepressants should be continued for 6 months after symptomatic recovery (Paykel and Priest 1992, Kasper 1997). There is still some uncertainty about the duration of prophylactic treatment in recurrent unipolar depression, although many believe that treatment should be continued indefinitely (BAP 1993). The situation is less clear for bipolar depression, where extending the duration of antidepressant treatment can precipitate hypomania or manic episodes, or contribute to 'cycle acceleration', in which affective episodes become progressively more frequent with time (Post 1992).

CONCLUSIONS

Although common and often serious, as well as disabling and long lasting, depression is frequently over-looked and managed rather poorly. Advances in the therapeutics of depression may have out-stripped increases in understanding of the aetiology and pathophysiology of the condition. Depressive syndromes may represent the clinical 'expression' of the progressive combination of genetic inheritance, particular patterns of early development, adversity in childhood, adolescence and early adult life, the experience of loss, and environment challenge; the symptoms and signs of depression are probably associated with changes in neuroendocrine status and neurotransmitter function – and with changes in psychological functioning – which maintain the condition, once established, and which may need to resolve before recovery can occur. While all these factors and variables require further investigation, much benefit would be gained from better use of existing pharmacological treatments and increased availability of particular psychological therapies. These changes can only occur through combining public education, professional training and socio-economic measures.

SUMMARY

Depressive disorders are common, often severe and usually associated with marked social and occupational impairment. Classificatory schemes vary, but there is general agreement on what constitutes a 'major' depressive episode. Depressive disorders are of multi-factorial origin: familial, biological, psychological and social variables are all important. Optimal management of depressed patients usually involves integrating psychological and pharmacological treatment approaches with practical social support. Public misunderstandings and variations in clinical practice together contribute to suboptimal outcomes in depression.

ACKNOWLEDGEMENTS

Thanks are due to Karen Middleton for secretarial assistance; to Alain Gregoire for tolerance and gentle persuasion; and to Judit Pasztor for her kindness and insights.

References

Abou-Saleh MT, Coppen AJ. Predictors of long term outcome of mood disorder on prophylactic lithium. Lithium 1990; 1: 27–35.

American Psychiatric Association. Diagnostic and Statistical Manual of Mental Disorders, 4th edn. Washington, DC: APA, 1994.

Anand A, Charney DS. Catecholamines in depression. In Honig A, van Praag HM (eds), Depression: Neurobiological, Psychopathological and Therapeutic Advances. Chichester: Wiley, 1997, pp. 147–178.

Anderson IM, Tomenson BM. Treatment discontinuation with selective serotonin re-uptake inhibitors compared with tricyclic antidepressants: a meta-analysis. British Medical Journal 1994; 310: 1433–1438.

Angst J. Epidemiology of depression. In Honig A, van Praag HM (eds), Depression: Neurobiological, Psychopathological and Therapeutic Advances. Chichester: Wiley, 1997.

Angst J, Merinkangas A, Scheidegger P, Wicki W. Recurrent brief depression: a new subtype of affective disorder. Journal of Affective Disorder 1990; 19: 87–98.

Baldwin DS, Hawley CJ, Abed R, Maragakis B, Cox J, Buckinham SA, Pover GH, Ascher A. A multicenter double-blind comparison of nefazodone and paroxetine in the treatment of outpatients with moderate-to-severe depression. Journal of Clinical Psychiatry 1996; 57 (suppl. 2): 46–52.

Baldwin DS, Rudge SE, Thomas SC. Dysthymia: options for pharmacotherapy. CNS Drugs 1995; 4: 422–431.

Baldwin DS, Sinclair JMA. Recurrent brief depression: 'nasty, brutish and short'. In Bhugra D, Munro A (eds), Troublesome Disguises: Underdiagnosed Psychiatric Syndromes. Oxford: Blackwell, 1997, pp. 226–240.

Berlanga C, Ortega-Soto MA. A 3-year follow up of a group of treatment-resistant depressed patients with a MAOI/tricyclic combination. Journal of Affective Disorders 1995; 34: 187–192.

Boyer W, Feighner JP. The utility of SSRIs in anxious depression. In Montgomery SA, den Boer JA (eds), SSRIs in Depression and Anxiety. Chichester: Wiley, 1998, pp. 101–113.

British Association for Psychopharmacology. Guidelines for Treating Depressive Illness with Antidepressants. Journal of Psychopharmacology 1993; 7: 19–23.

Brown GW, Adler Z, Bifulco A. Life events, difficulties and recovery from chronic depression. British Journal of Psychiatry 1988; 152: 487–498.

Brugha TS, Bebbington PE. The undertreatment of depression. European Archives in Psychiatry and Clinical Neuroscience 1992; 242: 1–3–108.

Byrne P. Stigma of mental illness. Changing minds, changing behaviour. British Journal of Psychiatry 1999; 174:1–2.

Checkley S. The management of resistant depression. In Checkley S (ed.), The Management of Depression. Oxford: Blackwell, 1998, pp. 430–457.

Cowen PJ, Smith KA. Serotonin and depression. In Honig A, van Praag HM (eds), Depression: Neurobiological, Psychopathological and Therapeutic Advances. Chichester: Wiley, 1997, pp. 129–146.

Cullberg J, Wasserman D, Stefansson CG. Who commits suicide after a suicide attempt? Acta Psychiatrica Scandinavica 1988; 77: 598–603.

Fonagy P, Roth A. What Works for Whom? A Critical Review of Psychotherapy Research. New York: Guildford, 1996.

Frank E, Kupfer DJ, Perel JM, Cornes C, Jaret DB, Mallinger AG, Thase ME, McEachran AB, Agrochocinski VJ. Three-year outcomes for maintenance therapies in recurrent depression. Archives in General Psychiatry 1990; 47: 1093–1099.

Guiness D. A guide to self-management. In Varma V (ed.), Managing Manic Depressive Disorders. London: Jessica Kingsley, 1997, pp. 165–178.

Harrington R (ed.). Epidemiology. In Depressive Disorders in Childhood and Adolescence. Chichester: Wiley, 1993.

Harris EC, Barraclough B. Suicide as an outcome for mental disorders. British Journal of Psychiatry 1997; 170: 205–228.

Hawton K, Arensman E, Townsend E, Bremner E, Feldman E, Goldney R, Gunnell D et al. Deliberate self-harm: systematic review of efficacy of psychosocial and pharmacological treatments in preventing repetition. British Medical Journal 1998; 317: 441–447.

Hirschfeld RMA, Shea MT. Personality. In Paykel E (ed.), Handbook of Affective Disorders. Edinburgh: Churchill Livingstone, 1992, pp. 185–194.

Hirschfeld RMA, Shea MT, Holzer CE. Personality dysfunction and depression. In Honig A, van Praag HM (eds), Depression: Neurobiolgical, Psychopathological and Therapeutic Advances. Chichester: Wiley, 1997, pp. 327–341.

Holmes C, Lovestone S. The molecular genetics of mood disorders. Current Opinions in Psychiatry 1997; 10: 79–83.

Isometsa ET, Lonnqvist JK. Suicide attempts preceding completed suicide. British Journal of Psychiatry 1998; 173: 531–535.

Kasper S. Long-term treatment of depression with antidepressants: evidence from clinical trials, prediction and practical guidelines. In Honig A, van Praag HM (eds), Depression: Neurobiological, Psychological and Therapeutic Advances. Chichester: Wiley, 1997, pp. 449–518.

Kasper S. The rationale for long-term antidepressant therapy. International Journal of Clinical Psychopharmacology 1993; 8: 225–235.

Kasper S, Stamenkovic M, Fischer G. Recurrent brief depression: diagnosis, epidemiology and potential pharmacological options. CNS Drugs 1995; 4: 222–229.

Kessler RC. Comorbidity of depression and anxiety disorders. In Montgomery SA, den Boer JA (eds), SSRIs in Depression and Anxiety. Chichester: Wiley, 1998, pp. 81–99.

Kessler RC, McGonagle KA, Zhao S, Nelson CB, Hughes M, Eshleman S, Wittchen H-V, Kender KS. Lifetime and 12-month prevalence of DSM-III-R psychiatric disorders in the United States: results from the National Comorbidity Survey. Archives in General Psychiatry 1994; 51: 8–19.

Meltzer H, Gill B, Petticrew M, Hinds K. The prevalence of psychiatric morbidity among adults living in private households. In OPCS Surveys of Psychiatric Morbidity in Great Britain, Report 1. London: OPCS Social Survey Division, 1995.

Mueller TI, Keller MB, Leon AC et al. Recovery after 5 years of unremitting major depressive disorder. Archives in General Psychiatry 1996; 53: 794–799.

Mynors-Wallis LM, Gath DM, Lloyd-Thomas AR, Tomlinson D. Randomised controlled trial comparing problem solving treatment with amitriptyline and placebo for major depression in primary care. British Medical Journal 1995; 310: 441–445.

Nolen WA, Zohar J, Amsterdam JD (eds), Refractory Depression: Current Strategies and Future Directions. Chichester: Wiley, 1994.

Ormel J, Tiemens B. Depression in primary care. In Honig A, van Praag HM (eds), Depression: Neurobiological, Psychopathological and Therapeutic Advances. Chichester: Wiley, 1997.

Paykel ES, Hart D, Priest RG. Changes in public attitudes to depression during the Defeat Depression Campaign. British Journal of Psychiatry 1998; 173: 519–522.

Paykel ES, Priest RG. Recognition and management of depression in general practice: consensus statement. British Medical Journal 1992; 305: 1198–1202.

Piccinelli M. Comorbidity of depression and generalised anxiety: is there any distinct boundary? Current Opinions in Psychiatry 1998; 11: 57–60.

Pirkis J, Burgess P. Suicide and recency of health care contacts. A systematic review. British Journal of Psychiatry 1998; 173: 462–474.

Post RM. Rapid cycling and depression. In Montgomery SA, Rouillon F (eds), Long-term Treatment of Depression. Chichester: Wiley, 1992.

Post RM, Frye MA, Denicoff KD, Kimbrell TA, Cora-Locatelli G, Leverich GS. Anticonvulsants in the long term prophylaxis of affective disorders. In Honig A, van Praag HM (eds), Depression: Neurobiological, Psychopathological and Therapeutic Advances. Chichester: Wiley, 1997, pp. 483–498.

Prien RF, Kocsis JH. Long-term treatment of mood disorders. In Bloom FE, Kupfer DJ (eds), Psychopharmacology: The Fourth Generation of Progress. New York: Raven, 1995, pp. 1067–1079.

Quitkin FM. The importance of dosage in prescribing antidepressants. British Journal of Psychiatry 1985; 147: 593–597.

Reid PD, Shajahan PM, Glabus MF, Ebmeier KP. Transcranial magnetic stimulation in depression. British Journal of Psychiatry 1998; 173: 449–452.

Robins LN, Locke BZ, Regier DA. Overview: psychiatric disorders in America. In Robins LN, Reiger DA (eds), Psychiatric Disorders in America. New York: Free Press, 1991, pp. 328–366.

Schou M. Lithium. In Honig A, van Praag HM (eds), Depression: Neurobiological, Psychopathological and Therapeutic Advances. Chichester: Wiley, 1997, pp. 473–482.

Schou M. Lithium Treatment of Manic-Depressive Illness. A Practical Guide. Freiburg: Karger, 1993.

Sclare P, Creed F. Life events and the onset of mania. British Journal of Psychiatry 1990; 156: 508–514.

Scott J. Predictors of non-response to antidepressants. In Nolen WA, Zohar J, Amsterdam JD (eds), Refractory Depression: Current Strategies and Future Directions. Chichester: Wiley, 1994, pp. 19–28.

Shepherd M, Cooper B, Brown AC, Kalton G. Psychiatric Illness in General Practice, 2nd edn. London: Oxford University Press, 1981.

Souery D, Lipp O, Matieu B, Mendlewicz J. Advances in the genetics of depression. In Honig A, van Praag HM (eds), Depression: Neurobiological, Psychopathological and Therapeutic Advances. Chichester: Wiley, 1997, pp. 297–309.

Souza FGM, Goodwin GM. Lithium treatment and prophylaxis in unipolar depression: a metranalysis. British Journal of Psychiatry 1991; 158: 666–675.

Thompson C, Baldwin DS, Tylee A. The defeat of depression: a European perspective. International Journal in the Methods of Psychiatric Research 1996; 6: S1.

Weiller E, Lecrubier Y, Maier W, Ustun TB. The relevance of recurrent brief depression in primary care: a report from the WHO Project on Psychological Problems in General health care conducted in 14 countries. European Journal of Archives in Psychiatry and Clinical Neuroscience 1994; 244: 182–189.

Wells KB, Stewart A, Hays RD et al. The functioning and well-being of depressed patients: results from the Medical Outcomes study. Journal of the American Medical Association 1989; 262: 914–919.

Wieck A, Kumar R, Hirst AD, Marks MN, Campbell IC, Checkley SA. Increased sensitivity of dopamine receptors and recurrence of affective illness after childbirth. British Medical Journal 1991; 303: 613–616.

World Health Organisation. The ICD–10 Classification of Mental and Behavioural Disorders: Clinical Descriptions and Diagnosis Guidelines. Geneva: WHO, 1992.

Further reading

Hale AS. ABC of mental health: depression. British Medical Journal 1997; 315: 43–46.

Healy D. The Antidepressant Era. Cambridge, MA: Harvard University Press, 1997.

Jamison KR. Touched with Fire: Manic-Depressive Illness and the Artistic Temperament. New York: Free Press, 1993.

Milligan S, Clare A. Depression and How to Survive it. London: Edbury, 1993.

Varma V (ed.). Managing Manic Depressive Disorders. London: Jessica Kingsley, 1997.

Wilkinson G, Moore B, Moore P. Treating People with Depression: A Practical Guide for Primary Care. Abingdon: Radcliffe Medical, 1999.

4

ANXIETY DISORDERS

Caroline Bell, Hugh Middleton, Pam Jezzard-Clark and David Nutt

INTRODUCTION

The anxiety disorders constitute a significant public health problem. They are common and patients are often seriously disabled. They are also associated with considerable comorbidity. Anxiety disorder patients have high rates of depression, substance abuse, marital disorder and financial dependency. Furthermore, they make up one of the most active groups of healthcare users, being responsible for a large proportion of consultations in primary care and a significant proportion of referrals to secondary services (Royal College of General Practitioners 1986, Goldberg and Huxley 1992).

Although anxiety disorders are many, these patients and their problems are poorly understood and continue to be managed in a wide variety of ways. To a considerable extent this is due to continuing conceptual controversy. Anxiety is a social as well as a psychiatric or medical construct and the traditional approach has been to regard those disabled by anxiety as individuals suffering an excessive degree of otherwise everyday human distress. They are, therefore, managed accordingly, by the provision of support, understanding and, where appropriate, sedation, but not necessarily with treatments of proven efficacy. The move towards defining specific anxiety disorders that might respond to more focal approaches to treatment is a recent development that might be dated from the publication of DSM-II (American Psychiatric Association 1968), but it only really gathered momentum with the publication of ICD–9 (World Health Organisation 1978) and DSM-III (American Psychiatric Association 1980). More than half the currently active UK medical workforce qualified before 1980 and public attitudes and expectations change even more slowly. Furthermore, the presence of co-morbidity, common risk factors and in some cases indistinguishable responses to treatment between patients with differing DSM and ICD diagnoses give continuing credence to the view that the anxiety disorders are but one manifestation of a more general 'neurotic syndrome' (e.g. Gelder 1986, Andrews 1990, Tyrer 1996). This is commonly recognized as a relative failure to manage 'stress' adaptively, and as a result tends to attract a wide variety of usually non-specific approaches to treatment. A recent investigation of provision for patients with anxiety disorder by a representative NHS trust revealed a wide variety of treatments, few truly evidence-based and little rationale behind selection (Ball et al. 1997).

This unsatisfactory state of clinical affairs contrasts quite starkly with research findings that support specific drug and psychological treatments for specific disorders. New pharmacotherapies such as the selective serotonin re-uptake inhibitors (SSRI) and buspirone, and older ones such as the tricyclic anti-depressants (TCA) have emerged as effective alternatives to the benzodiazepines. These developments have been paralleled by a similar growth in available psychological treatments particularly cognitive behaviour therapy (CBT). This period of progress seems set to continue with the rapid expansion of knowledge emerging from imaging studies about the brain circuits and transmitters regulating anxiety. Furthermore, increasing interest in the critical appraisal of NHS activities focuses attention upon the value and efficacy of treatments provided for common conditions such as morbid anxiety.

This chapter will consider the various anxiety disorders and give practical advice on their effective management. As the term 'anxiety' is often used in a very general way to encompass a broad range of symptoms and conditions, it is important to clarify exactly what the problem is. Time invested at the initial interview will reap benefits later – it allows a thorough history to be taken and a clear understanding of the patient's symptoms to be reached. This will allow the correct diagnosis to be made and the patient to feel understood, perhaps for the first time. Before any drug or psychological treatment starts patients need to be given a careful explanation of their condition including education about the nature of and the reasons for their anxiety, the likely time-course of response and any potential adverse effects.

Drug treatments

The choice of drugs available for use in anxiety are the anti-depressants (TCA, monoamine oxidase inhibitors (MAOI)/reversible inhibitors of monoamine oxidase (RIMA) and SSRI), benzodiazepines and other anxiolytics, e.g. buspirone. Their efficacy and time-course of action in the different disorders will be discussed separately, but their side-effect profiles and specific problems associated with their use are summarized in table 1.

Psychological treatments

The psychological treatment most proven in the treatment of anxiety is CBT. The term 'cognitive' actually comprises a number of more discrete psychological

DRUG	SIDE-EFFECTS AND INTERACTIONS	TOXICITY IN OVERDOSE	ANXIETY EXACERBATION	ONSET OF ACTION
TCA	Dry mouth, blurred vision, constipation, water retention, sedation, weight gain, sexual dysfunction	Dangerous	Early in treatment, i.e. first 1–2 weeks	4–6 weeks
MAOI	Weight gain, postural hypotension, sexual dysfunction. Interaction tyramine containing foods, interaction drugs, e.g. pethidine, sympathomimetics	Dangerous	Less tendency	4–6 weeks
RIMA	Headache, nausea, dizziness. Interaction drugs, e.g. pethidine, sympathomimetics. Much less interaction with tyramine containing foods, therefore no diet restriction.	Safer	Less tendency	4–12 weeks
SSRI	Headache, nausea, dizziness, sexual dysfunction, agitation	Safer	Early in treatment, i.e. 1–2 weeks	4–6 weeks
Benzodiazepine	Sedation, cognitive impairment ataxia. Cross tolerance with other drugs, e.g. alcohol. Tolerance dependence, withdrawal	Safer in isolation	None	1–2 weeks
5-HT agonists, e.g. buspirone	Nausea, headache, dizziness	Safer	None	3–4 weeks

Table 4.1 – Characteristics of drugs used to treat anxiety disorders.

phenomena, such as attention, thinking, planning, memory, imagery and others, and it is barely surprising that the expression 'cognitive therapy' has become debased by the acquisition of an wide range of applications. The term first came into use in order that the shortcomings of a purely behavioural approach to psychopathology might be complemented and strengthened by acknowledgement of the extent to which 'an individual's affect and behaviour are largely determined by the way in which he structures the world' (Beck et al. 1979). The cognitive model of psychopathology focuses attention on the extent to which fears and maladaptive behaviours can be attributed to idiosyncratic but internally consistent and comprehensible misperceptions, such that the core 'pathology' is a propensity to adopt specific maladaptive interpretations. Treatment aims to identify and modify the dysfunctional thoughts, assumptions and patterns of behaviour in the course of a limited number of focussed sessions.

THE CLASSIFICATION OF ANXIETY

Although there is no perfect way of categorizing the anxiety disorders, for practical purposes the diagnostic criteria of DSM-IV (American Psychiatric Association 1994) (Table 4.2) or ICD–10 (World Health Organisation International Classification of Disease) are generally used. Both systems divide anxiety into a series of sub-syndromes and provide clear operational criteria for each condition. Even though, at any one time, many patients will have symptoms from more than one syndrome, eliciting the primary diagnosis is important as this will influence the choice of treatment.

Below will be described the important features of each anxiety disorder according to DSM-IV criteria. This description will include a discussion of the epidemiology and the factors that help the clinician in the diagnostic process. We will then give a practical description of the use of medication and psychological treatments for each.

PANIC DISORDER

Panic attacks are very common, with at least 10% of the population experiencing at least one panic in their lifetime. The syndrome of panic disorder is a more serious and persistent condition characterized by recurrent attacks that significantly interfere with the patient's life. It is also common and has a lifetime prevalence of 3% (Kessler et al. 1994). The peak age of onset of panic disorder is in the third decade and there is a

- Panic disorder with or without agoraphobia
- Agoraphobia without a history of panic disorder
- Specific phobia
- Social phobia
- Obsessive–compulsive disorder
- Post-traumatic stress disorder
- Acute stress disorder
- Generalized anxiety disorder

Table 4.2 – Anxiety disorders in DSM-IV and ICD–10.

consistent female preponderance. The usual course of the disorder is chronic with periods of waxing and waning. Co-morbidity particularly with depression, suicide and drug and alcohol abuse (as a consequence of self-medication) is very common. Health concerns are also prominent. The nature of the symptoms is often somatic (table 3) and as a consequence patients are often convinced that the problem is physical and seek help from a variety of specialists through, for example, accident and emergency, cardiac, respiratory, neurology, gastroenterology and ENT departments. They are often unnecessarily and extensively investigated and in fact are one of the highest users of general medical services. Effective management is, therefore, crucial not only for the patient but also for the health service in general – it reduces demand on other services and is clearly cost effective.

Panic attacks are discrete periods of intense fear accompanied by a variety of somatic and cognitive symptoms (Table 4.3). They are very frightening and have a big impact on the patient – the first one is usually clearly remembered and patients dread and fear the next. They can be spontaneous (occurring 'out of the blue') or be situationally bound as the panic attacks become associated with specific situations. Particularly problematic are places from which escape may be difficult, e.g. buses, trains, motorways, or where help may be hard to find, e.g. busy supermarkets. The fear of this characteristic cluster of situations and the consequent avoidance it causes is called agoraphobia ('fear of the market place'). It can result in patients becoming housebound, as more and more situations are avoided, and is often one of the most disabling features of panic disorder. Some patients find being accompanied by someone helps others find even the support of an inanimate object, e.g. a pram, beneficial.

• Palpitations or pounding heart
• Sweating
• Trembling
• Sensation of shortness of breath
• Feeling of choking
• Chest pain
• Nausea or abdominal distress
• Feeling dizzy or light-headed
• Paraesthesia
• Chills or hot flushes
• De-realisation or depersonalization
• Fear of dying or having a heart attack
• Fear of losing control or going crazy

Table 4.3 – Symptoms of a panic attack.

Making the diagnosis

The key to making the diagnosis is a good history. This needs to include all symptoms of the panic attack, what the patient thinks is the worst thing that could possibly happen, when and where the first one occurred, and what situations precipitate them. From this other disorders can be differentiated without the need for extensive investigations (Table 4.4).

Treatment

Education is an early and important component of treatment. As panic disorder patients characteristically interpret their symptoms as evidence of their being at risk of a sudden medical disaster, alternative explanations and provision of a credible rationale for the course that is going to be followed are important first steps. Treatment then aims to improve the three core symptoms of panic disorder – panic attacks, anticipatory anxiety and avoidance.

Drug treatments

The era for the drug treatment of panic and agoraphobia dates from the 1960s with observations that the tricyclic antidepressant, imipramine and the monoamine oxidase inhibitors produced significant improvements in patients with anxiety (Sargant and Dally 1962, Klein 1964). Since then treatments have diversified and there are now four main classes of drug treatment available.

Tricyclic antidepressants (TCA)

Imipramine and clomipramine have been the most studied antidepressants of the TCA class. Efficacy for both has been repeatedly demonstrated in controlled trials with response rates of 60–70% being reported (Modigh 1987). The time-course over which symptoms improve is typically a reduction in panic attacks first after 4–6

- Other psychiatric disorders, e.g. social phobia, GAD, PTSD
- Substance use/abuse, e.g. alcohol withdrawal, caffeinism, amphetamine abuse
- Medical conditions, e.g.:
    - Hyperthyroidism
    - Asthma
    - Cardiac arrhythmias
    - Labyrinthitis
    - Phaeochromocytoma
    - Temporal lobe epilepsy

Table 4.4 – Differential diagnosis of panic attacks.

weeks, followed later by reductions in anticipatory anxiety and avoidance. The dose range of medication is wide, e.g. imipramine 25–300 mg/day, with some patients responding to low doses but most requiring doses in the higher range.

Monoamine oxidase inhibitors (MAOI) and reversible inhibitors of monoamine oxidase (RIMA)

Most controlled trials have used the MAOI, phenelzine and have demonstrated efficacy in treating panic and related disorders (Sheehan et al. 1980). The dose required is unclear but it again seems that doses in the higher range are necessary.

RIMA, e.g. moclobemide, may represent an effective alternative to the MAOI although so far there has only been one study which has demonstrated efficacy (van Vliet et al. 1991).

Specific serotonin reuptake inhibitors (SSRI)

Controlled trials have demonstrated efficacy in panic disorder for all the SSRI, zimelidine (now withdrawn) (Evans et al. 1986), fluvoxamine (den Boer and Westenberg 1987), paroxetine (Lecrubier et al. 1997), sertraline (Gorman et al. 1994), citalopram (Wade et al. 1997) and fluoxetine (Schneier et al 1990). Paroxetine has been the most comprehensively studied with dose ranging and short- and long-term trials, i.e. 48 weeks (Lecrubier et al. 1997). As a consequence it was the first SSRI to be licensed for panic disorder, and was followed by citalopram. The response rate and time-course of symptom improvement with SSRI is similar to that seen with the TCA and possibly more rapid (Lecrubier et al. 1997). Doses required for successful treatment are again high, e.g. 40 mg paroxetine (Dunbar et al. 1995).

Debate has centred around the relative roles of the serotonergic and noradrenergic systems in the efficacy of the antidepressants in panic disorder. The TCA, imipramine and clomipramine block the reuptake of both 5-HT and NA and response tends to correlate more with the plasma concentration of the parent compound (serotonergic) than that of major metabolite (noradrenergic) (Mavissakalian and Perel 1989). Although there have been reports of other antidepressants being effective, the general trend suggests that noradrenergic agents, e.g. maprotiline are less effective than serotonergic agents (den Boer and Westenberg 1988).

Benzodiazepines

Although benzodiazepines have long been known to be effective in reducing generalized anxiety it was not until the 1980s that they were demonstrated to be effective in panic disorder. Large, multi-centre, controlled studies showed approximately equivalent efficacy to the TCA over 8 weeks of treatment (CNCPS 1992). The main difference between the drugs was the quicker onset of action of the benzodiazepines (within 1 week) (Figure 4.1). Alprazolam was the first benzodiazepine to be studied, but subsequent work has confirmed efficacy for other benzodiazepines,

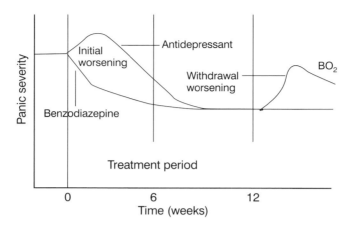

Figure 4.1 – Time course of panic treatment

e.g. lorazepam, clonazepam and diazepam (JohSnson et al. 1995). The doses required are again high, e.g. 4–6 mg alprazolam (equivalent to 40–60 mg diazepam). The problems associated with the benzodiazepines (discussed above) are well known and have considerably limited their use. Benzodiazepines are, however, very effective anxiolytics and do have a role in the management of short-term anxiety exacerbation and in some patients on a longer basis if other treatments have failed.

β-Blockers

β-Blockers are widely prescribed for the treatment of panic attacks despite the fact that controlled trials do not demonstrate efficacy (Munjack et al. 1989). The only situations where they do appear to have a role is in performance anxiety (e.g. for musicians).

5-HT$_{1a}$ agonists

Although effective in the treatment of generalized anxiety disorder 5-HT$_{1a}$ agonists, e.g. buspirone, are not effective in panic disorder (Sheehan et al. 1990).

Psychological treatment

Panic disorder is the anxiety disorder for which cognitive/behavioural psychotherapy has been tested most exhaustively. Four trials of cognitive/behavioural therapy based on the 'Oxford' model (Clark 1986) have demonstrated its superiority over control psychological treatments (Beck et al. 1992, Clark et al. 1994, Öst and Westling 1995, Arntz and van den Hout 1996). One of these (Clark et al. 1994) also made comparisons with drug treatment (imipramine) and found psychological treatment to be superior, especially at longer term follow up. A different form of cognitive/behavioural therapy for panic (panic control treatment) has been developed in the USA where it has been shown to be superior to control psychotherapies (Barlow et al. 1989), and alprazolam (Klosko et al. 1990). In a third (Black et al. 1993), fluvoxamine proved more effective than a shortened version of panic control treatment, even though this was more effective than placebo.

The essential feature of the cognitive/behavioural approach to panic disorder is an *a priori* acknowledgement that the disorder is driven by the propensity to make specific catastrophic interpretations of identifiable sensations. Palpitations might be interpreted as evidence of an impending heart attack, breathlessness as evidence of impending suffocation, dizziness as evidence of impending collapse, de-realisation as evidence of impending madness, nausea as evidence of impending incontinence, and so on. Individual patients generally subscribe to one or at most two such 'catastrophic' misinterpretations.

Questionnaires can be used to tease out interpretations, fears and patterns of avoidance. They can also be used to tease out 'safety' behaviours, e.g. if provoked to anxiety by dizziness because their misinterpretation is that it signals collapse, a panic disorder patient might hold on to furniture to prevent themselves from falling. As a result, the learning experience will be 'The only reason I did not collapse was because I took steps to stop it happening' rather than 'It was not going to happen anyway', and thus the misinterpretation is maintained. In essence, treatment involves identifying these cognitive/behavioural stereotypes and assisting patients to dismantle them. Psychological treatment proceeds with exposure to situations previously avoided and the deliberate dismembering of risk-reducing rituals. Relapse is related to the success with which misinterpretations are extirpated and risk-reducing rituals eliminated. Ideally, a patient should not be considered fully recovered unless it is clear their behaviour is entirely fluid and flexible with respect to such concerns.

Agoraphobia

Agoraphobia generally occurs as part of the panic disorder picture described above although pure agoraphobia without panics is found in some (predominantly female) patients. This presentation may in fact represent a disorder more related to specific phobias than panic disorder.

SPECIFIC PHOBIA

Phobias are common in childhood and often outgrown. Depending on the criteria used a lifetime prevalence of about 10% is reported with consistently higher rates being found in females. The peak age of onset depends on the subtype as shown in Table 4.5.

The essential feature of a specific phobia is a marked and persistent fear of a circumscribed object or situation. Exposure causes extreme anxiety and sometimes even panic. The object or situation is avoided as much as possible and there is marked anticipatory anxiety if the patient knows they have to encounter it. Patients know

- Animal or insect, e.g. spider, snakes
  generally childhood onset

- Natural environment, e.g. thunder, water, heights
  generally childhood onset

- Blood–injury, e.g. fear seeing blood or injections
  highly familial associated with vasovagal (fainting)
  response

- Situational, e.g. tunnels, lifts, flying, driving
  bimodal peak age onset – childhood and mid–20s
  overlap with panic disorder and agoraphobia

Table 4.5 – Subtypes of phobias.

the fear is irrational, e.g. spider phobics know the spiders they are terrified of cannot actually harm them, but this does not reduce the anxiety. The phobia, although limited to a specific area, can cause considerable distress and significant interference with the rest of their life, e.g. someone with a worm phobia cannot walk on grass or mud and cannot go out when it is raining.

Making the diagnosis

The diagnosis is not usually in doubt because patients are fully aware of what the feared stimulus is and they do not usually have other co-morbid conditions.

Drug treatment

Although there have been few controlled trials, and none of newer drugs, it is generally accepted that these conditions do not respond to drug treatment unless they occur secondary to another anxiety disorder or depression.

Psychological treatment

There is considerable evidence for the short-term efficacy of exposure therapy for animal and insect phobias where the phobic object can be manipulated with relative ease. Manipulating the natural environment is not so easy, but height phobia can be treated with success using buildings, ladders, scaffolding, etc. Blood–injury phobia appears to have a different psychophysiological background from the other specific phobias and is generally more resistant to treatment. Nevertheless, those disabled by needle phobia, frequently presenting as a disabling fear of medical consultations or hospitals, can be aided. Situational phobias are generally specific examples of agoraphobic avoidance and assessment should attempt to identify whether the difficulty began with a spontaneous panic attack. Fears of enclosure or the inability to escape suggest such an aetiology, which in turn suggests optimal treatment should be directed towards fears of panic. Flying phobia can be due to fears of enclosure, or of height phobia, and appropriate assessment enquiries will establish which. The former is best treated as a variant of panic disorder with agoraphobia, the latter as height phobia although the services of a flight simulator and true air travel will probably be needed to complete full exposure hierarchy.

Occasionally simple education and advice about self-help can benefit such patients. Others require an appropriate, skilled therapeutic alliance that focuses upon the need to work through an exposure hierarchy, documented homework and continuing practice and confrontation. The success of exposure therapy depends upon true habituation to the phobic stimulus or situation and failure follows when patients are enabled, encouraged or allowed to distract themselves during exposure. This principle illuminates the need for a graded hierarchy of exposures, beginning with one the patient can just about tolerate. There must be evidence of arousal at the beginning of exposure, exposure must continue until this has reduced and it is helpful if a therapist is available to encourage patients' engagement with the phobic object. The use of relaxation techniques during exposure is controversial. The goal should be to enable patients to discover that the phobic object or situation is not dangerous, rather than to develop techniques which mitigate their unpleasantness.

SOCIAL PHOBIA

The condition of social phobia has been described for over 2000 years but is only recently that it has become clearly established as a diagnosis in its own right. The main reason for this is that sufferers and clinicians have tended to view the symptoms as an enduring part of the personality and, therefore, not particularly amenable to treatment by drugs.

In the 1960s, when the term 'social phobia' was first introduced it was considered to be a relatively rare disorder but with the increasing sophistication of diagnostic criteria its prevalence has become clearer. At any one time 3% of the population are thought to be suffering from social phobia with lifetime prevalence rates of about 10% being quoted. The peak age of onset is the mid-to-late teens and the sex ratio in most clinical studies is equal (Schneier et al. 1992). The considerable impairment social phobia causes is because it impacts on almost every area of normal life. Patients are more likely to be poorly educated, not to progress in their careers and to be living alone. Co-morbidity is common particularly with depression, suicidal ideation, alcohol and drug abuse (often starting as an attempt at self-medication but resulting in up to 25% of social phobics being alcohol-dependent) (Davidson et al. 1993). In most cases the symptoms of social phobia precede those of the co-morbid disorder.

The essential feature of social phobia is the fear of scrutiny by other people, particularly in performance situations when patients feel they will be the centre of attention and will do something humiliating or embarrassing. The situations that provoke this fear and are avoided can be quite specific, e.g. fear of public speaking or be of a much more generalized nature involving fear of most social interactions, e.g. participating in small groups, eating, writing or working in front of others and speaking to people in authority or of the opposite sex (Table 4.6). Exposure to the feared situation almost invariably provokes anxiety with symptoms similar to those experienced by patients with panic attacks. Interestingly, some seem to be particularly prominent, i.e. blushing, tremor, sweating and a feeling of 'drying up' when talking. These are all noticeable to someone else and serve to compound the problem.

Making the diagnosis

Again, the key to making the diagnosis is a clear history. This needs to include what the focus of the fear is, what symptoms are experienced, what situations precipitate anxiety and whether being accompanied makes things better (in contrast with patients suffering agoraphobia, patients with social phobia often find having someone with them exacerbates the problem). The distinction between social phobia and avoidant personality disorder is often difficult. Avoidant personality disorder is conceived of as a condition in which disability has arisen from excessive sensitivity to rejection, disapproval or criticism. Social phobia is conceived of as a condition in which disabling avoidance has arisen because of an unwillingness to brave situations where there is a risk of public exposure or ridicule.

Treatment

Education is again a key part of treatment and perhaps more so than with the other disorders as many sufferers will never have even heard of the condition. They, therefore, need a careful explanation of the nature of the disorder, the symptoms and the treatment strategies.

- Public speaking
- Eating or drinking in public
- Writing, using the telephone or working while being watched
- Participating in groups
- Talking to people in authority
- Asking someone out for a date

Table 4.6 – Typical anxiety-provoking situations in social phobia.

Drug treatment

MAOI and RIMA

The rationale for the use of MAOIs in this condition developed from observations of similarities between social phobia and atypical depression particularly complaints of being hypersensitive to criticism and rejection. Since then the MAOI have been studied in double-blind controlled trials and have consistently demonstrated positive results. Most have used phenelzine and have reported response rates of 64–82% (review Pollack and Gould 1996). The RIMA moclobemide has been compared with phenelzine and shown to be equally effective, although phenelzine had a faster onset of action (Versiani et al. 1992). Moclobemide tends, however, to have fewer side-effects and to be better tolerated than traditional MAOI. A multi-centre placebo-controlled study with moclobemide has recently been completed and has confirmed its efficacy in social phobia (International Multicentre, Clinical Trial Group on Moclobemide in Social Phobia 1997)

TCA

TCAs do not appear to be effective in social phobia although early studies with clomipramine in patients with mixed anxiety conditions including social phobia did show clear benefits.

SSRI

Increasing clinical experience, several case reports and open studies have suggested that the SSRIs may be effective in the treatment of social phobia (review Pollack and Gould 1996). Placebo-controlled studies are currently underway which will provide more definitive evidence for their efficacy in this condition.

Benzodiazepines

Some high potency benzodiazepines have been reported to be effective in social phobia but in general the evidence for their use is not as strong as for the MAOI or RIMA (review Pollack and Gould 1996). In some resistant or unresponsive cases they may be required to treat anxiety which is incapacitating.

β-Blockers

β-Blockers continue to be widely used for the treatment of social phobia. Early studies did suggest efficacy but these have not been confirmed by later controlled studies (Liebowitz et al. 1992). Their only place is in the treatment of specific performance anxiety in, for example, musicians when management of the tremor is crucial.

Psychological treatments

Psychological approaches to social phobia are less well developed than those for panic disorder and the specific phobias. This reflects the recency with which social phobia has become acknowledged as a disorder in its own right. Psychological approaches range from social skills training through formal exposure techniques to more recent and conceptually sophisticated cognitive/behavioural therapies (Wells and Clark 1997). Reviews of the short- (van Dyck 1996) and long-term (Juster and Heimberg 1995, Scholing and Emmelkamp 1996, Taylor 1996) effects of these approaches reveal significant superiority over placebo and other treatments, of approaches involving exposure and/or cognitive restructuring. Methodological difficulties (Heimberg and Liebowitz 1996) have so far inhibited direct comparisons with drug treatment.

Patients with social phobia see themselves as being at particular risk of making a display of incompetence in the company of others. Understandable social anxieties such as 'I don't know what to say', 'I'll shake and lose control', 'What if I sweat' or 'What if I get anxious' are elaborated as images of stupidity, loss of control, frankly perspiring or a gibbering wreck. Attention to one's own behaviour draws attention away from others', and impairs appraisal of others' views of the situation. Furthermore, safety or risk-reducing behaviours accompany; for instance, avoiding conversation, avoiding cups and saucers, wearing particular clothes or excessive deodorant, controlling movements or hiding the face, and these have the effect of further limiting appraisal of the real possibility of humiliation. In essence, treatment involves dismantling associations between these appraisals of exaggerated risk, their associated catastrophizing and safety or risk-reducing behaviours. Direct feedback on social performance in the form of audio- or video-recordings can be particularly useful. Challenging situations and behaviours should be sought out; social behaviour is generally very conformist and imagined humiliation-provoking events are rare. An example of use in someone concerned about being noticed because they are clumsy might be to encourage them actually to spill a drink in a bar, and discover how little others notice.

OBSESSIVE-COMPULSIVE DISORDER (OCD)

Until recently OCD was considered a rare condition with a poor prognosis. This situation arose because of a combination of factors; the secretive nature of the disorder; the fact that patients did not tend to seek help from psychiatrists; and that many of the available treatments were of limited benefit. Things, however, changed in the 1980s. The Epidemiologic Catchment Area survey in the USA produced the striking finding that OCD was 50–100 times more prevalent than had previously been believed. It was found to have a lifetime prevalence of 2.5% (Robins and Regier 1991), a figure that has since been validated by subsequent studies in diverse cultures. OCD is equally common in males and females. It usually begins in adolescence with an earlier age of onset for males than females. The majority of patients follow a course that waxes and wanes with exacerbations at times of stress. Co-morbidity is common particularly with depression (two-thirds of patients with OCD have a lifetime history of depression) and other anxiety disorders. OCD seems to be part of a spectrum of related disorders including eating disorders, trichotillomania (compulsive hair pulling), onychophagia (compulsive nail biting), hypochondriasis, dysmorphophobia (preoccupation with some bodily defect) and paraphilias. Schizophrenia and Gilles de la Tourette's syndrome (involving chronic and frequent motor tics) are also closely associated (35–50% of patients with Gilles de la Tourette's have OCD and 20–30% of patients with OCD have current or past tics).

Obsessions are persistent ideas, thoughts, impulses or images that are experienced as intrusive and inappropriate and cause marked anxiety or distress. The patient recognizes that they are the product of their own mind not an outside force, and that they are unreasonable. Nowadays the most common themes for obsessions involve contamination, repeated doubts, the need to have things in a particular order, aggressive impulses and sexual imagery, although years ago religious and blasphemous ideas were more prominent. Exposure to the fear results in anxiety which the patient then attempts to suppress or neutralize by some other thought or action (often in a quite magical way), e.g. someone with doubts about having turned the lights off attempts to neutralize the anxiety by checking that it is off seven times.

Compulsions are repetitive behaviours (e.g. hand washing, checking) or mental acts (e.g. counting, repeating words silently) that the person feels driven to perform. They are usually associated with obsessions as an attempt to reduce anxiety produced by them, e.g. a patient with a fear of contamination will try to reduce the distress by repeated hand washing often until their skin is raw. The compulsions are often very ritualistic and must be performed in a set way to have the desired effect, which can result in patients starting the compulsions over and over again until the exact ritual has been achieved.

Patients often initially try to resist the obsessions or compulsions, but this causes such mounting tension and anxiety that they have to give in. As the disorder progresses the desire to resist tends to abate and the obsessions and compulsions are incorporated into daily living. They still, however, cause marked distress and often take over the patient's life, e.g. spending several hours each morning in the bathroom performing complex washing rituals. The obsessions or compulsions may be performed secretly but often draw in others members of the family, e.g. by getting someone else to do the checking for them.

Making the diagnosis

OCD is classified as an anxiety disorder in DSM-IV but as a separate condition in ICD–10. This reflects the European view that where anxiety and OCD coexist, the diagnostic criteria for OCD should take precedence.

The features that need eliciting from the history include the focus and intensity of the fear (is it an excessive worry or an obsession, is it of a particular situation, is it a preoccupation with appearance, is it delusional), presence or family history of tics and the presence of co-morbid disorders.

Drug treatment

TCA

The first breakthrough in the drug treatment of OCD came in 1967 with a report of the efficacy of clomipramine in 16 patients. It was not until the 1980s and 1990s, however, that large well-controlled studies were published which confirmed this efficacy (Clomipramine Collaborative Study 1991). In most studies the response of OCD symptoms was independent of any concurrent depressive symptomatology, and treatment at high dose for at least 10 weeks was required. Clomipramine is the most effective of the TCAs (Zohar and Insel 1987) and, as a consequence, is the only one licensed for the treatment of OCD. It is also the most serotonergic which lends support to the serotonin hypothesis of OCD and the idea that serotonin re-uptake seems to be crucial to the anti-obsessive efficacy of antidepressants.

SSRI

The use of more selective serotonergic agents in OCD developed from the clomipramine studies described above. Controlled studies have shown that the SSRI are more effective than placebo and as effective as clomipramine with 40–60% of patients responding. High doses are again required (e.g. paroxetine 40–60 mg/day, fluoxetine 20–60 mg/day) for a long duration, i.e. 10–12 weeks and are generally better tolerated than clomipramine. Fluoxetine, paroxetine and fluvox-amine have all been comprehensively studied and are licensed for the treatment of OCD. Studies with the other SSRI, sertraline and citalopram have also suggested efficacy but have not yet been licensed in the UK.

MAOI

A few studies have demonstrated efficacy for the MAOI in OCD particularly where panic symptoms coexist but the evidence for them is weaker than for clomipramine and the SSRIs.

Benzodiazepines

Benzodiazepines should not be used as the first line treatment of OCD but a few open studies have shown that they may have a use in some resistant cases.

Neuroleptics

The addition of neuroleptics, e.g. haloperidol, seems beneficial in patients with coexistent tics (or a family history of tics) suggesting a role for the dopamine system in this group.

Others

Augmentation strategies (e.g. lithium, tryptophan, or buspirone) aimed at modifying serotonin function have also been tried in resistant cases with variable success.

Psychological treatment

Patients with OCD are frequently quite difficult to help. Very often patients build a life around their obsessions and it is the demands of others, disrupted by the compulsive behaviour, that prompt a request for help. This limits the readiness with which patients engage and, therefore, the eventual efficacy of treatment.

Behavioural approaches to OCD have a long history and the best established and most well known is Marks' exposure with response prevention (Marks 1987). Treatment is based on a model of the disorder in which the anxiety-relieving effects of a compulsive act are seen to be rewarding and responsible for amplifying the anxiety-provoking effects of not carrying out the compulsive act in provoking situations. It takes a form very similar to that of graded exposure in the treatment of specific phobia. A hierarchy is drawn up from a tolerable but nevertheless anxiety-provoking stimulus that would normally elicit the compulsion to the most demanding. With therapist's support and through practice patients are enabled to habituate to each stimulus up the hierarchy whilst desisting from their compulsion.

Shortcomings of this approach have led to conceptual and practical developments, in particular an increased focus upon intrusive thoughts (e.g. Salkovskis 1985). Obsessions are viewed as naturally occurring intrusive thoughts that have acquired undue salience because of efforts to suppress them. Intrusive thoughts are considered to be unwanted and, therefore, properly suppressed because thoughts and the possibility of related actions are at times indistinguishable; thus, an undesirable intrusive thought such as 'I might harm the children' is indistinguishable from the undesirable risk, 'I might harm the children'. Suppressing the thought, therefore, becomes safety or risk-reducing behaviour, but as wilful thought suppression is inherently counter-productive, the obsession becomes intensified and other more ritualistic compulsions are recruited. Treatment involves helping the patient to dismember the association between the occurrence of intrusive thoughts and the possibility of an unwanted event actually occurring: 'I am worrying that I might harm the children' can be distinguished from 'I might harm the children'.

POST-TRAUMATIC STRESS DISORDER (PTSD)

The lifetime prevalence rates of PTSD in the community ranges from 1 to 14% with higher rates in populations at risk, e.g. the military. It can occur at any age and there is no clear sex difference. The disorder can have a huge impact on patients' lives leading to marital conflict and job loss. Co-morbid depression and alcohol and drug abuse (again often starting as self-medication) are common.

The essential feature of PTSD is the development of characteristic symptoms following exposure to an extreme traumatic stressor. The persons initial response often involves intense fear, helplessness or horror and is associated with character-istic symptoms including persistent re-experiencing of the traumatic event, persistent avoidance of stimuli associated with the trauma, numbing of general responsiveness, and persistent symptoms of increased arousal. To make the diag-nosis the full symptom picture must be present for at least 1 month (to distinguish it from acute stress disorder). Events that can cause it include direct personal expe-rience of threatened death or physical injury (e.g. military combat, physical or sexual assault, being held hostage, natural disasters, serious road traffic accident); witnessing the death or injury of another person; learning about the death or injury of a family member or close friend.

Making the diagnosis

In taking a history the association with a traumatic event is usually obvious although it should be remembered that some patients find it so painful to discuss the disturbing memories that they will try to avoid this.

Treatment

The treatment of this condition is poorly researched; there have been few properly controlled trials and almost all have been of relatively short duration and conducted on patients a long time after the causative incident; which may explain the poor outcome (review Nutt et al. 1995). An important issue is when to start treatment, but unfortunately this question has not yet been clearly addressed. Sooner is probably better, since delay may result in abnormal learned behaviour patterns becoming established, increased avoidance and inappropriate self-medication. Successful treatment has, however, been reported decades after the original trauma.

Drug treatment

Benzodiazepines

It has been noted that head trauma with unconsciousness seems to protect against road traffic induced PTSD (Mayou et al. 1993) and on this basis it may be that sedative drugs (especially those with amnesic properties, e.g. benzodiazepines) have a similar effect. They have not, however, been widely used because of fears of tolerance, dependence and problems on withdrawal although compared with alcohol, the most commonly used self-medication, they are much safer. The studies that have been done have reported that benzodiazepines improve some of the core symptoms of PTSD, e.g. intrusive memories, re-experiencing, nightmares and increased arousal.

TCA

There have only been three double-blind placebo controlled studies with TCA which have suggested modest improvements in doses up to 300 mg/day given for at least 8 weeks (Davidson et al. 1990). It may be that longer-term treatment may produce enhanced effects but further studies are needed.

SSRI

It has been suggested that SSRI may be effective although again there have been few studies and no double-blind placebo controlled trials. The ones that have been performed have shown that they reduce explosive behaviour, re-experiencing, increased arousal and avoidance (Nagy et al. 1993). As with other anxiety disorders high doses seem to be required.

MAOI and RIMA

The evidence from trials with MAOI is mixed. Two double-blind placebo controlled trials have been performed one showing improvements the other not. The RIMA have not been formally investigated and until these have been done their usefulness cannot be established.

Mood stabilizers

Carbamazepine has been shown to improve hostility, impulsivity and intrusive symptoms in seven of 10 Vietnam War veterans (Lipper et al. 1986). Other mood stabilizers, e.g. lithium, valproate and lamotrigine, have also been shown to improve some symptoms, e.g. hyperarousal, insomnia and impulsivity.

Other medication

Buspirone has been reported to be effective in an open study but no controlled studies have been performed. Case reports have suggested efficacy for cyproheptadine in alleviating nightmares which can be an extremely debilitating feature of PTSD. α2 Agonists, e.g. clonidine decrease noradrenergic tone and have also been reported to result in improvements in measures of arousal and intrusive experiences in Vietnam veterans.

Psychological treatments

PTSD arises when the nature and intensity of an event exceeds the individual's capacity to incorporate it into their global understanding. As a result it lies dormant, a psychological spectre threatening untold disruption if unleashed. From a psychological perspective PTSD is the result of impaired processing. Related psychological phenomena include repression, denial, dissociation and retrieval-inhibition. This conceptual framework provides a rationale to treatment which is essentially that of 'working through'. Patients are encouraged to reconstruct and review the traumatic event, bringing about emotional processing (Foa et al. 1989) which could well be the behavioural manifestation of changes in central noradrenergic activity implicated in some of the drug treatments. The validity of this approach is supported by empirical findings; e.g. the prevention of PTSD among female assault victims (Foa et al. 1995). For a review of the efficacy of different treatment approaches see Solomon et al. (1992).

An important aspect of PTSD is the frequency with which further disability arises from other, co-morbid problems. The core behavioural feature is psychological avoidance (denial, dissociation or repression) so it is barely surprising that co-morbid alcohol and/or drug abuse is common. Furthermore, there are high rates of co-morbid depression and in persistent cases individuals can build a life around their history of trauma as was the case for many of the Vietnam veterans. All or any of these can and do limit the readiness with which patients engage with psychological treatment. The therapeutic focus is undoubtedly reliving (processing) the trauma and this should be pursued. If co-morbidity prevents this, patient and therapist should not become embroiled in a futile search for a less painful alternative. More recent reviews of treatment for PTSD emphasize the need for a multi-dimensional approach (e.g. Shaley et al. 1996).

ACUTE STRESS DISORDER

The essential feature of acute stress disorder is the development of characteristic anxiety, dissociative and other symptoms that occur within 1 month of an extreme traumatic stress (similar to that described in PTSD). Although some distress and anxiety is normal and in many ways an understandable reaction to what has happened, it is the persistence or severity of the symptoms that warrants making the diagnosis. In some patients the anxiety and distress gradually resolves, but in others, for no clear reason, it evolves and develops into the more persistent condition of PTSD.

Making the diagnosis

The differential diagnosis of acute stress disorder includes a normal response to such an event and PTSD. These are differentiated by the severity of the symptoms and their duration.

Treatment

The aim of treatment is to reduce the distressing symptoms and to prevent them becoming established. Again there has been little controlled study of this area and as a result there are no established guidelines for treatment.

Drug treatment

Benzodiazepines

The benzodiazepines work quickly and are particularly useful for the anxiety and sleep disturbance common in acute stress disorder. In some patients a short course will promote sleep and help to minimize mental rehearsal of the trauma that may lead to long-term problems. There is the risk, however, that once started on a benzodiazepine some will find it hard to stop so their use should be reserved for patients in extreme distress.

Psychological treatments

By definition this is an exaggerated response to identifiable stress. It differs from PTSD not only in terms of the shorter delay after trauma, but also in terms of the nature of the response the trauma has provoked. Acute stress reactions are characteristically florid disturbances of behaviour, often including conversion phenomena, which can be understood as chaotic and maladaptive attempts to process the trauma.

Acute stress disorder is usually short-lived. Psychological aspects of management amount to support, provision of structured and safe surroundings, and reassurance of patient and relatives that the difficulty will pass. Hospital admission is sometimes necessary in extreme cases.

GENERALIZED ANXIETY DISORDER (GAD)

GAD is common with a lifetime prevalence of 5%. In epidemiological studies the sex ratio is about two-thirds female. It typically begins in the third decade and tends to run a chronic course with exacerbations at times of stress. Co-morbid disorders particularly depression and panic are common (Rickels et al. 1993). Patients with GAD often complain of somatic symptoms and like patients with panic disorder consequently seek and undergo extensive physical investigations.

The essential feature of GAD is chronic anxiety and worry. To the non-sufferer the focus of the worry often seems to be trivial, e.g. getting the housework done or being late for appointments, but to the patient it is persistent and disabling. The anxiety is often associated with other symptoms that include restlessness, difficulty concentrating, irritability, muscle tension and sleep disturbance, which may complicate the presentation.

Making the diagnosis

In establishing the diagnosis it is important to exclude other anxiety disorders particularly panic disorder and medical conditions, e.g. hyperthyroidism and caffeinism.

It is also important to take a careful history of the symptoms experienced in particular whether they are predominantly psychic or somatic as this determines response to particular drug treatments.

Drug treatment

Benzodiazepines

Historically benzodiazepines have been seen as the most effective treatment for GAD. They act rapidly with maximal effects being seen within the first 2 weeks and are especially effective at reducing anxiety, sleep disturbance and somatic symptoms. Patients like taking them because they are so effective and because they are well tolerated. The choice of benzodiazepine is determined by several factors particularly the half-life of the drug (longer acting ones may have sustained effects but are associated with the risk of accumulation especially in the elderly), and their onset of action (drugs with slower onset have less reinforcing potential). Although tolerance can occur studies have actually reported no dose escalation over many years (Rickels 1986). The problems of dependence and withdrawal may be of more concern in view of the long-term treatment that is often required in GAD. The risks of self-medication with, e.g. alcohol, should not, however, be ignored as this causes many more problems.

5-HT$_{1a}$ Agonists

Buspirone was the first non-benzodiazepine to demonstrate efficacy in GAD (Rickels 1982) but is generally less effective and slower in action than benzodiazepines and tends to cause insomnia rather than sedation. Its advantages over the benzodiazepines are that it does not seem to cause dependence or withdrawal reactions and does not interact with alcohol. It appears to be less effective in patients who have previously received benzodiazepines and is, therefore, probably best used in benzodiazepine naive patients.

TCA

A number of studies have shown that TCA are effective in GAD (Kahn et al. 1986). Compared with benzodiazepines they have a slower onset of action and tend to be less well tolerated by patients, but they are not associated to the same extent with the problems of dependence and withdrawal.

SSRI

It is likely that the SSRI might be similarly beneficial with fewer side-effects than the TCAs. No controlled studies have as yet been carried with SSRI although our clinical experience suggests that they are helpful.

MAOI and RIMA

MAOIs are effective in mixed anxiety states and may well be effective in GAD. No formal studies have, however, been performed although the recent availability of RIMAs suggest their use for this specific disorder should be re-evaluated.

β-Blockers

β-Blockers are widely used in the UK for GAD (although almost nowhere else in the rest of the world) despite the evidence that they do not reduce psychic anxiety and only have effects on some of the somatic not the psychological symptoms (Tyrer and Lader 1967).

Antipsychotics

Low dose antipsychotics are occasionally used in GAD with some success although most of the work dates from the 1950s and 1960s before benzodiazepines became widely available. In general they are less effective than benzodiazepines (Weiss et al. 1977) and are associated with the risk of tardive dyskinesia with chronic use.

In view of the chronic nature of GAD, a delayed response is not as critical as with acute situational anxiety. This taken together with the drawbacks of long-term benzodiazepine use suggest a sensible approach (especially in benzodiazepine naive patients) is to start with a reasonable trial of buspirone for 6–8 weeks at least a dose of 30 mg/day. The dose should be built up gradually over 2–3 weeks to minimize any unwanted actions and patients should be warned not to expect an immediate benefit. Those not responding should probably be tried with an antidepressant (TCA or SSRI) again for a reasonable period, i.e. 8 weeks at full therapeutic dose. In patients who remain unresponsive or in those with a previous long history of benzodiazepine use benzodiazepines may be the only medication that provide any relief. In this group of patients they can be used as the sole treatment, although attempts to switch to buspirone or an antidepressant should be made before coming to this decision. In patients with co-morbid depression an antidepressant should be used as the first line treatment.

The duration of treatment depends on the nature of the underlying illness. If symptoms are intermittent, i.e. triggered by anxiety-provoking situations, then intermittent benzodiazepines for a few weeks may be sufficient to treat these exacerbations. More typically, GAD requires longer-term treatment over 6–8 months with gradual tapering of medication after this. In some patients this will be sufficient, but in others it will not and their symptoms return. This group of patients often experiences severe, unremitting anxiety and requires maintenance medication with antidepressants or benzodiazepines in an analogous way to the long-term use of drugs for the treatment of epilepsy. If medication is not prescribed these patients will treat themselves and using the most widely accessible easily available anxiolytic alcohol. Since alcohol is highly toxic to many body systems, clinically supervised benzodiazepine use is definitely preferable.

Psychological treatment

To date GAD has enjoyed far less theoretical exploration than the other anxiety disorders. This probably reflects the fact that it has been seen as something of a 'dustbin' category; the anxious patients that are left over when those with panic attacks, obsessions, avoidance behaviour or a history of trauma have been excluded. The predominant feature of such patients is that they suffer worry. Worry is a defining feature of anxiety, morbid or otherwise. GAD is the anxiety disorder in which worry plays a particularly prominent part.

Focal cognitive/behavioural therapy for GAD has been shown to be superior to other forms of psychological management (Butler et al. 1991). Subsequent theorizing and practical investigations have led to the development of a positive psychological formulation of GAD, as a disorder in which the central feature is misinterpretation and misuse of worry as a coping mechanism (Wells 1995). Although it is still in early stages of development, a treatment based on this model and taking very much the same form as treatments for the other anxiety disorders is supported by questionnaire data and is under further development (Wells 1997).

HEALTH SERVICE POLICY IN RELATION TO THE ANXIETY DISORDERS

Only a small proportion of patients with anxiety receive specialized assessment and treatment. A conservative estimate of the overall point prevalence of disorders fulfilling formal diagnostic criteria for one or more of the anxiety disorders is 3.2% (Eaton 1995). One mental health service covering a catchment area of some 300 000 people was found to have less than 900 loosely defined anxiety disorder patients under its care at a defined point in time (Ball et al. 1997). When screening questionnaires are used considerable disparities between apparent morbidity, general practitioners' detection rates and referral rates emerge. In one study, 33% patients attending a primary care facility expressed a morbidly significant level of anxiety by questionnaire, but only half of these were recognized as 'cases' and provided with relevant treatment by their practitioners (Fifer et al. 1994). These findings are similar to those for a wider range of psychiatric disorders that consistently reveal a case detection rate of about 50% (compared with questionnaire data), and a rate of onward referral to specialized services of about 25% of those detected (Goldberg and Huxley 1992, Fink et al. 1995, Munk-Jorgensen et al. 1997). This background has striking implications for the development of public health policy in this area. On the one hand only between 10 and 12% of those with conspicuous morbidity find their way to specialized services; on the other hand, little is known about the value of making provision for the excluded majority. Treatment trials are largely confined to carefully selected samples of those referred to specialized services. Not only is it difficult to extrapolate from selected samples to a wider population, but also decisions about management, such as whether to refer in the first place, appear to be made in a complex and poorly understood manner (Joukamaa et al. 1995, Goldberg and Gater 1996, Sleath et al. 1997). Until much more is known about the severity, natural history and response to treatment of the majority of cases of anxiety disorder which are neither referred nor investigated it is unrealistic to develop a comprehensive public health policy for these conditions. Nevertheless, the literature allows a few generalizations about drug and psychological treatments for anxiety disorders and the development of specific disorder-related psychotherapies offers a model of how a comprehensive approach might develop.

COMMON THEMES IN THE DRUG TREATMENT OF ANXIETY DISORDERS

The dose of medication, particularly antidepressants required for the effective treatment of anxiety is typically higher than that needed for antidepressant effect. It also takes longer for improvements to be seen, usually at least 4–8 weeks rather than the 2–3 week's delay seen in depression. Both are important points and emphasize the need to maintain the patient on as high a dose as can be tolerated for at least 8 weeks before changing medication. Patient education is crucial in obtaining this cooperation.

Anxiety exacerbation in panic disorder is dose-related and is reported in at least 20% of patients started on antidepressants (probably less with MAOI). It can lead to patients stopping treatment and, therefore, needs to be carefully managed. This can be achieved by an explanation of what may happen, starting the antidepressant at a very low dose, e.g. 10 mg paroxetine or imipramine, and/or using a high potency benzodiazepine, e.g. clonazepam 0.5 mg bd as required for 2–3 weeks.

The duration of treatment is often a tricky issue as fewer studies have been done. The prevailing tendency, derived from concerns over the benzodiazepines, has been to use short courses of treatment, usually for 6–10 weeks but for many anxiety states this is not long enough to maximize response. Our clinical practice is to apply the same rules as used in the treatment of depression. Thus, for the first episode patients are treated for at least 8 months and then medication is tailed off over a further 4–8 weeks if the patient is in remission. Patients with recurrent illness are treated for 1–2 years to enable them to learn and put into place psychological approaches to their problems. In some cases, however, illnesses are lifelong with maintenance treatment being justified on the grounds of it having a significant effect on patients well-being and functioning. This is a decision reached after careful assessment of the risks and benefits involved.

Co-morbidity with depression, other anxiety disorders and substance abuse is very common and usually warrants treatments aimed at both conditions, e.g. panic disorder and depression is best treated with an antidepressant.

The combination of medication with psychological techniques is almost always the most beneficial approach especially in resistant cases. Often, patients are seen who are so incapacitated by their anxiety that they are quite unable to participate in any group or individual work. Improvements from medication allows them actually to attend and then use the appropriate techniques and approaches.

COMMON THEMES AMONG PSYCHOLOGICAL APPROACHES TO THE ANXIETY DISORDER

The psychological emphasis of this chapter has been on behavioural and cognitive/behavioural approaches to the anxiety disorders. This is because that is the approach best supported by empirical evidence. Unfortunately, the requisite psychotherapeutic skills are not widely available; furthermore, other psychological treatments are in use including anxiety management, self-help groups and manuals, and more interpretive and/or forms of psychotherapy.

The term 'anxiety management' conveys the impression of anxiety as something that arises for unexplained reasons and which has to be managed. The importance of full exposure to psychophysiologically arousing stimuli in emotional processing is well established (e.g. Foa and Kozak 1986). Thus, the development of distraction, relaxation and other 'anxiety management' techniques can, and not infrequently does, lead to a palliative rather than therapeutic outcome.

Anxiety management has become popular because it lends itself to a didactic, group approach facilitating provision for a relatively large number of patients by a relatively small number of practitioners. Unfortunately there has been little formal evaluation of this approach, but its apparent economy encourages its use. Individual anxiety management does lead to therapeutic gain (Butler et al. 1987) but effect sizes are much smaller than those obtained by more selective and focused treatments (e.g. Clark et al. 1994). The main continuing reasons for relying upon anxiety management in planning and organizing services are that it is relatively cheap and that most services are unable to provide an alternative.

Self-help groups and manuals, some of which are beginning to be produced in computerized form, are another popular low-cost approach to treating anxiety disorders. There is evidence that they can be effective although their very nature mitigates against formal evaluation. The underlying basic concepts supporting treatment of morbid anxiety are not complex and are readily communicated. Self-help groups suffer the same criticisms as professionally organized anxiety management groups. Manuals and computer programmes may well help some but they cannot (yet) personalize formulation to the extent that is often necessary to win full engagement. Furthermore, those disabled by morbid anxiety who have turned to the NHS for help deserve a professional approach, which must include review of the efficacy of whatever course they might be following. Thus, it is not enough to 'prescribe' self-help; it is important to review whether it is working, and if it is not, a more determined approach should be considered.

Anxiety disorder patients often evoke supportive, interpersonal, psychodynamic or even crisis intervening responses. There are many reasons for seeking assistance with emotional distress where symptoms of anxiety are prominent. Clear assessment should distinguish between those who might benefit from crisis management, interpersonal counselling, longer-term psychodynamic psychotherapy, treatment for depression or other interventions, and those who are suffering an anxiety disorder. If and when a clear and specific anxiety disorder is identified, treating this will best serve the patient, rather than providing more symptomatic intervention directed at secondary, often interpersonal, consequences. If an anxiety disorder is not identified then a more interpersonal, pscho-dynamic or supportive approach might be helpful if services are available.

Finally there are those with an anxiety disorder who, for reasons of age, tranquillizer dependence, or limitations of personality or intellect, cannot engage with and benefit from otherwise appropriate treatment. These have to be recognized and supported with appropriately adjusted expectations of success.

FUTURE DEVELOPMENTS

NHS Trusts, general practitioners and health authorities are under considerable pressure to provide psychotherapeutic as well as psychopharmacological services for patients with psychiatric disorder. Research findings show that the only unequivocally effective form of psychological treatment for anxiety disorder is cognitive/behavioural psychotherapy. Providing this requires sufficiently precise and detailed assessment and appropriate psychotherapeutic skills. Such practitioners are relatively rare and tend to be fairly senior and expensive. Furthermore, it is probable though not proven that a considerably greater number of patients might benefit from this approach than currently have access to it.

In theory this should not deter investment. Where economic analyses have been carried out the untreated anxiety disorder patients are costly (Katon et al. 1996), and investment in treating panic disorder has proved to be highly cost-efficient (Salvador-Carulla et al. 1995). In practice, the considerable new investment needed to fulfil this promise across the NHS is unlikely to become available until it is starkly clear that such benefits operate locally. A more realistic approach is to embark upon an attempt to refine and improve provision by existing services.

Traditionally cognitive–behavioural psychotherapy has been provided by those with special qualifications and a relatively high level of training experience. On the other hand, as research continues to refine and identify the essential 'active ingredients' of treatment, it is becoming increasingly easy for the less highly trained and experienced to acquire the ability to carry out an effective intervention.

Treatment for panic disorder has reached this point. A realistic first step towards incorporating optimal treatment for anxiety disorders into the activities of ordinary NHS services would be to enable practitioners (medical, nursing or other), to recognize panic disorder patients as they enter the service and to divert them to treatment by a specialist group such as nurses who have acquired specific skills in this area. In a community setting this might involve committing one experienced and appropriately interested nurse from each community mental health team (CMHT) to the treatment of panic disorder patients. Other members of the CMHT are trained to identify panic disorder patients among referrals, as are those receiving referrals at related day hospitals and outpatient clinics. Such patients are directed to the sector 'Panic nurse' for individual treatment along the lines of the 'Oxford' model, supported by questionnaires and regular individual supervision.

This approach acknowledges the research findings and provides a way of incorporating a newly developed treatment of proven efficacy into every day clinical practice. It does not and cannot address the issue from a public health perspective. The estimated prevalence of panic disorder is about 1.5% (Eaton 1995) and the detection and referral rate in primary care is about 10% (Goldberg and Huxley 1992, Fifer et al. 1994). Thus, a catchment area of 100 000 people should give rise to about 150 referred panic disorder patients, considerably more than a single therapist could absorb even if they were doing this full-time. Thus, even if this small proportion of the theoretical population-based morbidity due to panic disorder were to be identified for such treatment, the numbers involved are such that a significant increase in resources would be needed. Such demands for further resources compete with others, for supportive counselling, improved supervision of the chronically disabled and, of course, with demands from medicine and surgery. Proper provision and the widespread use of the best available proven methods of treatment for anxiety disorders can only be expected (if at all) after full debate about health service priorities and public expectations of psychiatry. Providers may wish to contribute to this debate by developing a first-rate practice where its parameters are established, even though this might focus and reduce the range of clients they provide for. Such services would then exemplify what can be achieved given appropriate public commitment.

References

American Psychiatric Association. Diagnostic and Statistical Manual of Psychiatric Disorders, 2nd edn. Washington, DC: APA, 1968.

American Psychiatric Association. Diagnostic and Statistical Manual of Psychiatric Disorders, 3rd edn. Washington, DC: APA, 1987.

American Psychiatric Association. Diagnostic and Statistical Manual of Psychiatric Disorders, 4th edn. Washington, DC: APA, 1994.

Andrews G, Stewart G, Morris-Yate A, Holt P, Henderson S. Evidence for a general nekurotic syndrome. British Journal of Psychiatry 1990; 157: 6–12.

Arntz A, van den Hout M. Psychological treatments of panic disorder without agoraphobia: cognitive therapy versus applied relaxation. Behaviour Research and Therapy 1996; 34: 113–121.

Ball L, Blore D, Dunn H et al. Provision for anxiety disorder patients by a representative community mental health trust. Psychiatric Bulletin 1997 (submitted).

Barlow DH, Craske MG, Cerny JA, Klosko JS. Behavioural treatment of panic disorder. Behaviour Therapy 1989; 20: 261–282.

Beck AT. Cognitive Therapy and the Emotional Disorders. New York: International Universities Press, 1976.

Beck AT, Sokol L, Clark DA, Berchick B, Wright F. Focused cognitive therapy for panic disorder: a crossover design and one year follow-up. American Journal of Psychiatry 1992; 147: 778–783.

Black DW, Wesner R, Bowers W, Gabel J. A comparison of fluvoxamine, cognitive therapy and placebo treatment of panic disorder. Archives of General Psychiatry 1993; 50: 44–50.

Den Boer J, Westenberg H. Effect of a serotonin and noradrenaline uptake inhibitor in panic disorders; a double-blind comparative study with fluvoxamine and maprotiline. International Journal of Clinical Psychopharmacology 1988; 3: 59–74.

Den Boer J, Westenberg H, Kamerbeek W. Effects of SSRI in anxiety disorders; a double-blind comparison of fluvoxemine and clomipramine. International Journal of Clinical Psychopharmacology 1987; 2: 21–32.

Butler G, Cullingham A, Hibbert G, Klimes I, Gelder M. Anxiety management for persistent generalised anxiety. British Journal of Psychiatry 1987; 151: 535–542.

Butler G, Fennell M, Robson P, Gelder M. Comparison of behaviour therapy and cognitive behaviour therapy in the treatment of generalised anxiety disorder. Journal of Consulting and Clinical Psychology 1991; 59: 167–172.

Clark DM. A cognitive approach to panic. Behaviour Research and Therapy 1986; 24: 461–470.

Clark DM, Salkovskis PM, Hackmann A et al. A comparison of cognitive therapy, applied relaxation and imipramine in the treatment of panic disorder. British Journal of Psychiatry 1994; 164: 759–769.

Clomipramine Collaborative Study Group. Clomipramine in the treatment of patients with OCD. Archives of General Psychiatry 1991; 48: 730–738.

Davidson et al. Journal of Clinical Psychopharmacology 1993.

Dunbar G, Steiner M, Oakes R et al. A fixed dose study of paroxetine (10 mg, 20 mg, 40 mg) and placebo in the treatment of panic disorder. European Journal of Neuropsychopharmacology 1995; 5: 361 (abst P5–27).

Eaton WW. Progress in the epidemiology of the anxiety disorders. Epidemiologic Reviews 1995; 17: 32–38.

Evans L, Kenardy J, Schneider P, Hoet H. Effect of a selective serotonin re-uptake inhibitor in agoraphobia with panic attacks. Acta Psychiatrica Scandinavica 1986; 73: 49–53.

Fifer SK, Mathias SD, Patrick DL et al. Untreated anxiety among adult primary care patients in a health maintenance organization. Archives of General Psychiatry 1994; 51: 740–750.

Fink P, Jensen J, Borgqukist L et al. Psychiatric morbidity in primary public healthcare: a Nordic multi-centre investigation Part I. Method and prevalence of psychiatric morbidity. Acta Psychiatrica Scandinavica 1995; 92: 409–418.

Foa EB, Kozak MJ. Emotional processing and fear: exposure to corrective information. Psychological Bulletin 1986; 99: 20–35.

Foa EB, Hearst-Ikeda D, Perry KJ. Evaluation of a brief cognitive–behavioural program for the prevention of chronic PTSD in recent assault victims. Journal of Consulting and Clinical Psychology 1995; 63: 948–955.

Foa EB, Steketee G, Rothbaum BO. Behavioural/cognitive conceptualizations of post-traumatic stress disorder. Behaviour Therapy 1989; 20: 155–176.

Gelder MG. Neurosis: another tough old word. British Medical Journal 1986; 292: 972–973.

Goldberg D, Gater R. Implications of the World Health Organization study of mental illness in general healthcare for training primary care staff. British Journal of General Practice 1996; 46: 483–485.

Goldberg F, Huxley P. Common Mental Disorders. London: Tavistock/Routledge, 1992.

Gorman J. Poster presented at XIXth CINP, Washington, DC, 27 June–1 July, 1994 poster 94–015.

Heimberg RG, Liebowitz MR. Issues in the design of trials for the evaluation of psychosocial treatments for social phobia. International Clinical Psychopharmacology 1996; 11 (suppl. 3): 55–64.

International Multicentre Clinical Trial Group on Moclobemide in Social Phobia 1997.

Joukamaa M, Sohlman B, Lehtinen V. The prescription of psychotropic drugs in primary healthcare. Acta Psychiatrica Scandinavica 1995; 91: 359–364.

Juster HR, Heimberg RG. Social phobia: Longitudinal course and long-term outcome of cognitive–behavioural treatment. Psychiatric Clinics of North America 1995; 18: 821–842.

Kahn RJ, McNair DM, Lipman RS et al. Imipramine and chlordiazepoxide in depressive and anxiety disorders. Archives of General Psychiatry 1986; 43: 79–85.

Katon W, Rosenbaum JF, Gorman JM et al. Panic disorder: relationship to high medical utilization, unexplained physical symptoms and medical costs. Journal of Clinical Psychiatry 1996; 57: 11–22.

Klein DF. Delineation of two drug responsive anxiety syndromes. Psychopharmacologica (Berlin) 1964; 5: 397–408.

Klosko JS, Barlow DH, Tassinari R, Cerny JA. A comparison of alprazolam, and behaviour therapy in the treatment of panic disorder. Journal of Consulting and Clinical Psychology 1990; 58: 77–84.

Lecrubier Y, Bakker A, Dunbar, Judge R and Collaborative Paroxetine Panic Study Investigators. A comparison of paroxetine, clomipramine and placebo in the treatment of panic disorder. Acta Psychiatrica Scandinavica 1997a; 95 2: 145–152.

Lecrubier Y, Judge R and Collaborative Paroxetine Panic Study Investigators. Long-term evaluation of paroxetine, clomipramine and placebo in panic disorder. Acta Psychiatrica Scandinavica 1997b; 95 2: 153–160.

Liebowitz MR, Schneier FR, Campeas R et al. Phenelzine vs atenolol in social phobia; a placebo controlled comparison. Archives of General Psychiatry 1992; 49; 290–300.

Lipper S, Davidson J, Grady TA et al. Preliminary study of carbamazepine in PTSD. Psychosomatics 1986; 27: 849–854.

Marks IM, Hodgson P, Rachman S. Treatment of obsessive compulsive neurosis by *in-vivo* exposure. A two-year follow-up and issues in treatment. British Journal of Psychiatry 1975; 127: 349–364.

Mavissakalian M, Perel IM. Imipramine dose response relationship in panic disorder with agoraphobia. Archives of General Psychiatry 1988; 46: 127–131.

Mayou R, Bryant B, Duthie R. Psychiatric consequences of road traffic accidents. British Medical Journal 1993; 307: 647–651.

McNally RJ. New developments in cognitive–behaviour therapy. Current Opinions in Psychiatry 1995; 8: 395–399.

Michelson D, Lydiard RB, Pollack MH, Tamura RN, Hoog SL, Tepner R, Demitrack MA, Tollefson GD and the Fluxetine Panic Disorder Study group. American Journal of Psychiatry 1998; 155: 213–218.

Modigh K. Antidepressant drugs in anxiety disorders. Acta Psychiatrica Scandinavica 1987; 76 (suppl. 335): 57–71.

Munk-Jorgensen P, Fink P, Brevik JI et al. Psychiatric morbidity in primary healthcare: A multi-centre investigation. Part II. Hidden morbidity and choice of treatment. Acta Psychiatrica Scandinavica 1997; 95: 6–12.

Nagy LN, Morgan CA, Southwick SM et al. Open prospective trial of fluoxetine for PTSD. Journal of Clinical Psychopharmacology 1993; 13: 107–113.

Noyes R, Garvey MJ, Cook BL et al. Problems with tricyclic antidepressant use in patients with panic disorder or agoraphobia: results of a naturalistic follow up study. Journal of Clinical Psychiatry 1989; 50: 163–169.

Nutt DJ, Bell CB, Potokar JP. Drug treatment of chronic anxiety. In Lader MH and Ancill R (eds), Pharmacological Management of Chronic Psychiatric Disorders. London: Baillière's Clinical Psychiatry, International Practice and Research, 1995, chapter 4: 565–559.

Öst LG, Westling B. Applied relaxation vs cognitive therapy in the treatment of panic disorder. Behaviour Research and Therapy 1995; 33: 145–158.

Pohl RB, Wolkow RM, Clary CM. Sertraline in the treatment of panic disorder: a double-blind multicenter trial. American Journal of Psychiatry 1998; 155: 9: 1189–1195.

Pollack MH, Gould RA. The pharmacotherapy of social phobia. International Journal of Clinical Psychopharmacology 1996; 11 (suppl. 3); 71–75.

Rickels K, Downing R, Schweizer E. Antidepressants for the treatment of GAD. Archives of General Psychiatry 1993; 50: 884–895.

Rickels K, Schweizer E. Benzodiazepines for the treatment of panic attacks; a new look. Psychopharmacology Bulletin 1986; 22: 93–99.

Rickels K, Weisman K, Norstad N et al. Buspirone and diazepam in the treatment of anxiety; a controlled study. Journal of Clinical Psychiatry 1982; 43: 81–86.

Robins LN, Regier DA. Psychiatric Disorders in America: The Epidemiologic Catchment Area Study. New York: Free Press, 1991.

Royal College of General Practitioners, Office of Population Censuses and Surveys, Department of Health and Social Services. Morbid Statistics from General Practice, Third National Study, 1981–1982. London: HMSO, 1986.

Salvador-Carulla L, Segui J, Fernandez-Cano P, Canet J. Assessment of costs distribution and cost-offset after diagnosis of panic disorders. In Racagni G, Mendlewicz J (eds), Current Therapeutic Approaches in Panic and other Anxiety Disorders, 1995.

Sargant W, Dally P. Treatment of anxiety states by antidepressant drugs. British Medical Journal 1962; i: 6–9.

Schneier FR, Johnson J, Hornig CD, Liebowitz MR, Weissman MM Social phobia: comorbidity and morbidity in an epidemiologic sample. 1992; 49(4): 282–286. Archives of General Psychiatry 1992; 49: 282–289.

Schneier F, Liebowitz M, Davies S et al. Fluoxetine in panic disorder. Journal of Clinical Psychopharmacology 1990; 10: 119–121.

Scholing A, Emmelkamp PMG. Treatment of generalised social phobia: results at long-term follow-up. Behaviour Research and Therapy 1996; 34: 447–452.

Shaley AY, Bonne O, Eth S. Treatment of post-traumatic stress disorder: a review. Psychosomatic Medicine 1996; 58: 165–182.

Sheehan DV, Ballenger JC, Jacobsen G. Treatment of endogenous anxiety with phobic, hysterical and hypochondrical symptoms. Archives of General Psychiatry 1980; 37: 51–59.

Sheehan DV, Raj AB, Sheehan KH, Soto S. Is buspirone effective for panic disorder? Journal of Clinical Psychopharmacology 1990; 10: 3–11.

Sleath B, Svarstad B, Roter D. Physician vs patient initiation of psychotropic prescribing in primary care settings: a content analysis. Social Science and Medicine 1997; 44: 541–548.

Soloman SD, Gerrity ET, Muff AM. Efficacy of treatments for post-traumatic stress disorder: an empirical view. Journal of the American Medical Association 1992; 268.

Taylor S. Meta-analysis of cognitive–behavioural treatments for social phobia. Journal of Behaviour Therapy and Experimental Psychiatry 1996; 27: 1–9.

Tyrer P. Comorbidity of consanguinity. British Journal of Psychiatry 1996; 168: 669–672.

Van Dyck R. Non-drug treatment for social phobia. International Clinical Psychopharmacology 1996; 11 (suppl. 3): 65–70.

Van Vliet I, Westenberg H, Den Boer J. The efficacy of a reversible MAO inhibitor, brofaromine, in panic disorder. Biological Psychiatry 1991; 29 (suppl.): 266S–267S.

Versiani M, Nardi A, Mundum F. Pharmacotherapy of social phobia – a controlled study with the reversible MAOI (RIMA), moclobemide and phenelzine. British Journal of Psychiatry 1992; 161: 353–360.

Wade AG, Lepola U, Koponen HJ et al. The effect of citalopram in panic disorder. British Journal of Psychiatry 1997 (in press).

Weiss BL. Controlled comparison of trifluoperazine and chlordiazepoxide in the treatment of anxiety. Current Therapy and Research; 1977; 22: 635–643.

Wells A. Cognitive Therapy of Anxiety Disorders. Chichester: Wiley, 1997: 200–235.

Wells A. Meta-cognition and worry: a cognitive model of generalised anxiety disorder. Behavioural and Cognitive Psychotherapy 1995; 23: 301–320.

Wells A, Clark DM. Social phobia: a cognitive approach. In Davey DCL (ed.), Phobias: A Handbook of Description, Treatment and Theory. Chichester: Wiley, 1997.

Zohar J, Insel TR. OCD; psychobiological approaches to diagnosis, treatment and pathophysiology. Biological Psychiatry 1987; 22: 667–687.

5

EATING DISORDERS

Janet Treasure and Simone Fox

INTRODUCTION

The eating disorders, anorexia nervosa and bulimia nervosa are frequently discussed in tandem and generalized statements are made about both of them. Although there is a degree of overlap and a variety of additional syndromes (eating disorder not otherwise specified (EDNOS), binge-eating disorder, atypical eating disorder) in the peripheries, the core features of both disorders are distinguishable.

Descriptions of restricting anorexia nervosa date back over several centuries and the typical disorder is by no means limited to Westernized cultures. On the other hand, bulimia nervosa was only 'discovered' in the last quarter of the twentieth century and although it has overtaken anorexia nervosa as the most common eating disorder in the West, there are many pockets of the world where it does not exist.

The topic of this book is severe mental illness. Although this term is frequently used, as is its alternative, serious, the terms are rarely defined. It is probable that anorexia nervosa fits into this category no matter what niceties of definition are used. Indeed, Goldberg and Gourney (1997) place anorexia nervosa in the category of severe mental disorder using the criteria of an illness that is unlikely to remit spontaneously, which is associated with major disability and whose care will usually involve both the primary and the community mental health teams. Although anorexia nervosa is a relatively rare disorder it has a large impact on the individual and on health services. The illness begins early in life and then runs a chronic course with high levels of morbidity and disability, leading to premature death in over one-fifth of cases. High technology (medical intensive-care units) or high-intensity (psychiatric inpatient units) treatments are often used. The threshold for high intensity care varies greatly throughout the world. The management of anorexia nervosa is uncertain. There is very little evidence upon which to base treatment decisions. In the world as a whole probably less than 300 patients with anorexia nervosa have been entered into randomized controlled treatment trials. Drugs do not have a significant place in treatment.

Bulimia nervosa should probably not be classified as severe, although a subgroup of the illness, which merges into borderline personality disorder spectrum, may do. Bulimia nervosa is a heterogeneous disorder including as it does many normal adolescents who experiment with dieting and weight control through to women who latch onto the behaviour to create a sense of identity and coherence in their lives. These are women who have experienced a childhood filled with adversity and abuse and reach adulthood with an Axis II disorder and a propensity to develop a variety of Axis I disorders such as, depression, alcohol abuse, substance abuse as well as bulimia nervosa. It is this group of patients who fail to respond to the short-term treatments that have been developed (about 70%) and remain symptomatic in the follow-up period (the longest so far is 10 years). These groups often use and/or need a high level of resources. For the most part their needs are equivalent to those of all patients with severe personality disorders who come for psychiatric help but there are specific aspects in terms of childcare and physical health that need to be addressed.

ANOREXIA NERVOSA

Needs and services

Countries with sophisticated health services that can accurately ascertain cases tend to be consistent in finding that the incidence of anorexia nervosa lies between 5–7 per 100 000 of the total population (Hoek 1993, Turnbull et al. 1996). The modal duration of the illness is 6 years (Herzog et al. 1997). This means that anorexia nervosa is one of the top three common chronic illness in teenage girls (Lucas et al. 1991) alongside asthma and obesity. Not all cases present for treatment. Although a higher proportion of cases of anorexia nervosa compared with bulimia nervosa get through the filters and reach specialist care this by no means reflects their own motivation to get help but rather the fact that their problem is more overt (Hoek 1993). The prevalence of anorexia and bulimia nervosa within the various levels of healthcare is shown in Table 5.1.

LEVEL OF MORBIDITY	CHARACTERISTIC OF FILTER BULIMIA		ANOREXIA
1. Community		370	1500
	>filter 1: illness behaviour		
2. Total in primary care		260	1050
	>filter 2: detection of disorder		
3. Conspicuous in primary care		160	170
	>filter 3: referral to psychiatrist		
4. Total psychiatric patients		127	87
	>filter 4: admission to psychiatric beds		
5. Psychiatric in-patients only			

Table 5.1. One-year period prevalence rates per 100,000 young females at different levels of care.

Unlike most other psychiatric conditions in which the use of inpatient beds is rapidly decreasing admission rates for anorexia nervosa in many countries are increasing (Williams and King 1987, Munk-Jorgensen et al. 1995). A 5-year follow-up survey of 112 patients in New Zealand after their first hospital admission for anorexia nervosa found that 48% were re-admitted on more than one occasion (Mackenzie and Joyce 1990). Only patients with schizophrenia or organic disorders exceeded the cumulative length of stay in hospital.

A major factor shaping care is economics. Health rationing is biting everywhere. The costs of psychiatric inpatient treatment alone in Denmark are £1.2 million per 1 million population (Nielsen et al. 1997) and this does not include outpatient and daycare programmes and somatic inpatient care. In the USA, inadequate insurance or managed care is decreasing the length of admissions. However, clinicians are questioning the wisdom of this policy. A recent report suggested that the outcome of the group who were discharged at a lower weight because of financial reasons was poorer than those who completed their treatment in that 50% were likely to be re-admitted later (Baran et al. 1995).

Insight into illness

One of the frustrating and puzzling aspects of anorexia nervosa is the patient's lack of concern about the severity of their illness and the dangerousness of their behaviour. This leads to marked resistance to treatment. Some would argue that this feature suggests that the illness should be categorized as a psychotic disorder and indeed in South America and Sweden this is so. These patients concerns about food and shape are parodies of our cultural angst. (Interestingly the overactivity of anorexia nervosa a century ago was explained by the need to rush around and do charity work.) A recent study compared the beliefs held by patients with anorexia nervosa with patients with schizophrenia and people who held religious beliefs. The form of these three types of beliefs differed: the beliefs of those with schizophrenia were similar to perceptually based beliefs as if the 'imagination has been crystallized into reality', whereas the thoughts in anorexia nervosa were ideas that has been imbued with emotions, consequences and associations, 'reality expanded by fantasy' (Jones and Watson 1997).

The course

In describing the impact of any psychiatric illness it is important to review the course over time. Many research groups have attempted this task from a variety of different settings. Fortunately there has been a remarkable degree of uniformity in the outcome measures used which have for the most part been the Morgan and Russell (1975) scales. This is good in that it allows for comparisons across studies but bad in that the scales were developed in the 1970s and so do not have the advantage of new methodologies and were not designed to take into account the changes in diagnostic criteria which have emerged over time. The Morgan and Russell scales measure the patients adjustment along five dimensions:

- nutritional status
- menstrual function
- mental state
- psychosexual adjustment
- socio-economic adjustment

Two categories of outcome are measured: (1) general outcome based on body weight and endocrine function (Table 5.2); and (2) clinical dimensions and general prognosis (for this each of the five dimensions was expressed on a 12-point scale and the average outcome scale calculated as the mean of scores on five scales).

Although short-term recovery in terms of weight gain is commonly achieved after inpatient treatment, the relapse rate is high. The likelihood of stable recovery increases with time. Presented, therefore, are the results of the outcome studies grouped into time intervals, 2–5 years (Table 5.3), 5–10 years (Table 5.4) and over 10 years (Table 5.5). The series of Morgan and Russell (1975) and that of Theander (1985) have been followed up at intervals over 20 years. The papers detailing outcome of a minimum of 25 cases have been collated. The papers have been ranked in the tables according to the age at presentation, as this is one of the main variables that has been found to predict outcome (Steinhausen 1995). The production of uniform descriptors of the cases has also been attempted.

Most of the series are of cases that had inpatient treatment. Thus, it is uncertain how representative these are as a degree of referral and selection bias would have

---

Good outcome

Weight maintained within 15% of average body weight (ABW) according to actuarial tables; regular menstrual cycles. (In males regular sexual activity, intercourse or masturbation replaces the latter.)

Intermediate outcome

Weight maintained within 15% of ABW but amenorrhoea persists. (In males intermittent or no sexual activity.)

Poor outcome

Weight less than 15% below ABW or bulimic symptoms

Weight was expressed as a percentage ABW as defined from the Metropolitan Life Tables (1959).

Table 5.2

been present. The intensity of treatment given during the index admission varied from a minimum of 2 weeks (Kriepe et al. 1989) to 9 months. Also the content and model of treatments used were diverse, ranging from tube feeding to psychodynamic treatment. Additional treatment, which is usually given after the index admission, has not always been recorded.

The study of Gilberg et al. (1994) is exceptional as it is of cases detected by screening the total 1-year age cohort from a Swedish town and so includes community as well as clinical cases. This unique sample warrants a detailed examination. All cases had fulfilled DSM-III-R criteria for anorexia nervosa at some stage of their life although at the time when they entered the study some were in the process of recovery. The mean BMI at the first examination was 18.3 kg/m^2 whereas the minimum BMI was 14.9 kg/m^2. Many of these cases (23/51, 45%) were not referred to the treatment services. In the series as a whole 41% were in the good outcome category at 5 years follow-up. This is a somewhat lower than in studies of similar aged groups who had more intensive forms of treatment. (The definition of treatment used in this study was having received therapy on at least eight occasions over 8 months.) Of the 15 in the poor outcome category, five had not received any treatment; and in the group of 15 with the best outcome, three had had no treatment. A subgroup with severe obsessive, ritualistic and social interaction problems had the worst outcome. There is little obvious difference in terms of clinical details between cases from this sample and from cases referred to special clinics apart from their weight at assessment referred to above. One difference may be in the time-course. Clinical samples had a longer duration of illness.

Short-term outcome

Outcome from 2 to 5 years is shown in table 3. Apart from the Morgan and Russell (1975) series in which the average age is 21, all of the other series followed up in this short time frame were young adolescents. The adolescent group appeared to have a better outcome (47% in the good outcome category) than the older group (39% good outcome).

Intermediate range outcome (5–9 years)

The results of outcome from between 5 and 9 years are shown in table 4. This series of papers contains the outcome from studies including children, adolescents and older patients. The outcome of two series from children was relatively good with over 50% in the good outcome categories. The series from Great Ormond Street also had one-third in the poor outcome category but this may be because this National UK centre is referred more severe cases. The range of good outcome in the adolescent groups was from 48 to 72% with less than 24% in the poor outcome category. Interestingly the Swedish study discussed above with about 50% of cases

Authors	Date	No. of subjects	Age at 1st presentation	Age at F-Up	Complete	F-Up duration	Duration of treatment	Previous hospital admission	Weight before	Amenorrhea at F-Up	Good M&R	Intermediate M&R	Poor M&R	Mortality
Jarman et al.	1991	43 all F	14	18.3	74%	4.3								
Cantwell et al.	1977	33 32F 1M	14.1	19.7	79%	4.9	9.5 mo							0
Van der Ham	1994	25	16		100%	4			43kg	4(16%)	47%	43%	10%	
Greenfield et al.	1991	40 all F	16.3	20.8	75%	4.6	2 days							
Morgan and Russell	1975	41 38F 3M	21.5 21.5		100% 100%	10 Apr	<3mo-51% 3-6mo-34% 6mo-15%	49%		15(42%)	39%	27%	29%	0

Table 5.3 – Outcome 2–5 years.

Study	Date	No. of subjects	Age at 1st presentation	Age at F-Up	Complete	F-Up duration	Duration of treatment	Duration of illness at presentation	Weight before	Weight after	Amenorrhea at F-Up	Good M&R	Intermediate	Poor M&R	Mortality
Hawley	1985	21 17F 4M	11.5	20.2	86%	8.7		0.7 yrs			Reg. per 60 Irreg. 20%	50%	33%	17%	0
Bryant-Waugh et al.	1988	48 33F 15M	11.7	20.8	62%	7.2	?		87% score less than 80%	92%		58%	6%	36%	2
Remschmidt et al.	1987	36	14.5			7.8	22.3 wks								
Martin	1985	25	14.9		100%	5.1 2.6-6.8	11 mo	7 yrs	45%	95%	10%	76%	16%	8%	
Jenkins	1987	21 all F	15	21.4	86%	6 3.25-12	6.2 mo		68%	94%		48%	19%	24%	
Steinhauser	1993	60 57F 3M	15.7	20.9	83%	5	13.9 wks		14.1 BMI	19.4 BMI	36%	68%	18%	14%	4 (6.65%)
Kreipe et al.	1989	55	16?	22.7	89%	6.7	min 2 wks		72.10%	96.10%	20%				1
Gillberg et al.	1994	51	16.1	21	100%	6.7			18.3 BMI	21.2 BMI	4 (8%)	41%	35%	24%	
Santosa et al.	1987	55 all F	17.7		73%	6.8		1.6 yrs	28.20% waste		21%	Excellent 37.50%	Improved 25% Symptomatic 17.50%	poor 5%	2
Touyz and Beumont	1984	49 47F 2M	19	27	69%	8.5	6-8 wks	2 yrs	75.20%		4 (8%)	37%	18%	10% incl. 2 dead	2
Hall et al.	1984	50 all F	20.1	25.7	92%	8	2.5 yrs		73.90%	91.80%	9%	36%	36%	26% incl. 2 dead	2
Morgan et al.	1983	41 38F3M				5		2	63.30%			39%	27%	29%	5%
Hall and Crisp	1979	105 all F	20.8		97%	5.9		3.54 yrs	68.10%	89.80%	9 (9%)	48%	30%	20%	2
Burns and Crisp	1984	1984 all M	27	21.6		100% 20-Feb	8	3.75 yrs	68%	86.60%	44% no sexual act.	44%	26%	30%	0

Table 5.4 – Anorexia Nervosa Outcome 5-10 years.

ascertained from the community had fewer cases in the good outcome category and a larger proportion in the intermediate outcome. This was in spite of the fact that their average weight at the time of ascertainment was higher than the other two groups. It is difficult to interpret these findings. One possibility is that specialist treatment for this age group may improve the outcome. The proportion of patients in the good outcome category in the older age group ranged from 36 to 48%.

Long-term outcome (after 10 years)

The outcome after 10 years is shown on table 5.5. The case studies in these series were similar in that the age at presentation was 19 with 3-year duration and a similar degree of weight loss. The range of good outcome or recovery was between 30 and 53% with the percentage in the poor outcome category or dead ranging from 19 to 25% after 10 years. The studies with a very long follow-up (Theander 1985, Ratnasuirya et al. 1991) had a mortality rate of 17 and 18% respectively, with 20 and 6% in the poor outcome category.

Mortality

Anorexia nervosa has the highest death rate of any psychiatric illness: in males twice that of patients with schizophrenia; for females four times as high (Sullivan 1995, Nielsen et al. 1998). In the UK there are on average 25 deaths each year with anorexia nervosa recorded on their death certificates, but this will be a gross underestimate as deaths from suicide or medical co-morbidity may not have 'anorexia' recorded. Also some coroners do not allow anorexia nervosa to be used as a cause of death and prefer the euphemism of self-neglect.

A recent meta-analysis of 42 studies found that the crude mortality rate of anorexia nervosa was 5.9%. The aggregate mortality rate has been estimated as 0.56% per year (Deter and Herzog 1994, Sullivan 1995). This is similar to the findings based upon a register study in Denmark (Moller-Madson et al. 1996, Nielsen et al. 1998). The standardized mortality rate after a mean of 7.8 years following inpatient treatment was 9.1%.

The factors that have been found to predict overall prognosis (duration of illness, age of onset (older poorer), severity of weight loss and number of previous admissions) are also associated with a higher mortality. Deter and Herzog (1994) found that the standardized mortality rate (SMR) was 9.1% for patients admitted for the first time and 14.4% for the group as a whole. Patton (1988) found a 15-fold greater mortality rate if the weight was less than 35 kg. Both a low weight (less than 60% of average body weight) and low serum albumin were strong predictors of later mortality (Herzog et al. 1992). The SMR of patients who were first admitted over the age of 20 years was significantly higher than that of younger patients (17 versus 6) (Moller-Madson et al. 1996). A worrying trend in the latter study was for the SMR to show an

Authors	Date	No. of subjects	Age at 1st presentation	Age at F-Up	Complete	Duration of treatment	F-Up duration	Duration of illness	Weight before	Weight after	Amenorrhea at F-Up	Recovered	Good M&R	Intermediate M&R	Poor M&R	Mortality
Tolstrup et al.	1985	151 140 F 11M	19	31 (16-63)	80%	12 mo	12.5 4.0-22	2.4	68%	84%			40%	29%	19%	6%
Eckert et al.	1995	76 all F	20	28	100%		10	3	31.1 kg	18.5 BMI	15%	25%	28%	34%	13%	6.60%
Deter and Herzo	1994	84 (all F)	20.7	32.5	78.6%		11.8		13.3 BMI	19.6 BMI	14.90%		40.50%	25%	10.70%	11%
Ratnasuriya et al.	1991	41 38F 1M	21.5	40.9	100%		20.2	3.7	64.28%	80.40%	27%		30%	33%	20%	17.50%
Theander	1985						33 15						76% 63%	1% 17%	6% 7%	18% 13%

Table 5.5 – Anorexia Nervosa Outcome 10+ years.

increase in the later time cohorts (SMR 1970–74 = 11; 1980–84 = 19). This, in combination with the increased re-admission rates, suggests the condition has become more severe in recent times.

Cause of death

In Sullivan's 1995 meta-analysis of causes of mortality, 89 (54%) of the deaths could be attributed to the medical complications of an eating disorder, 44 (27%) to suicide and 31 (19%) to unknown or other causes. In the Danish case register study, half the deaths were from the physical complications of anorexia nervosa the others were from suicide (Moller-Madson et al. 1996). In Patton's series the most common form of death in the anorexic group was suicide (6/11) usually from a drug overdose (Patton 1988).

Psychosexual function

The cases of anorexia nervosa from the Swedish case control study had significantly lower global scores in psychosexual adjustment than the comparison group (Table 5.6). This was most marked in terms of actual behaviour rather than attitudes. About 12% of the anorexic group had a negative attitude to menstruation. Fertility is reduced in women who have suffered from anorexia nervosa. In part this is due to suboptimal recovery. However, some women conceive despite maintaining their weight at suboptimal levels (Namir et al. 1986). Others may conceive after being given hormonal fertility treatment. After a follow-up of 12.5 years in a Danish study, the fertility rate in 140 women with anorexia nervosa was only one-third that expected (Brinch et al. 1988). The perinatal mortality rate was 6-fold higher than expected and the birth weight was lower than average. In a study in which pregnant women with anorexia nervosa were followed prospectively the infants grew slowly

	AN (N = 51)	Comparison
Median range score of socio-economic state	9 (3–12)	11.5 (6–12)
Median range on psychosexuual adjustment	11 (2–12)	12 (7–12)
Many close and superficial friends	26 (51%)	42 (82%)
Social activities: mixes well out of the family	27 (53%)	45 (82%)

Table 5.6 – Psychosocial functioning 5 years after the diagnosis of anorexia nervosa (AN) (data from Gillberg et al. 1992).

in utero especially in the last trimester (Treasure and Russell 1988). The longer term effects of undernutrition on the developing foetus have not been delineated as no one series has been large enough to address this issue. However, one can perhaps draw some lessons from the outcome of people who were conceived during the Dutch famine during World War II. This population has a higher rate of schizophrenia, schizoid personality disorder and neurological defects (Hoek et al. 1996, Susser et al. 1996).

Apart from the physical consequences of undernutrition there are also concerns about the ability of mothers with anorexia nervosa to feed their children. There has been one report of a mother with anorexia nervosa who failed to feed her infant who died after 10 weeks (Smith and Hanson 1972), but this case was atypical. Subgroups of children presenting with growth retardation in The Netherlands were found to have mothers with anorexia nervosa. The mothers were presumed to be underfeeding their children (van Wezel-Meijler and Wit 1989). Russell et al. (1998) describe a series of eight mothers with anorexia nervosa. Nine children suffered some degree of food deprivation: with severe reduction in weight for age in six cases and height for age in seven. Long-term treatment of one mother resulted in catch up growth of the two sons.

General parenting deficits have been observed in patients with anorexia nervosa in association with high levels of marital conflict (Woodside and Shekter-Wolfson 1990).

Psychiatric co-morbidity

Depressive features, which are in part an epiphenomenon of the starvation state, are often seen in conjunction with anorexia nervosa. Obsessive phenomena are also common and these are also exaggerated by weight loss. Significant psychiatric co-morbidity is seen at follow-up but it usually occurs in those who have continuing eating disorders. The most frequent disorders present at follow-up are anxiety disorders (43%) and affective disorders (30%) (Halmi et al. 1991, Smith et al. 1993). In the Swedish community study a significantly higher proportion of the anorexic group had an abnormal mental state at follow up (24/51 anorexics versus 6/51 controls.

Personality features

Patients with anorexia nervosa are commonly said to be perfectionist with obsessional personalities (Vitousek and Manke 1994). Gillberg and colleagues suggest that one-third of patients with anorexia nervosa have an 'empathy' disorder (Gillberg and Rastam 1992, Gillberg et al. 1995). The working definition of empathy disorder is either social difficulties involving problems in understanding other peoples perspectives, thoughts and feelings or that the subject relates in a non-reciprocal, fashion to the examiner. Ritualistic behaviours and obsessive compulsive phenomenon are associated with this subgroup (Rastam 1992). Svinivasagam et al. (1995) report that perfectionism as well as an obsessive need for symmetry and exactness persists after long-term recovery from anorexia nervosa.

Physical co-morbidity

Medical problems occur in two-thirds of patients with poor outcome and one-third of those who have a good outcome (Herzog et al. 1997). Osteoporosis (14%) and kidney problems (10%) predominate. In the Swedish case control study four of the group with anorexia nervosa had experienced trauma related fractures. None of the comparison group had this feature. This suggests that bone fragility is increased in the group with anorexia nervosa as both groups were exposed to similar levels of trauma. This group also report persistent dysdiadochokinesis in 20% of the patient group. More of those exhibiting this phenomenon were in the poor outcome group. Recent studies suggest that there may be long-term effects on the brain. Lambe et al. (1997) reported that even after recovery there were persistent grey matter volume deficiencies.

Psychosocial functioning

The quality of life in patients with anorexia nervosa is very poor (Keilen et al. 1994). These patients become extremely socially isolated with low levels of emotional and practical support (Tiller et al. 1996). The Swedish case control study found that the socio-economic status was significantly reduced in the anorexic group although employment status did not differ (table 3). In addition to this impoverished social life they have difficulties gaining independence from their family. The converse of this is that families are involved in providing long-term care, which is a large burden.

Treatment

Inpatient treatment is regarded as standard practice (APA 1993) despite its high cost and its debatable efficacy (McKenzie and Joyce 1990, Crisp et al. 1991). In the short-term, inpatient treatment leads to full recovery of weight but in the majority of cases these changes are not maintained. Several studies have addressed the issue of additional outpatient therapy to prevent relapse after inpatient treatment. In adolescents, family therapy, given during the year following in-patient treatment, prevented relapse, whereas individual therapy was more effective in older patients (Russell et al. 1987). There was a trend for the effect after one year to persist over 5 years of follow-up (Eisler et al. 1997).

Simultaneously with these developments in relapse prevention there has been an interest in developing treatments to prevent admission. The types of therapy and patient considered eligible for outpatient therapy vary widely. In the USA, the threshold for resorting to inpatient care is low, i.e. a body mass index of less than 16 kg/m² (Garner and Needleman 1997) or 20% weight loss (APA 1993). In contrast, in the UK and some other European countries admission is reserved for the severely ill with a body mass index of less than 13 kg/m² (Treasure and Szmukler 1995, van Furth 1998). Not only are outpatient approaches cheaper, but also it has been suggested that they may lead to better long-term outcome (Morgan et al. 1983, Beumont et al. 1993).

There have been very few clinical trials that evaluate outpatient psychotherapies for this debilitating disorder. Those that have been accomplished have had very low power and selected samples. Crisp et al. (1991) attempted to compare the effectiveness of inpatient care with outpatient treatment. The interpretation of the study is difficult as 60% of those allocated to inpatient treatment refused this approach despite being offered no other form of treatment. Nevertheless, the outcome of all patients and the subgroup who complied with treatment was no better in those allocated to inpatient treatment than for those given outpatient treatment. These results need to be tempered by the fact that those allocated to inpatient treatment were older and with a longer duration of illness and a lower mean weight, all of which are factors known to be associated with a poor prognosis. An important conclusion from these results is that patients with good prognostic features can be managed with outpatient treatment.

Several small studies complement the findings of Crisp et al. reported above in that they have shown that outpatient treatment alone can be effective in adult anorexia nervosa (Hall et al. 1987, Channon et al. 1989, Brambilla et al. 1995a, b, Treasure et al. 1995). A variety of models of treatment was used: nutritional counselling, dynamic psychotherapy, cognitive behavioural therapy, behavioural therapy, cognitive analytical therapy and pharmacotherapy,. New models of treatment such as motivational enhancement therapy have been developed (Treasure and Ward 1997).

The new models of care for anorexia nervosa aim to produce a service which is more equitable, with care being more carefully adjusted to need. It is probable that patients with severe chronic anorexia nervosa will need longer types of intensive care. Halfway houses or hostels may be appropriate for this rehabilitation phase. In a pilot project we have found that if the staff in the hostel have special training they can provide the aftercare needed for the group with a severe chronic course. This approach needs to be explored further, otherwise the combination of exhaustion of medical funding, repeated attempts at short-term treatment and the existential despair of living with a chronic severe illness can lead to a malignant course.

BULIMIA NERVOSA

Needs and services

The incidence of bulimia nervosa has been rapidly increasing since its description in 1979. Less than 20 years later the annual incidence was found to be over 14 per

100 000 total population (Turnbull et al. 1996) with a lifetime prevalence of 1.8% (Wade et al. 1996). The illness does not appear to have been present in older cohorts (Kendler et al. 1991, Wade et al. 1996). This suggests that it is a new late twentieth-century phenomenon.

A variety of services has been developed for bulimia nervosa but there is little evidence that high intensity care such as inpatient or day patient care has a better outcome than short-term psychotherapy (Treasure 1997).

The course

The outcome of the larger studies is shown in the tables. This compliments the information given in a recent review (Keel and Mitchell 1997).

There is much less variability in the case mix and although the form of treatment varies greatly in intensity from short outpatient treatment to inpatient treatment the outcome remains very similar in that about 50% have recovered by 1 year and this proportion remains stable over time. In contrast, the course in one-third of cases is punctuated by relapses.

Mortality

The mortality of bulimia nervosa is lower than that of anorexia nervosa at about 0.3% in the larger studies followed over time. Two of these were from suicide (Mitchell and Eckbert 1987, Maddocks et al. 1992) and the other was from a side-effect of medication (a hypertensive crisis in a patients on a monamine oxidase inhibitor) (Fallon et al. 1988).

Prognostic factors

Few prognostic factors have been replicated across studies. However, several groups have found that those who either have multiple forms of impulsive behaviour or show the features of borderline personality have a worse prognosis. In contrast, comorbidity with other mental illnesses does do not appear to be related to outcome.

Psychosexual function

Lacey and Smith (1987) reported on the outcome of pregnancies in a small series of cases with bulimia nervosa. They found a higher than expected number of complications. Mothers with bulimia nervosa also have difficulty feeding their children. Lacey and Smith reported that 15% of mothers in their series reported attempting to 'slim down' their babies. Stein and Fairburn (1989) described five mothers with difficulties feeding their children. Stein et al. (1994) then developed an elegant observational method for mothers with eating disorders ascertained from a community based epidemiological study. A total of 34 women were recruited, who during the postnatal year had experienced bulimia nervosa (n = 6) eating disorder not otherwise specified (12) or subthreshold eating disorders (16). The infants of mothers with eating disorders tended to be lighter than controls and the infant weight was found to be related to the amount of conflict during mealtimes (measured objectively by video recording) and the mothers concerns about her own shape.

Psychological co-morbidity

About one-third of patients with bulimia nervosa have either a premorbid history of obesity or a family history of obesity. This is a specific risk factor for the bulimic disorders (Fairburn et al. 1997, 1998). Depression, substance abuse and alcoholism are commonly associated with bulimia nervosa.

Physical co-morbidity

Problems with teeth are very common in bulimia nervosa as they become eroded and prone to caries as a result of vomiting or drinking acidic drinks (Milosevic 1999). Osteoporosis has been found in bulimia nervosa but it is usually linked to a previous episode of anorexia nervosa (Newman et al. 1989).

Psychosocial functioning

Patients with bulimia are dissatisfied with their social network and describe a large discrepancy between their ideal and perceived levels of support (Thelan et al. 1990, Tiller et al. 1996).

Forensic problems

Stealing is common in bulimia nervosa (Mitchell and Boutacoff 1986). For the most part this is food but other items can be involved (for a review, see Krahn et al. 1991).

Treatment

In contrast to anorexia nervosa there has been a cornucopia of randomized controlled trials evaluating treatment for bulimia nervosa (Wilson and Fairburn 1998). Cognitive behavioural treatment is effective for about one-third of the patients treated (Schmidt 1998, Wilson 1999). However, the standard research designs leave many questions unanswered. How many of those who responded could have been managed with fewer resources? How can services be made more cost-effective? What can be done to improve the efficacy? It is also uncertain whether the conclusions drawn from randomized controlled trials can be generalized to service delivery as many of the patients who present for treatment are complex and would be excluded from many such trials (the range of percentage exclusion from psychotherapy trials is 0–39% and from drug trials is 0–47%; Mitchell et al. 1997).

One attempt to produce a cost-effective approach has been to offer a series of treatments increasing in intensity. This model of sequential care was recommended in the Royal College of Psychiatrists Report (1991). Several alternative models have been described (Garner et al. 1986, Fairburn and Peveler 1990, Fairburn et al. 1992, Tiller et al. 1993, Garner and Needleman 1997). One advantage is that resources are not squandered. Those who respond to a minimal intervention are 'filtered out'. One possible adverse effect of sequential treatment is that it can lead to the experience of failure, which may lower the already fragile self-esteem and damage the therapeutic alliance.

A variety of low intensity models of treatment has been developed and evaluated. These involve a variety of methods for disseminating knowledge and skills while fostering a degree of self-help and therapeutic collaboration.

A group psycho-educational intervention of five 90-min lectures (total of 7.5 h) with an emphasis on symptom management was developed in Canada and examined in a quasi-experimental design (Davis et al. 1990, Olmsted et al. 1991). This produced a 20% abstinence rate from binge eating. The minimal intervention was as effective as a more intensive treatment in the less severely affected subgroup.

Huon (1985) evaluated an intervention that involved sending seven monthly instalments from a self-help programme to 90 subjects with DSM-III bulimia. The active treatments were more effective than the waiting list group. This approach has been continued using books which include education, with cognitive, behavioural and motivational elements, for example 'Getting Better Bit(e) by Bit(e)' (Schmidt and Treasure 1993). These have been found to be effective (Schmidt et al. 1993, Treasure et al. 1994) and can reduce the number of therapy sessions given either in sequential models of care (Treasure et al. 1996) or as adjuncts in models of guided self-care (Thiels et al. 1998). A different self-care manual as part of guided self-care has also been found to be effective in an open study of bulimia nervosa (Cooper et al. 1996). These forms of minimal treatment appear to be of particular usefulness in the treatment of binge eating disorder (Carter and Fairburn 1998).

Medication with antidepressants is less effective (with abstinence rates of 20–30%) and therapeutic gains are less well maintained than those of psychotherapy for bulimia nervosa are (for a review, see Mayer and Walsh 1998). There is, however, some evidence to suggest that combinations of the two summate.

Many of the individuals who fail to respond to short-term therapy have personality difficulties and may require longer forms of psychotherapy. There is work in progress to identify forms of treatment with greater efficacy in this subgroup. Thus, there are adaptations of CBT such as a focus on motivation, or interpersonal issues or upon the negative evaluation and shame about self. Alternatively integrative therapies such as cognitive analytical therapy (Ryle 1990) or schema focused therapy (Young 1990) or Linehans (1993) dialectical behavioural therapy are being tested. The more severely disturbed patients may require treatment lasting 1 year or longer. Even so the outcome is far from satisfactory (Johnson et al. 1987, 1990, Herzog et al. 1991, Tobin 1993).

Conclusions

- Anorexia nervosa has a severe effect on the individual as it runs a long course (on average 6 years), starts during a critical phase of development, and is associated with additional psychological and physical problems. The mortality rate is higher than for any other psychiatric condition.

- Anorexia nervosa places a large burden upon families and healthcare providers. The standard treatment recommendations require expensive and scarce inpatient treatment resources. Different models of care have not yet been fully evaluated although they may be as effective.

- There is an opportunity to provide a more equitable model of care for anorexia nervosa, which matches treatment intensity to patient need. Many studies have consistently found that certain factors such as age of onset, duration of illness and severity of weight loss are important prognostic factors.

- A large proportion of cases of bulimia nervosa has persistent psychosocial impairment and physical complications.

- Evidence suggests that a range of intensities of treatment may also be necessary for bulimia nervosa. Cases with co-morbidity such as diabetes mellitus or personality disorder will need long-term help.

References

American Psychiatric Association. Practice guidelines for eating disorders. American Journal of Psychiatry 1993; 50: 212–228.

Baran S-A, Weltzin TE, Kaye WH. Low discharge weight and outcome in anorexia nervosa. American Journal of Psychiatry 1995; 152: 1070–1072.

Beumont PJV, Russell JD, Touyz S. Treatment of anorexia nervosa. Lancet 1993; 341: 1635–1640.

Brambilla F, Draisci A, Peirone A et al. Combined cognitive behavioral, psychopharmacological and nutritional therapy in eating disorders. 1. Anorexia nervosa – restricted type. Neuropsychobiology 1995a; 32: 59–63.

Brambilla F, Draisci A, Peirone A et al. Combined cognitive behavioral, psychopharmacological and nutritional therapy in eating disorders. 2. Anorexia nervosa – binge-eating purging type. Neuropsychobiology 1995b; 32: 64–67.

Brinch M, Isager T, Tolstrup K. Anorexia nervosa and motherhood: reproduction pattern and mothering behaviours of 50 women. Acta Psychiatrica Scandinavica 1998; 77: 611–617.

Bryant Waugh R, Knibbs J, Fosson A, Kaminski Z, Lask B. Long term follow-up of patients with early onset anorexia nervosa. Archives in Diseases of Childhood 1988; 63: 5–9.

Burns T, Crisp, AH. Outcome of anorexia nervosa in males. British Journal of Psychiatry 1984; 145: 319–325.

Cantwell DP, Sturzenberger S, Burrogh J, Salkin B, Green JK. Anorexia nervosa: an affective disorder. Archives in General Psychiatry 1997; 34: 1087–1093.

Carter JC, Fairburn CG. Cognitive behavioural self help for binge eating disorder: a controlled effectiveness study. Journal of Consulting and Clinical Psychology 1998; 66: 616–623.

Channon D, De Silva P, Hemsley D, Perkins R. A controlled trial of cognitive behavioural and behavioural treatment of anorexia nervosa. Behavioural Research Therapy 1989; 27: 529–535.

Cooper PJ, Coker S, Fleming C. An evaluation of the efficacy of supervised cognitive behavioural self-help for bulimia nervosa. Journal of Psychosomatic Research 1996; 40: 281–287.

Crisp AH, Norton K, Gowers S, Halek C, Bowyer C, Yeldham D, Levett G, Bhat A. A controlled study of the effect of therapies aimed at adolescent and family psychopathology in anorexia nervosa. British Journal of Psychiatry 1991; 159: 325–333.

Davis R, Olmsted MP, Rockert W. Brief group psychoeducation for bulimia nervosa: assessing the clinical significance of change. Journal of Consulting and Clinical Psychology 1990; 58: 882–885.

Deter HC, Herzog W. Anorexia nervosa in a long-term perspective: results of the Heidelberg–Mannheim study. Psychosomatic Medicine 1994; 56: 20–27.

Eckert ED, Halmi KA, Marchi P, Grove W, Crosby R. Ten-year follow-up of anorexia nervosa: clinical course and outcome. Psychological Medicine 1995; 25: 143–156.

Eisler I, Dare C, Russell GFM, Szmukler G, Le Grange D, Dodge E. A five year follow-up of a controlled trial of family therapy in severe eating disorder Archives in General Psychiatry 1997; 54: 1025–1030.

Fairburn CG, Agras WS, Wilson GT. The research on the treatment of bulimia nervosa. Practical and theoretical implications. In Anderson GH, Kennedy SH (eds), Biology of Feast and Famine. San Diego: Academic Press, 1992, pp. 317–340.

Fairburn CG, Doll HA, Welch SL, Hay PJ, Davies BA, O'Connor ME. Risk Factors for Binge eating disorder. Archives in General Psychiatry 1998; 55: 425–432.

Fairburn CG, Peveler RC. Bulimia nervosa and a stepped care approach to management. Gut 1990; 31: 1229–1222.

Fairburn CG, Welch SL, Doll HA, Davies BA, O'Connor ME. Risk Factors for bulimia nervosa: a community based case control study. Archives of General Psychiatry 1997; 54: 509–517.

Fallon B, Foote B, Walsh BT, Roose SP. 'Spontaneous' hypertensive episodes with monamine oxidase inhibitors. Journal of Clinical Psychiatry 1998; 49: 163–165.

Fettes PA, Peters JM. A meta analysis of group treatments for bulimia nervosa. International Journal of Eating Disorders 1992; 11: 97–110.

Garner DM, Garfinkel PE, Irvine MJ. Integration and sequencing of treatment approaches for eating disorders. Psychotherapy and Psychosomatics 1986; 46: 67–75.

Garner DM, Needleman LD. Sequencing and Integration of Treatments. In Garner DM, Garfinkel PE (eds), Handbook of Treatment of Eating Disorders. New York: Guilford, 1997, pp. 50–66.

Gillberg C, Rastam M, Gillberg IC. Anorexia nervosa: physical health and neurodevelopment at 16 and 21 years. Development in the Medicine of Child Neurology 1994; 36: 567–575.

Gillberg IC, Rastam M, Gillberg C. Anorexia nervosa 6 years after onset: Part I. Personality disorders. Comprehensive Psychiatry 1995; 36: 61–69.

Gillberg IC, Rastam M. Do some cases of Anorexia Nervosa reject underlying autistic like cauditives. Behavioural Neurology 1992; 5: 27–32.

Goldberg D, Gourney K. The General Practitioner, the Psychiatrist and the Burden of Mental Health Care. Maudsley Discussion paper No 1. London: Chapman & Hall, 1997.

Greenfeld DG, Anyan WR, Hobart M, Quinlan DM. Insight into illness and outcome in anorexia nervosa. International Journal of Eating Disorders 1991; 10: 101–109.

Hall A, Crisp AH. Brief psychotherapy in the treatment of anorexia nervosa. British Journal of Psychiatry 1987; 151: 185–191.

Hall A, Slim E, Hawker R, Salmond C. Anorexia nervosa: long-term outcome in 50 female patients. British Journal of Psychiatry 1984; 145: 407–413.

Halmi KA, Eckert E, Marchi P, Samugnara V, Apple R, Cohen. Comobidity of psychiatric diagnosis in anorexia nervosa. Archives in General Psychiatry 1991; 48: 718.

Hartmann A, Herzog T, Drinkman A. Psychotherapy of bulimia nervosa: what is effective? A meta-analysis. Journal of Psychosomatic Research 1992; 36: 159–167.

Hawley RM. The Outcome of anorexia nervosa in younger subjects. British Journal of Psychiatry 1985; 146: 657–660.

Herzog T, Hartmann A, Sandholz A, Stammer H. Prognostic factors in outpatient psychotherapy of bulimia. Psychotherapy and Psychosomatics 1991; 56: 48–55.

Herzog W, Deter HC, Fiehn W, Petzold E. Medical findings and predictors of long-term physical outcome in anorexia nervosa – a prospective, 12-year follow-up study. Psychological Medicine 1997; 27: 269–279.

Herzog W, Rathner G, Vandereycken W. Long-term course of anorexia nervosa: a review of the literature. In Herzog W, Deter HC, Vandereycken W (eds), The Course of Eating Disorders: Long-term Follow-up Studies of Anorexia and Bulimia Nervosa. Berlin: Springer, 1992, pp. 15–29.

Herzog W, Schellber D, Deter H-C. First recovery in anorexia nervosa patients in the long-term course: a discrete-time survival analysis. Journal of Consulting and Clinical Psychology 1997; 65: 169–177.

Hoek HW, Susser E, Buck KA, Lumey LH, Lin SP, Gorman JM. Schizoid personality disorders after prenatal exposure to famine. American Journal of Psychiatry 1996; 153: 12.

Hoek HW. Review of the epidemiological studies of eating disorders. International Review of Psychiatry 1993; 5: 61–74.

Hsu LKG, Crisp AH. Outcome of anorexia nervosa. Lancet 1979; i: 61–65.

Huon G. An initial validation of a self help program for bulimia. International Journal of Eating Disorders 1985; 4: 573–588.

Jarman FC, Rickards WS, Hudson IL. Late adolescent outcome of early onset anorexia nervosa. Journal of Paediatrics and Child Health 1991; 27: 221–227.

Jenkins ME. An outcome study of anorexia nervosa in an adolescent unit. Journal of Adolescence 1987; 10; 71–81.

Johnson C, Tobin DL, Dennis A. Differences in treatment outcome between borderline and non borderline bulimics at one-year follow-up. International Journal of Eating Disorders 1990; 9: 617–627.

Johnson WG, Carrigan SA, Mayo LL. Innovative treatment approaches to bulimia nervosa. Special Issue. Recent Advances in Behavioural Medicine. Behaviour Modification 1987; 11: 373–388.

Jones E, Watson JP. Delusion, the overvalued idea and religious beliefs: a comparative analysis of their characteristics. British Journal of Psychiatry 1997: 170: 381–386.

Keel PK, Mitchell JE. Outcome in bulimia nervosa. American Journal of Psychiatry 1997; 154: 313–321.

Keilen M, Treasure T, Schmidt U. Quality of life measurements in eating disorders, angine, and transplant candidates: are they comparable? Journal of the Royal Society of Medicine 1994; 87: 245–249.

Kendler KS, McLean C, Neal M, Kessler R, Health A, Eaves L. The genetic epidemiology of bulimia nervosa. American Journal of Psychiatry 1991; 148: 1627–1637.

Krahn DD, Nairn K, Gosnell BA, Drewnowski A. Stealing in eating disordered patients. Journal of Clinical Psychiatry 1991; 52: 112–115.

Kriepe RE, Churchill BR, Strauss J. Long-term outcome of adolescents with anorexia nervosa. American Journal of Diseases in the Child 1989; 143: 1322–1327.

Lacey JH, Smith G. Bulimia Nervosa: the impact of pregnancy on mother and baby. British Journal of Psychiatry 1987; 150: 777–781.

Laessle RGZ, Soettl C, Pirke K. Meta-analysis of treatment studies for bulimia. International Journal of Eating Disorders 1987; 6: 647–653.

Lambe EK, Katzman DK, Mikulis DJ, Kennedy SH. Cerebral gray matter volume deficits after weight recovery from anorexia nervosa. Archives of General Psychiatry 1997; 54: 537–542.

LeGrange D, Eisler I, Dare C, Russell GFM. Evaluation of family therapy in anorexia nervosa: a pilot study. International Journal of Eating Disorders 1992; 12: 347–357.

Linehan MM. Skills Training Manual for Borderline Personality Disorder. New York: Guilford, 1993.

Lucas AR, Beard CM, O'Fallon WLM, Kurland LT. 50-year trends in the incidence of anorexia nervosa in Rochester, Minnesota: a population based study. American Journal of Psychiatry 1991; 148: 917–922.

Maddocks SE, Kaplan AS, Woodside DB, Langdon L. Two year follow-up of bulimia nervosa. The importance of abstinence as the criterion of outcome. International Journal of Eating Disorders 1992; 12: 133–141.

Martin FE. The treatment of outcome of anorexia nervosa in adolescents: a prospective study and give year follow-up. Psychiatry Research 1985; 19: 509–514.

McKenzie JM, Joyce PR. Hospitalisation for anorexia nervosa. International Journal of Eating Disorders 1990: 11: 235–241.

Milosevic A Eating disorders – a dentist's perspective. European Eating Disorder Review 1999; 7: 103–111.

Mitchell JE, Boutacoff LI. Laxative abuse complicating bulimia. Medical treatment implications. International Journal of Eating Disorders 1986; 5: 325–334.

Mitchell JE, Eckbert ED. Scope and significance of eating disorders. Special Issue: Eating Disorders. Journal of Consulting and Clinical Psychology 1987; 55: 628–634.

Mitchell JE, Maki DD, Adson DE, Ruskin BS, Crow S. The selectivity of inclusion and exclusion criteria in bulimia nervosa treatment studies. International Journal of Eating Disorders 1997; 22: 243–252.

Moller-Madsen S, Nystrup J, Nielsen S. Mortality in anorexia nervosa in Denmark during the period 1970–1987. Acta Psychiatrica Scandinavica 1996; 94: 454–459.

Morgan HG, Russell GFM. Value of family background and clinical features as predictors of long-term outcome in anorexia nervosa: a four-year follow up study of 41 patients. Psychological Medicine 1975; 5: 355–371.

Morgan HG, Purgold J, Wellbourne J. Management and outcome in anorexia nervosa a standardised prognostic study. British Journal of Psychiatry 1983; 143: 282–287.

Munk-Jorgensen P, Moller-Madsen S, Nielsen S, Nystrup J. Incidence of eating disorders in psychiatric hospitals and wards in Denmark 1970–1993. Acta Psychiatrica Scandinavica 1995; 92: 91–96.

Namir S, Melman KN, Yager J. Pregnancy in restrictor type an: a study of 6 women. Journal of Eating Disorders 1986; 5: 838–845.

Newman MM, Halmi KA. Relationship of bone density to estradiol and cortisol in anorexia nervosa and bulimia. Psychiatry Research 1989; 29: 105–112.

Nielsen S, Moller-Madsen S, Isager T, Jorgensen J, Pagsberg K, Theander S. Standardised Mortality in eating disorders – a quantitative summary of previously published and new evidence. Journal Psychosomatic Research 1998; 44: 413–434.

Nielsen S, Moller-Madsen S, Nystrup Journal. Utilisation of psychiatric beds in the treatment of ICD–8 eating disorders in Denmark 1970–1993: a register study. European Psychiatry 1996; 11 (suppl. 4), 220s.

Olmsted MP, Davis R, Rockert W, Irvine MJ, Eagle M, Garner DM. Efficacy of a brief group psychoeducational intervention for bulimia nervosa. Behavioural Research Therapy 1991; 29: 71–83.

Paganinihill A, Henderson VW. Oestrogen replacement therapy and risk of Alzheimer disease. Archives of Internal Medicine 1996; 156: 2213–2217.

Palmer RL, Treasure JL. Providing specialised services for anorexia nervosa. British Journal of Psychiatry (in press)

Patton GC. Mortality and eating disorders. Psychological Medicine 1988; 18: 947–951.

Rastam M. Anorexia nervosa in 51 Swedish adolescents: premorbid problems and comorbidity. Journal of American Academy of Child and Adolescent Psychiatry 1992; 31: 819–829.

Ratnasuriya RH, Eisler I, Szmuckler GI, Russell GF. Anorexia nervosa: outcome and prognostic factors after 20 years. British Journal of Psychiatry 1991; 158: 495–502.

Remschmidt H, Muller H. Satinare gewichts-ausgangsdaten und langzeitprognose der anorexia nervosa. Z Kinder-Jugendpsychiat 1987; 15: 327–341.

Remschmidt H, Wienand F, Wewet C. Der Langzeitverlauf der anorexia nervosa. Monatssehr Kinderheilkd 1988; 136: 726–731.

Royal College of Psychiatrists. Eating Disorders. Council Report CR14. London: Royal College of Psychiatrists, 1992.

Russell GFM, Treasure JL, Eisler IE. Mothers with anorexia nervosa who underfeed their children: their recognition and management. Psychological Medicine 1998; 28: 93–101.

Ryle A. Cognitive Analytic Therapy: Active Participation in Charge. Chichester: Wiley, 1990.

Santosa P, Gavaretto G, Canton G. Anorexia nervosa in Italy: clinical features and outcome in a long-term follow-up study. Psychopathology 1987; 20: 8–17.

Schmidt U, Tiller J, Treasure J. Self-treatment of bulimia nervosa: a pilot study. International Journal of Eating Disorders 1993; 13: 273–277.

Schmidt U, Treasure J. Getting Better Bit(e) by Bit(e): A Survival Kit for Sufferers of Bulimia Nervosa and Binge Eating Disorder. Hove: Lawrence Erlbaum, 1993.

Schmidt U. Treatment of bulimia nervosa. In Hoek HW, Treasure JL, Katzman MA (eds), The Integration of Neurobiology in the Treatment of Eating Disorders. New York: Wiley, 1998.

Smith C, Feldman SS, Nasserbakht A, Steiner H. Psychological characteristics and DSM-III-R Diagnoses at 6-year follow-up of adolescent anorexia nervosa. Journal of the American Academy of Child and Adolescent Psychiatry 1993; 32: 1237–1245.

Smith SM, Hanson R. Failure to thrive and anorexia nervosa. Postgraduate Medical Journal 1972; 48: 382–384.

Stein A, Fairburn CG. Children of mothers with bulimia nervosa. British Medical Journal 1989; 23: 777–778.

Stein A, Woolley H, Cooper SD, Fairburn CG. An observational study of mothers with eating disorders and their infants. Journal of Child Psychology and Psychiatry and Allied Disciplines 1994; 35: 733–748.

Steinhausen HC. Treatment and outcome of adolescent anorexia nervosa. Hormone Research 1995; 43: 168–170.

Steinhausen NC, Seidel R. Outcome in adolescent eating disorders. International Journal of Eating Disorders 1993; 14: 487–496.

Sullivan PF. Mortality in anorexia nervosa. American Journal of Psychiatry 1995; 152: 1073–1074.

Susser E, Neugebauer R, Hoek HW, Brown AS, Lin S, Labovitz D, Gorman JM. Schizophrenia after prenatal famine. Archives in General Psychiatry 1996: 53: 25–31.

Svinivasagam NM, Kaye WH, Plotnicov KH, Greeno C, Weltzin TE, Rao R. Persistent perfectionism, symmetry and exactness after a long term recovery from anorexia nervosa. American Journal of Psychiatry 1995; 152: 1630–1634.

Theander S. Outcome and prognosis in anorexia nervosa and bulimia: some results of previous investigations, compared with those of a Swedish long-term study. Journal of Psychiatric Research 1985; 19: 493–508.

Thelan MH, Farmer J, McLaughlin Mann L, Pruitt J. Bulimia and interpersonal relationships: a longitudinal study. Journal of Counselling Psychology 1990; 37: 85–90.

Thiels C, Schmidt U, Treasure J, Garthe R, Troop N. Guided self change for bulimia nervosa incorporating a self-care manual. American Journal of Psychiatry 1998; 155: 947–953.

Tiller J, Schmidt U, Treasure J. Treatment of bulimia nervosa. International Review of Psychiatry 1993; 5: 75–86.

Tiller JM, Sloane G, Schmidt U, Troop N, Power M, Treasure JL. Social support in patients with anorexia nervosa and bulimia nervosa. International Journal of Eating Disorders 1996; 21: 31–38.

Tobin DL. Psychodynamic treatment and binge eating. In Fairburn CG, Wilson GT (eds), Binge Eating, Nature Assessment and Treatment. New York: Guilford, 1993, pp. 97–122.

Tolstrup K, Brinch M, Isager T, Nielsen S, Nystrup J, Severin B, Olesen NS. Long-term outcome of 151 cases of anorexia nervosa. Acta Psychiatrica Scandinavica 1985; 71: 380–387.

Touyz SW, Beumont PJV. Anorexia nervosa. A follow-up investigation. Medical Journal of Australia 1984; 18 August: 219–222.

Treasure JL, Russell G. Intrauterine growth and neonatal weight gain in anorexia nervosa. British Medical Journal 1988; 296: 1038.

Treasure JL, Schmidt U, Troop N, Tiller J, Todd G, Turnbull SJ. Sequential treatment for bulimia nervosa incorporating a self-care manual. British Journal of Psychiatry 1996; 168: 94–98.

Treasure JL, Szmukler GI. Medical and Surgical Complications of Chronic Anorexia Nervosa. In Szmukler GI, Dare C, Treasure JL (eds), The Eating Disorders: Handbook of Theory Treatment and Research. 1995, pp. 197–220.

Treasure JL, Todd G, Brolly M, Tiller J, Nehed A, Denman F. A pilot study of randomised trial of cognitive analytical therapy versus educational behavioural therapy for adult anorexia nervosa. Behaviour Research and Therapy 1995; 33: 363–367.

Treasure JL, Troop NA, Ward A. An approach to planning services for bulimia nervosa. British Journal of Psychiatry 1997; 169: 551–554.

Treasure JL, Ward A. A practical guide to the use of motivational interviewing in anorexia nervosa. European Eating Disorder Review 1997a; 5: 102–114.

Treasure JL, Ward A. Cognitive analytical therapy in the treatment of anorexia nervosa. Clinical Psychology and Psychotherapy 1997b; 4: 62–71.

Treasure JL. Psychological treatment of eating disorders. In Tantum D (ed.), Clinical Topics in Psychotherapy. London: Gaskell and Royal College of Psychiatrists, 1998, pp. 117–143.

Turnbull S, Ward A, Treasure JL, Jick H, Derby L. The demand for eating disorder care an epidemiological study using the General Practice Research Database. British Journal of Psychiatry 1996; 169: 705–712.

Van der Ham T, van Stein DC, van Engeland H. A four year prospective follow-up study of 49 eating disorder adolescents: differences in the course of illness Acta Psychiatrica Scandinavica 1994; 90: 229–235.

Van Furth EF. The treatment of anorexia nervosa. In Hoek HW, Treasure JL, Katzman M (eds), Neurobiology of Eating Disorders. Chichester: Wiley, 1998, pp. 307–322.

Van Wezel-Meijer G, Wit JM. The offspring of mothers with anorexia nervosa: a high risk group for under nutrition and stunting? European Journal of Paediatrics 1989; 149: 130–135.

Vitousek K, Manke F. Personality variables and disorders in anorexia nervosa and bulimia nervosa. Special Issue: Personality and Psychopathology. Journal of Abnormal Psychology 1994; 103: 137–147.

Wade TH, Abrahams S, Treloar SA, Martin NA, Tiggermann M. Assessing the prevalence of eating disorders in the Australian twin population. Australia and New Zealand Journal of Psychiatry 1996; 30: 845–851.

Whitbread J, McGown A. The treatment of bulimia nervosa. What is effective? A meta-analysis. Indian Journal of Clinical Psychology 1994; 21: 32–44.

Williams P, King M. The 'epidemic' of anorexia nervosa: another medical myth? Lancet 1987; i: 205–207.

Wilson GT, Fairburn CG. Treatments for eating disorders. In Nathan PE, Gorman JM (eds), A Guide to Treatments That Work. New York: Oxford University Press, 1998, pp. 501–530.

Wilson GT. Treatment of bulimia nervosa: the next decade. European Eating Disorders Review 1999; 7: 77–83.

Woodside DB, Shekter-Wolfson LF. Parenting by patients with anorexia nervosa and bulimia nervosa. International Journal of Eating Disorders 1990; 9: 303–309.

Young J. Cognitive Therapy for Personality Disorders: A Schema Focused Approach. Sarasota: Professional Resource Press, 1990.

6

SOMATOFORM DISORDERS

Christopher Bass

INTRODUCTION

One of the most important innovations in the third edition of the American Psychiatric Association's Diagnostic and Statistical Manual of Mental Disorders (DSM-III 1980) was its introduction of a new class of psychiatric syndrome called somatoform disorders. The essential features are 'physical symptoms suggesting physical disorder for which there are no demonstrable organic findings or known physiological mechanisms and for which there is positive evidence, or a strong presumption, that the symptoms are linked to psychological factors or conflicts'. The ICD–10 (1992) followed the American lead. Unfortunately, despite the close collaboration in the preparation of ICD–10 and DSM-IV, differences have arisen between the two classifications of somatoform disorders (Table 6.1).

The major differences are: (1) conversion disorder is classified separately in ICD–10 and grouped instead with 'dissociative disorders'; (2) ICD–10 does not include a category of 'body dysmorphic disorder' – such cases are classified as a variant of hypochondriacal disorder instead; (3) neurasthenia (chronic fatigue syndrome) is included in the ICD–10 not as a somatoform disorder but as a separate category (F48.0); and (4) ICD–10 but not DSM-IV includes 'somatoform autonomic dysfunction' as a form of somatoform disorder. Common characteristics of somatoform disorders are shown in table 2 (Benjamin and Bridges 1994).

Although the diagnostic categories shown in table 1 have the appearance of being relatively homogeneous, this is illusory. The concept of somatoform disorder is fraught with serious difficulties for the following reasons: (1) many of the defining concepts, such as number of somatic symptoms and hypochondriacal attitudes, are better described in dimensional rather than categorical terms; (2) some somatoform disorders are so chronic and enduring (especially hypochondriasis and somatization disorder) that it would make more sense to classify them as personality disorders (Axis 2) than as mental state disorders (Axis 1) (Tyrer et al. 1990,

DSM-IV (1994) SOMATOFORM DISORDERS	ICD–10 (1992) NEUROTIC, STRESS RELATED AND SOMATOFORM DISORDERS
Conversion disorder	(F44) Dissociative and conversion disorder (F45) Somatoform disorders
Somatization disorder	.o Somatization disorder
Undifferentiated somatoform disorder	.1 Undifferentiated somatoform disorder
Hypochondriasis	.2 Hypochondriacal disorder
No specific category	.3 Somatoform autonomic dysfunction
Somatoform pain disorder	.4 Persistent somatoform pain disorder
Body dysmorphic disorder	No specific category (included in 45.2) (F48) Other neurotic disorders
No specific category	.o Neurasthenia (fatigue syndrome)

Table 6.1 – Comparison of the DSM-IV (1994) and ICD–10 (1992) classifications of somatoform and related disorders.

1999); (3) most patients have clinical features that fit criteria for several diagnostic categories simultaneously, e.g. conversion disorder and somatization disorder (Mayou et al. 1995).

The somatoform disorders should be distinguished from **somatization**, which is a term used to describe the variety of processes that lead patients to seek medical help for bodily symptoms which are attributed to organic disease but have no relevant organic basis (Murphy 1990). This is best seen as a **process** rather than a discrete disorder, and it can be acute, subacute or chronic (more than 6 months). Once it is chronic it becomes a somatoform disorder; these essentially chronic disorders are the subject of this chapter. As the concept of somatoform disorders has been in use for nearly two decades, the work cited in this chapter relates mainly to the DSM-IV. Nevertheless, it is relevant to the ICD–10 and has influenced its compilers.

- Excessive use of medical and surgical services
- Failure to be reassured by 'negative findings'
- 'Doctor and hospital-shopping'
- Reluctance to recognize the relevance of psychological factors
- Mutual hostility between patients and their doctors

Table 6.2 – Common characteristics of patients with somatoform disorders.

CONVERSION DISORDER

An essential difference between conversion disorder (CD) and other somatoform disorders is that 'an alteration or loss of physical functioning' is required for the diagnosis, i.e. it is not diagnosed on the basis of symptom complaints alone. There are difficulties, however, with the definition of CD. First, it is implied that physical disorder must be excluded, but neurological co-morbidity is high: deciding which symptoms are accounted for by organic disease and which are not can be difficult. Second, it is stated that a temporally related psychological stressor should be identified, but in practice this is often impossible to establish. In many cases no conflicts are uncovered at the time of presentation. Finally, although the process should be unconsciously mediated, in practice it can be difficult to distinguish between this and factitious or simulated illness.

The one year prevalence of CD in the community has been estimated to be 0.3% (Faravelli et al. 1997). Although one-third of neurological inpatients have no organic explanation for their physical complaints (Ewald et al. 1994), only about 1% are thought to exhibit symptoms of CD (Marsden 1986).

A high level of psychiatric co-morbidity has been noted in most studies, with depression (38–50%) and anxiety (10–16%) being responsible for most of this (Crimlisk et al. 1998). There is also a high incidence of personality disorders in CD as well as somatization disorder. Patients with the latter disorder usually develop conversion symptoms, e.g. aphonia, monoplegia, at some stage during the course of their chaotic and chronic 'illness careers'.

Outcome findings in CD depend to some degree on the setting: tertiary referral centres tend to attract patients with chronic or intractable conditions. Better outcome is associated with short or acute onset, early improvement during a hospital admission (Couprie et al. 1995) and the presence of an Axis I diagnosis such as depression (Crimlisk et al. 1998). When symptoms have become chronic, however, or the patient has a co-existing personality disorder there is much less chance of improvement (Mace and Trimble 1996, Crimlisk et al. 1998).

The risk of overlooking organic pathology when making a diagnosis of CD has attracted considerable attention but has almost certainly been exaggerated. Recent technological advances, especially in neuro-imaging, have dramatically improved the likelihood of accurately diagnosing organic neurological disorders, As a consequence the rate of misdiagnosis is now accepted to be in the region of 5% (Crimlisk et al. 1998).

Some of these patients can become profoundly disabled and dependent on state benefits. In a recent study of such patients who had become wheelchair dependent, Davison et al. (1999) found that all were receiving benefits and there was a considerable burden on their carers. These patients often find their way into neurology rehabilitation services, where many receive respite care. There is a lack of appropriate treatment facilities for patients with CD: a 'psychosomatic' ward on a general hospital site staffed by mental health and general nurses is the most satisfactory treatment environment, but few such resources exist in the UK (see Chapter 14). Therapeutic efforts need to be co-ordinated: it is not helpful if psychological issues and conflicts are dealt with by the 'psychological' team, and the physical rehabilitation and physiotherapy are addressed by other workers (often on a different site).

BODY DYSMORPHIC DISORDER

Patients who present with excessive concern about a trivial or non-existent physical abnormality, which they believe renders them misshapen or ugly, have long been recognized, but never satisfactorily classified. The concern may vary in intensity from a mild sensitivity, through a preoccupation sufficient to motivate requests for corrective surgery, to an unshakeable belief held with delusional conviction.

DSM-III-R (1987) introduced the new category of Body Dysmorphic Disorder to cover the middle part of this range. The body image disturbance of anorexia nervosa and the gender dysphoria of transsexualism are specifically excluded, as are beliefs about deformity of **delusional** intensity, which are classified with delusional disorder, somatic type (F22.0 in ICD–10). In practice, however, the distinction between a delusion and an over-valued idea of deformity may be difficult, especially if there is some degree of deformity, and the clinician has to make a judgement about whether the concern shown is excessive. Regrettably, neither DSM-IV nor ICD–10 criteria guide the clinician in judging what is excessive concern. Such judgements are not medical but aesthetic and are likely to vary between doctors.

Despite these nosological complexities there has been considerable interest in BDD. The author of a recent book on the subject claims that it may affect as many as 2% of the US population (Phillips 1996). In a recent British survey of 50 cases three-quarters of the sample was female and there was a high degree of co-morbidity. The most common Axis I diagnoses were either a mood disorder (26%), social phobia (16%) or obsessive–compulsive disorder (6%). Twenty-four percent had made a suicide attempt in the past and personality disorders were present in 72% of patients. The authors concluded that BDD was associated with high rates of co-morbid psychiatric morbidity and was a chronic handicapping disorder (Veale et al. 1996a). Even higher rates of co-morbid disorders were found in an American study of 30 cases: 93% had an associated lifetime diagnosis of a major mood disorder, 33% a psychotic disorder and 73% an anxiety disorder. Furthermore, 97% avoided usual social and occupational activities, and 30% had been housebound (Phillips et al. 1993).

The psychiatrist's role is liaison with general practitioners and surgeons in an attempt to avoid unnecessary surgery, which carries iatrogenic risks and serves merely to maintain the preoccupation. Serotonin re-uptake inhibitors are effective in some patients with BDD, including those with the delusional disorder variant (Phillips et al. 1998). In a recent pilot randomized controlled trial of cognitive behavioural therapy there were significant changes in the treated group after 12 weeks on specific measures of BDD and depressed mood (Veale et al. 1996b). Clearly more studies are warranted in this field.

HYPOCHONDRIASIS

The central feature of hypochondriasis – a belief, held with less than delusional conviction, that one has a serious physical disease, is common to ICD–10 and DSM-IV, as well as earlier definitions (Gillespie 1928). A key criterion for the diagnosis, however, is that the fear or belief 'persists despite appropriate medical evaluation and reassurance'.

The prevalence of hypochondriacal concerns in the general population is unknown. In a recent study the prevalence of hypochondriasis (DSM-IV) in primary care was 3% (Escobar et al. 1998). Patients with this disorder had higher levels of medically unexplained symptoms (abridged somatization) and were more impaired in their physical function than patients without the disorder. Barsky et al. (1990a) reported a 6-month prevalence of DSM-III-R hypochondriasis in a sample of general medical outpatients of between 4.2 and 6.3%.

There is also evidence of considerable co-morbidity, especially with panic disorder (Barsky et al. 1994). Hypochondriacal patients with co-morbid panic disorder somatize more, report more social and occupational role impairment, and visit emergency departments more frequently than those without. Hypochondriacal symptoms can also occur in patients with depression and somatization disorder (Oxman and Barrett 1985). Noyes (1999) has recently reviewed the phenomenological overlap between hypochondriasis and several anxiety disorders.

Although there is undoubtedly evidence of transient as well as recurrent forms of the disorder (Barsky et al. 1990b), Tyrer et al. (1990) have argued that some hypochondriacal patients have a personality disorder (Axis 2) rather than a mental state disorder. Patients with this disorder have a very poor prognosis but extremely high health service use. They concluded that 'the natural history of neurotic symptoms in the presence of hypochondriacal personality disorder is one of a persistent, and possibly malignant, condition that shows virtually no tendency to spontaneous remission' (Tyrer et al. 1999). This is an important finding, which is borne out not only by anecdotal clinical experience, but also by recent findings from a study by Barsky et al. (1998). These authors carried out a 4–5-year prospective study of DSM-III-R hypochondriasis and found that although the patients showed a considerable decline in symptoms and improvement in role functioning over 4–5 years, two-thirds of them still met diagnostic criteria for the disorder.

Patients with hypochondriasis are very difficult, but not impossible, to treat. A recent innovative treatment based on a cognitive–behavioural techniques was recently shown to be effective in a controlled trial, but only one therapist was involved (Warwick et al. 1996). In a study that attempted to replicate and extend these findings, Clark et al. (1998) found that cognitive therapy was a specific treatment for hypochondriasis, but that behavioural stress management was also effective. It is worth noting that the study was restricted to patients willing to accept referral to a specialist psychological treatment unit (70% from GPs), and that the mean duration of the current episode of hypochondriasis was 4 years. Nevertheless, it represents an important advance.

SOMATIZATION DISORDER

The criteria for this disorder, which first appeared in DSM-III in 1980, are 'a history of many physical complaints or a belief that one is sickly, beginning before the age of 30 and persisting for several years'. In addition the patient must have at least 13 physical symptoms from a list of 35 specified in the manual. These are listed in six groups: pain, gastrointestinal, cardiopulmonary, conversion (pseudo-neuro-logical), sexual and female reproductive symptoms. For a symptom to count towards the diagnosis it must satisfy three criteria: there is no pathophysiological mechanism to account for the symptom; it has not occurred only during the panic attack; and it has caused the person to take medicine (other than over-the-counter pain medication), see a doctor or alter life-style.

These criteria may appear arbitrary to anyone unfamiliar with the recent history of the concept of hysteria in the USA. Hysteria used in the North American sense before 1980 referred to a chronic, persistent disorder characterized by multiple physical symptoms and a poor prognosis that occurred predominantly in women. To avoid the pejorative connotations of hysteria, the term Briquet's syndrome was introduced in 1970. This in turn was superseded by somatization disorder (SD) in 1980.

SD is included as one of the somatoform disorders in ICD–10 (F.45.0), but the diagnosis has attracted little attention from UK researchers. One possible expla-nation for this is a consequence of Slater's influential attack on the concept of hysteria (Slater 1965). In a 10-year follow-up study of patients admitted to a specialist neurological hospital with a diagnosis of hysteria, Slater found that over half the patients developed clear cut neurological or psychiatric conditions during follow-up. But examination of Slater's original series of 85 patients reveals that at follow-up there were 14 patients (17%) 'suffering from a lasting personality disorder who came somewhere near to satisfying the criteria proposed by Guze', i.e. what is currently known as SD. The neglect of SD in the UK has been regrettable, for reasons outlined below.

Data from the Epidemiological Catchment Area (ECA) Program suggest a lifetime prevalence for SD of between 0.1 and 0.4% (Swartz et al. 1986). However, this is probably a gross underestimate because the diagnosis can only be made after excluding physical pathology relevant to symptoms, and this information was not available in the ECA survey. The author believes that the diagnosis can only be established with any confidence by reviewing the patient's medical records from both primary care and the general hospital. This is a time-consuming but worthwhile endeavour, because once the diagnosis is made it has very important implications for management (see below).

The multi-axial classification in DSM-III provides a framework to consider the features associated with the diagnosis of SD. It commonly co-exists with other Axis I disorders, notably major depression, panic disorder and phobic disorders, especially agoraphobia. It has been viewed as itself more akin to a personality disorder (Axis II) than an episode of illness (Axis I), since it begins early in life and is by definition chronic. Recent support for this view was reported by Stern et al. (1993), who found that 72% of patients with SD had a personality disorder, compared with 30% of 'psychiatric' control subjects with anxiety and depression. Concurrent physical disorders (Axis III) occur in about half the patients and may well be iatrogenic, e.g. adhesions complicating a negative exploratory laparotomy for abdominal pain. Little is known about the relationship between life events (Axis IV) and presentation in somatization disorder, but anecdotal evidence suggests that they are important.

Many patients with this diagnosis have considerable functional disability (Axis V) in terms of work capacity, dependence on benefits, days in bed and mobility. Of a British sample of patients with SD, 10% was confined to wheelchairs (Bass and Murphy 1991). Golding et al. (1991) found that 83% of the men and 46% of the women with SD were rated as work disabled. Furthermore, men were more likely than women to report that a family member missed work because of the participant's illness or injury, suggesting that SD may be more disruptive of men's occupational and social functioning than women's. Indeed, in another study the self-rated physical functioning of patients with SD was even poorer than in patients suffering from chronic organic disease: SD patients spent an average of 7 days in bed each month (Smith et al. 1986).

Somatization disorder also has a disruptive effect on parenting: compared with matched patients with major depression, women with SD were twice as likely to have children with severe conduct disturbance and three times as likely to be 'poor parents', e.g. reported for child abuse (Zoccolillo and Cloninger 1985) (see Chapter 17).

For all these reasons establishing a diagnosis of SD should be considered as important (and complex) as making a diagnosis of schizophrenia. Somatization disorder generally lasts for a lifetime: at least in a proportion of patients with schizophrenia remissions are possible with modern treatment. British psychiatrists have failed to appreciate the importance of this chronic and enduring disorder. These patients constitute an enormous drain on the financial resources of health services, yet optimum management strategies have yet to be worked out. Effective interventions could lead to considerable cost savings, and there is an urgent need for more research in this disorder.

SOMATOFORM PAIN DISORDER

DSM-III (1980) established the category Psychogenic Pain Disorder, with criteria identical to conversion disorder, except that they are applied to the single symptom of pain. In DSM-III-R (1987) the term 'somatoform pain disorder' was introduced: this requires a 6-month history of persistent pain, in the absence of organic pathology sufficient to explain it. In ICD–10 (1992) there is an assumption of psychological causation. Psychosocial factors are certainly important in maintaining chronic pain, even though they may not have been aetiologically relevant.

These patients are much more likely to attend pain clinics than mental health services, and constitute a heterogeneous group. There is no reason to expect that patients with atypical facial pain or fibromyalgia have anything in common other than a complaint of pain, and lumping them together under a single diagnostic label does not help in identifying a cause or an appropriate treatment. The prevalence of co-morbid psychiatric disorders varies considerably according to treatment settings. The commonest diagnoses are affective disorders (depressive disorders are more common than anxiety disorders in patients with chronic pain), substance abuse (estimated to be about 10% of pain clinic attenders; Kouyanou et al. 1998), and personality disorders (Benjamin and Bridges 1994).

In addition to these high rates of lifetime and current psychiatric disorders in patients with chronic pain and fibromyalgia (chronic widespread pain of indeterminate cause), there is evidence of high service use and considerable functional disability. For example, in a recent US study patients with fibromyalgia had an average of 10 outpatient medical visits per year and were hospitalized at a rate of every one-third year because of pain (Wolfe et al. 1997a). More than 16% were in receipt of disability payments compared with 2.2% of the US population (Wolfe et al. 1997b), half were dissatisfied with their health and 59% rated their health as fair or poor (Wolfe et al. 1997c).

The mental health clinician's main concern should be in detecting (and minimizing whenever possible) the maintaining factors and reducing disability in patients with chronic pain, and instituting a management plan. This can be carried out either in the outpatient setting or, preferably, in a joint clinic run with a pain specialist. Most patients find this clinical arrangement acceptable, but few such clinics exist in the UK (Dolin and Stephens 1998).

UNDIFFERENTIATED SOMATOFORM DISORDER

By now it should be clear that the classification of the somatoform disorders remains inadequate, not only because of substantial overlap between individual somatoform disorders and between somatoform and other Axis I disorders, but also because of the difficulty separating some of these disorders from the normal range. Many patients present with features of more than one disorder, and cannot readily be 'fitted' into one category. Some report multiple unexplained symptoms, but not the requisite 13 necessary for a diagnosis of somatization disorder. The category undifferentiated somatoform disorder (USD) is intended in DSM-IV for this latter group, but it is a testament to the failure of the classificatory system that this supposedly residual category is actually by far the most common somatoform diagnosis in community surveys, being 150 times more prevalent than somatization disorder (Deighton and Nicol 1985, Escobar et al. 1987).

Because the criteria for USD are overly inclusive, attempts have been made to find a more valid and useful diagnosis. One suggestion has been multi-somatoform disorder or MSD, defined as three or more medically unexplained, currently bothersome physical symptoms plus a long (2 or more years) history of somatization. This has a prevalence of 8.2% in primary care and, compared with mood and anxiety disorders, is associated with comparable impairment in health-related quality of life, more disability days and clinic visits, and greater clinician-perceived patient difficulty (Kroenke et al. 1997). MSD appears to be a valid diagnosis and potentially more useful than the DSM-IV diagnosis of USD.

NEURASTHENIA (F48.0 IN ICD–10; BROADLY RESEMBLES CHRONIC FATIGUE SYNDROME)

There has been an explosive growth of both media and research interest in chronic fatigue syndrome (CFS) in the past 10 years or so. Wessely (1990) has argued that chronic fatigue or 'ME' is simply 'old wine in new bottles'. The old wine in question is neurasthenia, which was first described in the early nineteenth century and became one of the most common diagnoses in medicine a century or so ago. In recognition of the recent resurgence of interest in chronic fatigue, it has been retained in ICD–10 (F48.0), although it is classified with 'other neurotic disorders' rather than as a somatoform disorder. The central feature is fatigue, and two types are identified, depending on whether the fatigue is predominantly mental, or predominantly physical.

CFS is an important disorder because it is very common, often associated with psychiatric morbidity, and frequently disabling. In a British study carried out in primary care the point prevalence of CFS using the 1995 CDC criteria was 2.6%, falling to 0.5% if co-morbid psychological disorders were excluded (Wessely et al. 1997). The functional impairment is profound and associated with substantial impairment in work, social and home environments. Profoundly disabled and bed-bound patients often write about their experiences and attract media attention (Firth 1999). The disorder, therefore, represents a considerable public health and economic burden. There is evidence that the greater the impairment, the greater the psychological morbidity, although such observations do not imply causality (Working Party Report 1996).

SOMATOFORM DISORDERS: COUNTING THE COST

The personal and public costs of these chronic and disabling disorders are high and likely to remain so unless specialized rehabilitation services are developed. As resources for healthcare are limited, more detailed economic appraisals of services for patients with somatoform disorders are urgently required. Feldman deals with these issues in more detail in Chapter 14.

SUMMARY

I have attempted to describe the characteristics of a group of disorders that straddle both psychiatry and medicine. They are common, and may become chronic and disabling as well as placing a considerable burden on services. Because patients with these disorders more commonly present in non-psychiatric settings (primary care and the general hospital), general psychiatrists and healthcare providers often overlook them. This is regrettable because treatments have been introduced recently that have been shown to be effective. The dilemma for healthcare providers is that interventions need to be delivered at a relatively early stage in the evolution of the disorders, before iatrogenic and other factors lead to the development of disabilities and invalidism. This presents a challenge for both psychiatric and medical services which, regrettably, few at the present time appear to be meeting.

References

American Psychiatric Association Diagnostic and Statistical Manual of Mental Disorders, 3rd edn. Washington, DC: American Psychiatric Association, 1980.

Barsky AJ, Wyshak G, Klerman G, Latham K. The prevalence of hypochondriasis in medical outpatients. Social Psychiatry and Psychiatric Epidemiology 1990a; 25: 89–94.

Barsky A, Wyshak G, Klerman G. Transient hypochondriasis. Archives of General Psychiatry 1990b; 47: 746–752.

Barsky A, Barnett M, Cleary P. Hypochondriasis and panic disorder. Boundary and overlap. Archives of General Psychiatry 1994; 51: 918–925.

Barsky A, Fava J, Bailey E, Ahern D. A prospective 4–5 year study of DSM-III-R hypochondriasis. Archives of General Psychiatry 1998; 55: 737–744.

Bass C, Benjamin S. Management of chronic somatization. British Journal of Psychiatry 1993; 162: 472–480.

Bass C, Murphy M. Somatisation disorder in a British teaching hospital: the unnatural history of a non-disease. British Journal of Clinical Practice 1991; 45: 237–244.

Benjamin S, Bridges K. Do chronic somatizers have special needs? In Benjamin S, House A, Jenkins P (eds), Liaison Psychiatry: Defining Needs and Planning Services. London: Gaskell, 1994.

Clark DM, Salkovskis P, Hackmann A et al. Two psychological treatments for hypochondriasis. A randomised controlled trial. British Journal of Psychiatry 1998; 170: 218–223.

Couprie W, Wijdicks E, Rooijmans H, van Gijn. Outcome in conversion disorder: a follow-up study. Journal of Neurology, Neurosurgery and Psychiatry 1995; 58: 750–752.

Crimlisk H, Bhatia K, Cope H et al. Slater revisited: 6-year follow-up of patients with medically unexplained motor symptoms. British Medical Journal 1998; 316: 582–586.

Davison P, Sharpe M, Wade D, Bass C. 'Wheelchair' patients with non-organic disease: a psychological enquiry. Journal of Psychosomatic Research 1999 (in press).

Deighton C, Nicol A. Abnormal illness behaviour in young women in a primary care setting: is Briquette's syndrome a useful category? Psychological Medicine 1985; 15: 515–520.

Dolin S, Stephens J. Pain clinics and liaison psychiatry. Anaesthesia 1998; 53: 317–319.

Escobar JI, Burnam M, Karno M et al. Somatization in the community. Archives of General Psychiatry 1987; 44: 713–718.

Escobar JI, Golding JM, Hough RL et al. Somatization in the community. Relationship to disability and use of services. American Journal of Public Health 1987; 77: 837–840.

Escobar J, Gara M, Waitzkin H, Silver R, Holman A, Compton W. DSM-IV hypochondriasis in primary care. General Hospital Psychiatry 1998; 20: 155–159.

Ewald H, Rogne T, Ewald K, Fink P. Somatization in patients newly admitted to a neurological department. Acta Psychiatrica Scandinavica 1994; 89: 174–179.

Faravelli C, Salvatori S, Galassi F, Aiazzi L, Drei C, Cabras P. Epidemiology of somatoform disorders: a community survey in Florence. Social Psychiatry and Psychiatric Epidemiology 1997; 32: 24–29.

Firth S. Independent on Sunday, 28 March 1999, p. 4.

Gillespie R. Hypochondria: its definition, nosology and psychopathology. Guy's Hospital Report 1928; 78: 408–460.

Golding J, Smith GR, Kashner T. Does somatization disorder occur in men? Archives in General Psychiatry 1991; 48: 231–235.

Kouyanou K, Pither C, Wessely S. Medication misuse, abuse and dependence in chronic pain patients. Journal of Psychosomatic Research 1997; 43: 497–504.

Kroenke K, Spitzer R, de Gruy F et al. Multisomatoform disorder. An alternative to undifferentiated somatoform disorder for the somatizing patient in primary care. Archives of General Psychiatry 1997; 54: 352–358.

Mace C, Trimble M. Ten year outcome of conversion disorder. British Journal of Psychiatry 1996; 169: 282–288.

Marsden D. Hysteria – a neurologist's view. Psychological Medicine 1986; 16: 277–288.

Mayou R, Bass C, Sharpe M. Overview of epidemiology, classification, and aetiology. In Mayou R, Bass C, Sharpe M (eds), Treatment of Functional Somatic Symptoms. Oxford: Oxford University Press, 1995.

Murphy MR. Classification of the somatoform disorders. In Bass C (ed.), Somatization: Physical Symptoms and Psychological Illness. Oxford: Blackwell, 1990.

Noyes R. The relationship of hypochondriasis to anxiety disorders. General Hospital Psychiatry 1999; 21: 8–18.

Oxman T, Barrett J. Depression and hypochondriasis in family practice patients with somatization disorder. General Hospital Psychiatry 1985; 7: 321–329.

Phillips KA, McElroy S, Keck P et al. Body dysmorphic disorder: 30 cases of imagined ugliness. American Journal of Psychiatry 1993; 150: 302–308.

Phillips KA. The Broken Mirror: Understanding and Treating Body Dysmorphic Disorder. Oxford: Oxford University Press, 1996.

Phillips KA, Dwight MM, McElroy SL. Efficacy and safety of fluvoxamine in body dysmorphic disorder. Journal of Clinical Psychiatry 1998; 59: 165–171.

Report of a Joint Working Group of the Royal Colleges of Physicians, Psychiatrists and General Practitioners. Chronic Fatigue Syndrome. Council Report 54. London: Royal College of Psychiatrists, 1996.

Slater E. Diagnosis of 'hysteria'. British Medical Journal 1965; 1: 1395–1399.

Smith GR, Monson R, Ray D. Patients with multiple unexplained symptoms. Their characteristics, functional health, and healthcare utilisation. Archives of Internal Medicine 1986; 146: 69–72.

Stern J, Murphy MR, Bass C. Personality disorders in patients with somatisation disorder: a controlled study. British Journal of Psychiatry 1993; 163: 785–789.

Swartz M, Blazer D, George L, Landerman R. Somatization disorder in a community population. American Journal of Psychiatry 1986; 143: 1403–1408.

Tyrer P, Fowler-Dixon R, Ferguson B, Kelemen A. A plea for the diagnosis of hypochondriacal personality disorder. Journal of Psychosomatic Research 1990; 34: 637–642.

Tyrer P, Seivewright N, Seivewright H. Long-term outcome of hypochondriacal personality disorder. Journal of Psychosomatic Research 1999.

Veale D, Boocock A, Gournay K et al. Body dysmorphic disorder. A survey of 50 cases. British Journal of Psychiatry 1996a; 169: 196–201.

Veale D, Gournay K, Dryden W et al. Body dysmorphic disorder: a cognitive behavioural model and pilot randomised controlled trial. Behaviour Research and Therapy 1996b; 34: 717–729.

Warwick H, Clark DM, Cobb AM, Salkovskis P. A controlled trial of cognitive behavioral treatment of hypochondriasis. British Journal of Psychiatry 1996; 169: 189–195.

Wessely S. Old wine in new bottles: neurasthenia and ME. Psychological Medicine 1990; 20: 35–53.

Wessely S, Chalder T, Hirsch S, Wallace P, Wright D. The prevalence and morbidity of chronic fatigue syndrome: a prospective primary care study. American Journal of Public Health 1997; 87: 1449–1455.

Wolfe F, Anderson J, Harkness D et al. A prospective, longitudinal, multicentre study of service utilisation and costs in fibromyalgia. Arthritis and Rheumatology 1997a; 40: 1560–1470.

Wolfe F, Anderson J, Harkness D et al. Work and disability status of persons with fibromyalgia. Journal of Rheumatology 1997b; 24: 1171–1178.

Wolfe F, Anderson J, Harkness D et al. Health status and disease severity in fibromyalgia: results of a six-centre longitudinal study. Arthritis and Rheumatology 1997c; 40: 1571–1579.

World Health Organisation. Mental, behavioural, and developmental disorders. In International Classification of Diseases. Geneva: Division of Mental Health, 1992.

Zoccolillo M, Cloninger C. Parental breakdown associated with somatization disorder (hysteria). British Journal of Psychiatry 1985; 147: 446–448.

7

SEVERE MENTAL ILLNESS IN OLD AGE

Sarah Craig and Alistair Burns

All the world's a stage

And the men and women merely players:

They all have exits and their entrances:

And one man in his time plays many parts,

His acts being seven ages. As, first the infant,

Mewling and puking in the nurse's arms.

And then the whining schoolboy, with his satchel

And shining morning face creeping like snail

Unwillingly to school. And then the lover

Sighing like furnace, with a woeful ballad

Made to his mistress eyebrow. And then the soldier

Full of strange oaths and bearded like the pard

Jealous in honour, sudden and quick in quarrel,

Seeking the bubble reputation

Even in the cannon's mouth. And then the justice

In fair round belly with good capon lined

With eyes severe and beard of formal cut

Full of wise saws and modern instances;

And so he plays his part. The sixth age shifts

Into the lean and slippered pantaloon,

With spectacles on nose and perch on side;

His youthful hose, well safed, a world too wide,

For his shrunk shank; and his big manly voice

Turning again toward childish treble, pipes

And whistles in his sound. Last seen of all

That ends this strange eventful history,

His second childishness and mere oblivion,

Sans teeth, sans eyes, sans taste, sans everything

William Shakespeare (1600), *As You Like It*, Act 2, Scene 7

INTRODUCTION

The manager of the Imperial War Museum once said in a radio interview that, in marketing his establishment, he had the problem of trying to sell three of the most unpopular words in the English language. Old age psychiatry, dealing with mental health problems in elderly people, is not far behind. Attitudes towards ageing and older people are essentially negative, the relative worth of older people in western society is low and they are the butt of many jokes (Palmore 1971). These negative attitudes span society as a whole and include some professionals. The advent of the 'third age' with its associated learning objectives (Laslett 1989) places it between the second age of working and child bearing and the fourth age of increasing frailty and dependence, a modern equivalent of Shakespeare's Seven Ages of Man. Arguments for a functional rather than chronological approach to ageing have been advocated with attitudes defined in terms of current ability rather than achievement of a certain biological age. Retirement is perceived by many as a negative life event, the necessity for a person to retire at a predetermined biological age rather than coinciding with the onset of physical inability is unclear and a relatively recent phenomenon. In 1931, a quarter of men over 65 were economically active compared to 8% in 1991. In 1921 11% of people lived alone compared to 37% in 1993, the sex distribution being equal in 1931 but men outnumbering women 2:1 in 1993. Of people over the age of 65, 1.4% are in institutions, the number increasing to 27.6% of women and 15.6% of men over the age of 85.

Characteristics of older people

As a group, elderly people differ in three main ways from younger adults with regard to mental health problems, although there is common ground in the presentation and management of specific mental disorders. First, the elderly frequently present with physical problems, either as a symptom of mental illness or as a co-existing disorder. For this reason mental health problems are often missed as efforts to concentrate on physical symptoms often take priority. Second, it is often the older person's family who present the problem to health or social services and this can have an impact on compliance with treatment and the therapeutic alliance. Relationships within families, and different individual agencies may influence their presentation and ultimate management. Third, the ageing process is often devalued. It is a common belief that being old equates to ill health, both physically and mentally. 'There's nothing for him to look forward to' 'She's a lot to be depressed about', 'She forgets things because she's old', are all comments frequently made about elderly people.

Pathways to care

The main pathways to psychiatric care for older people are the general practitioner (GP), social services and geriatricians. GPs in the UK are now obliged to offer annual health checks to patients over 75 years and this should include an assessment of their mental state. At the very least, the checks should include questions such as 'Do you feel sad, depressed or miserable?' and 'Do you have any problems with your everyday memory?', as well as an objective assessment. Some practices prefer to use standardised tests such as the Geriatric Depression Scale and the Abbreviated Mental Test Score. It has been shown that mental conditions are rarely identified by practice nurses (Chew et al. 1994) and detection does not always lead to effective intervention. Good liaison between departments of geriatrics and old age psychiatry can facilitate identification of physical and mental disorders. The importance of continuing education, on both sides, cannot be underestimated. Care workers in social services looking after people in their own homes may be the first to identify problems, and are often in an ideal position to notice any change in normal functioning of their clients. Similarly, social services departments will carry out their own needs assessment when considering a client for care, which has the capacity to identify mental disorders. However, they need adequate training to do so.

Numbers of elderly people

Of the total world population (5544 million) in 1993, 6% are over the age of 65 (Mann 1996). This is different between developed and developing countries with comparative figures being 14% in Europe, 17% in the USA and only 3% in African countries. In the UK, by 2041, 11% of the over 60 population will be over 85 compared to 6% currently. Increased life expectancy accounts for the change, summarised in table 1.

There is an average increase of 1.8 years of life estimated for an 80 year old man in 2001 compared to 1961 and 2.5 years for women (OPCS 1991).

Table 7.1

EXPECTATION OF LIFE AT BIRTH		
Year of birth	**Males**	**Females**
1841	39	42
1881	47	52
1901	51	58
1921	61	68
1941	69.6	75.4
1961	73.6	79.1
1981	75.5	80.4
1991	76.0	80.8

From: OPCS (1991), National population projections 1989 based series PP2 No 17. London: HMSO. Quoted in Johnson and Falkingham (1992), p. 23.

Implications for Health and Social Services

Commonly stated requirements for adequate services include flexibility and excellent interdisciplinary communication, blurring of professional boundaries and that they be directed towards the care and benefit of the older person. The realities are that, despite many areas of excellent practice and the absolute dedication, professionalism and skill of individual practitioners, resources often are not directed towards older people, especially in the current climate which focuses much effort and money on younger acutely ill and usually psychotic patients. The scandals of the 1960s which prompted investigations into the care of elderly people, most often in hospital, and which led to the creation of the Hospital Advisory Service have long been forgotten and probably will not be repeated although there are occasional instances of neglect of elderly residents in nursing and residential homes.

Older people tend to be more severely disabled and this is particularly marked for those over the age of 85. Family support constitutes the main portion of care given to older people with fewer than half receiving statutory services and less than 10% entirely dependent on them. With less than 5% of people in long term care in the UK and the stated government policy of maintaining people in their own homes where possible, pressure on social services is likely to continue. Government documents such as the White Paper, Caring for People (Secretaries of State for Health and Social Security, 1989), The National Health Service and Community Care Act 1990 (DoH 1990) and the Carers (Recognition of Services) Act 1995 all underscore this direction of policy in relation to care of elderly people.

SPECIFIC MENTAL DISORDERS

DEPRESSION

Depression is often regarded as the inevitable consequence of ageing and the traditional associations of age with physical frailty, death of contemporaries and loss of socio-economic status fuels the belief that depression is understandable and therefore untreatable in older people.

Epidemiology

Generally, and in common with depression at any age, depressive symptoms are commoner than depressive illness. Rates of depressive illness in older people vary between 1 and 3% while those with depressive symptoms number between 10 and 15% (e.g. Gurland et al. 1983). Women are usually more affected than men but, in contrast to many other disorders there is no obvious age related increase in prevalence. Indeed, nonagenarians have lower rates of depression than people in their 60s and 70s (Lindesay et al. 1989). Not all depressive symptom clusters in older people can be neatly divided into these two categories. Other symptom profiles are becoming increasingly recognised, often coded into diagnostic criteria including adjustment disorder, dysthymia, the depression/dementia complex and, of particular relevance to older people, depression as a reaction to the presence of physical illness (Blazer and Williams 1980). Older people who are in residential care or in acute or rehabilitation medical wards have much higher rates of depression (e.g. 40% in residential care, Ames et al. 1988, up to 45% in medical inpatients, Jackson and Baldwin 1993). It may be that exclusion of this group of people from traditional community surveys has led to the relative underestimate of depression in older people.

Clinical features

DSM IV criteria (APA 1994) for major depressive illness include five or more of the following symptoms, present during the same two week period and representing a change from previous function:

- Depressed mood most of the day, nearly every day

- Markedly diminished interest or pleasure in all, or almost all activities

- Significant weight loss, or decrease or increase in appetite nearly every day

- Insomnia or hypersomnia

- Psychomotor agitation or retardation

- Fatigue or loss of energy

- Feelings of worthlessness or excessive or inappropriate guilt

- Diminished ability to think or concentrate, or indecisiveness

- Recurrent thoughts of death, suicidal ideation with or without a plan

In older people, the clinical presentation of depression can be very different, studies suggesting that somatic complaints, delusional ideation, agitation and 'confusion' may all be commoner in older people (Baldwin 1997) for an excellent review). Atypical depression is commonly present in the absence of complaints of depressed mood, most often consisting of a preoccupation with physical symptoms. This can prompt a detailed search for disease which, in itself, can reinforce a patient's negative beliefs. Steadily accruing numbers of normal investigations gradually increase the confidence of the doctor that the problem is primarily a depressive disorder. Often, a judgement has to be made in a situation where there is some physical disease present but is insufficient to account for the psychiatric state. Specifically, memory complaints can lead to an erroneous diagnosis of dementia and pain can give rise to injudicious surgical procedures. Other atypical presentations include neurotic complaints, deliberate self-harm attempts and recently developed alcohol excess (Baldwin 1997). Relationships within families are often detrimentally affected when a member becomes depressed.

The coexistence of depression and dementia deserves special mention. Depression is a recognised risk factor for Alzheimer's disease (Henderson et al. 1992) and the proportion of patients with dementia who have depression is far greater than that expected by chance (e.g. Burns et al. 1990). Some of the symptoms in DSMIV (APA 1994) can be seen to be similar to those of dementia e.g. poor memory and loss of concentration. The term 'pseudodementia' was originally used to describe the situation where symptoms suggestive of dementia turned out to be due to a (treatable) depressive illness. It is traditional teaching in old age psychiatry that it is a cardinal sin to miss a potentially treatable depression in the setting of a dementia but this will change as treatments become available for the commonest form of dementia, Alzheimer's disease. Patients with depression have evidence of cognitive impairment on neuropsychological tests, some of which revert to normal after treatment (e.g. Abas et al. 1990).

Aetiology

There are a number of aetiological factors in depression, many of them common to depression occurring in younger people. Predisposing factors include: lack of social support and lack of intimacy (Murphy et al. 1982); physical illness; premorbid personality; and changes in cerebral structure and function (i.e. evidence of organic brain changes, Pearlson et al. 1989). The genetic predisposition to late life depression is less than in younger people and life events in older people are associated with a depressive illness as they are in their younger counterparts (Murphy 1982). The contribution of vascular disease to depression is being recognized (Simpson et al. 1998).

Prognosis

The prognosis of depression in old age has been the subject of a meta-analysis (Cole 1990) who reported on over 1000 patients showing that while just over 40% were well at two year follow-up, this diminished to just over a quarter with further follow-up – the majority were either continuously unwell or experiencing relapsing illness. Studies of the prognosis of depression are bedevilled by differences in treatments given and until there are widely agreed standardised protocols for the treatment of depression in the elderly it will be difficult to compare studies.

Treatment

Antidepressants are the treatment of choice when a patient has a depressive illness. Guidelines for treating depression have been suggested which, although not specifically for elderly people, have implications in their treatment (British Association for Psychopharmacology 1993). A proportion of depressive symptoms tend to resolve spontaneously, particularly if there are obvious precipitants and it is often reasonable in this situation to review the patient and withhold treatment to assess whether symptoms resolve. It is not unknown to suggest a prescription for antidepressants, to review a patient a month later to find they are back to normal, to congratulate oneself on efficiency and skill of diagnosis only to find that due to an administrative failure, the patient has not actually had the tablets!

Considering the widespread use of antidepressants there is surprisingly sparse evidence of their efficacy in older patients. Gerson (1985) concluded that while drugs are better than placebo, a quarter improved on no treatment and that all anti-depressants have unwanted side effects. It would now be considered unethical to do a treatment trial of an antidepressant versus placebo and most of the newer drugs have been tested against older, mostly tricyclic, agents. It is probably true to say that most antidepressants have very similar efficacy profiles and major differences revolve round the nature and number of side effects of a particular drug. This is not the appropriate setting in which to review the immense body of, primarily pharma-ceutically sponsored, literature comparing different antidepressants and we will restrict ourselves to some general statements about prescribing these drugs for elderly people.

There is debate as to whether the new SSRIs should be the first choice of treatment (Katona 1994) and this will vary between old age psychiatrists. Many would contend that traditional tricyclics still have a place in the absence of relative contra-indication and often quite low doses of drugs (e.g. amitriptyline 10 mg three times a day) can give very effective symptomatic relief from depression without untoward side-effects. Side-effects of tricyclic antidepressants include postural hypotension, sedation and those related to its anticholinergic effect (dry mouth, constipation, urinary retention, cardiotoxicity, blurred vision and delirium). Side-effects of selective serotonin reuptake inhibitors include gastrointestinal effects (nausea, diarrhoea and weight loss), anxiety/agitation/insomnia and headaches. Lofepramine has relatively few side effects (because of markedly reduced cholinergic effects) but reports of disturbance in liver function have been made. Blood dyscrasias have been described with mainserin and trazodone has a marked sedative effect (this can be a positive advantage).

The adage of 'start low, go slow' (Baldwin 1997) should be followed. Patients with cardiovascular problems (especially postural hypotension and cardiac arrhythmias) should probably be started on one of the newer drugs as first choice. If the patient does not respond despite an adequate therapeutic dose given for at least 6 weeks (easier to say than to effect in clinical practice), then second line treatment would include changing to another class of drug or adding a second drug (such as an SSRI to a tricyclic or vice versa) or adding lithium. If compliance has been poor because of side-effects, an alternative form of a drug of the same class could be used. There is good evidence that drugs are effective in people with depression and dementia (e.g. Reifler et al. 1989) and patients with physical illness and depression (Evans 1993).

Optimum duration of treatment with antidepressants has yet to be precisely established. One recent study (Old Age Depression Interest Group 1993) suggested that continued treatment for two years was associated with a 2.5 times reduction of relapse rate in patients taking active drug (prothiaden) compared to placebo.

Electro Convulsive Therapy

Electro convulsive therapy (ECT) is well tolerated in older patients (Benbow 1989) and is regarded by some as the treatment of choice for patients with delusional depression (Baldwin 1988). It is said that patients with more endogenous features of depression respond better (delusions, vegetative symptoms, worthlessness, loss of interest, guilt) and it can be given safely to patients with a combination of dementia and depression (Benbow 1989, Godber et al. 1987).

Psychosocial treatments

These should not be underestimated or ignored in the treatment of elderly people. Clear precipitating or maintaining factors for which something can be done such as social isolation and poor accommodation should be identified and dealt with wherever possible. Formal support groups, cognitive and family therapy, and psychotherapy can be used with benefit (Ong et al. 1987, Yost et al. 1986, Benbow 1990) but should be regarded as adjuncts to treatment rather than replacing antidepressant therapy.

MANIA

Epidemiology

In comparison to depression, mania is relatively uncommon in older people but it does occur and is often unrecognised. It is usually seen in the setting of a bipolar affective disorder and only one in ten elderly people with mania have not had a previous history of depression. Older people with mania tend to have been older when they had their first illness (overwhelmingly an episode of depression) compared to younger people but when older people exclusively are studied there tends to be a bimodal distribution of mania with one peak in the late thirties and another in the early seventies (Broadhead and Jacoby 1990). Prevalence rates of mania are estimated as 0.1% in community surveys (for obvious reasons, a manic person will not remain unknown to the services for long) and about 6% of patients with known affective disorder (Weissman et al. 1988, Hopkinson 1964).

Aetiology

The main aetiological factors associated with bipolar disorder are described under depression. There have been a series of case reports suggesting that late onset mania is associated with organic brain changes but it is likely that some form of physical insult needs to be combined with an individual predisposition to affective disorder. An association between mania and senile dementia has been described as has an overactive, sometimes delirious subtype of dementia (presbyophrenia, Berrios 1985). Organic features have been found in up to 50% of older patients with mania (Broadhead and Jacoby 1990) but a diagnosis of senile dementia occurs in the minority. Mania post-stroke has been described with the suggestion that subcortical and right brain lesion might have a particular affinity to cause mania (Starkstein et al. 1991). Disorders of frontal lobe function can also give rise to manic-like states as suggested by Gustafson (1987).

Clinical features

The characteristic symptoms of mania are similar to those in younger people, i.e. elevated mood, increase in motor activity, irritability, increase in sexual drive, increased familiarity, profligate behaviour, overtalkativeness along with poor concentration and decreased sleep. Classifications recognise a number of subtypes, in particular hypomania and mania with the latter requiring complete disruption of work and social activities for diagnosis. Subtypes with and without psychotic features (delusions, hallucinations) have also been suggested. In elderly people, mood is as often irritable as euphoric. Pressure of speech is relatively rare and delusional ideas are usually of a persecutory, religious or grandiose nature. Post (1965) emphasised the garrulousness, slow flight of ideas and cognitive impairment often seen in elderly people with a diagnosis of delirium which is often mistaken for mania. The admixture of manic and depressive symptoms in old age may account for some of the differing phenomenology in older people. The prognosis of mania in old age is aligned with that of any associated depressive disorder and any underlying organic brain changes. Shulman et al. (1992) demonstrated a cumulative mortality rate of 35% 5 years after an episode of mania and of 70% after 10 years.

Treatment

The cornerstone of treatment in the acute phase is pharmacological – antipsychotics and lithium carbonate. The exact choice of drug depends on the preference and experience of an individual clinician and the severity of illness. For people with severe manic symptoms, haloperidol is probably still the treatment of choice but it must be used cautiously in view of antidopaminergic side-effects. Immobilisation of a patient from drug-induced Parkinsonism should not be mistaken for effective treatment and can cause delirium. Lithium is a safe treatment in the acute phase, after appropriate checking of renal function and establishment of normal thyroid function. Most clinicians would aim to have a level towards the lower end of the established therapeutic levels range. Carbamazapine and sodium valproate have also been tried with benefit and ECT can be used in extreme illness which is life threatening, often described in younger people as 'manic stupor'. Prophylactic management includes regular follow-up with the opportunity to detect early symptoms.

CONFUSIONAL STATES

Confusion invariably means different things to different professionals and the term acute or sub-acute confusional state is best replaced by the term delirium. Like dementia, delirium denotes a clinical syndrome for which there are many causes.

Epidemiology

This depends entirely on the population from which the sample is drawn. The prevalence in community samples is, understandably, low but as delirium is a condition which usually quickly comes to the attention of others, this is not surprising (Folstein et al. 1991, estimated 1%). Six percent of people in nursing homes have been estimated to suffer from delirium (Rovner et al. 1986). By far the highest rates are found in medical and surgical wards (up to 60%, Levkoff et al. 1991).

Aetiology

The aetiology of delirium is related to the physical disorders underlying the condition which are many and varied. Predisposing factors include increasing age, the presence of dementia, previous alcohol abuse and prolonged surgical procedures (Lipowski 1990, Whittaker 1989). An exhaustive list of all the possible causes of delirium is unhelpful and can be found elsewhere (e.g. Lipowski 1990), the commonest ones in clinical practice being urinary or respiratory infections, heart failure and carcinomatosis. Less common are transient ischaemic attacks, a large number of drugs some with anticholinergic actions, drug interaction or withdrawal from alcohol or benzodiazepines, metabolic imbalances such as renal or hepatic failure, hypoglycaemia and cerebral anoxia (Royal College of Physicians 1981).

Clinical features

The core dysfunction in delirium is an acute disturbance of brain function (compared to the chronic disturbance of dementia) of which disorder of attention and disorganised thinking are the primary changes. Impairment of consciousness traditionally was the cardinal feature of delirium but difficulties in its precise definition made it difficult to operationalise. Other features include a global disturbance of cognition, psychomotor disturbance in the sleep/wake cycle and the presence of psychiatric disorders (most often hallucinations, Lipowski 1990). The syndrome can be further characterised according to the level of alertness and psychomotor activity into hypoalert/hypoactive. Subjects with hypoalert delirium (so called 'quiet' delirium) are the most difficult to recognise as many of the positive behaviours are absent.

Prognosis

Delirium tends to start quickly and have a relatively short duration, almost always less than four weeks. Conventional teaching is that delirium lasts longer than commonly supposed in elderly people and an illness lasting many weeks should not exclude the diagnosis, although often dementia and delirium can occur together. The mortality is high, obviously related to the severity of the underlying physical illness, which underscores the need for accurate diagnosis.

Treatment

The two strands to treatment include discovery and treatment of the underlying cause and symptomatic control of agitation and psychiatric disturbance. Traditional teaching suggests that patients should be nursed in a well-lit room and in isolation. However, these may be unnecessary and there are no empirical data to support their use (Lindesay et al. 1990). Drug treatment of choice is haloperidol but care must be used because of a long half life and a tendency to cause extrapyramidal effects.

NEUROSIS

Neurosis in the elderly is an emerging area of importance with increasing evidence that the symptoms comprise a single syndrome whose exact symptom complex changes over time (e.g. Lindesay 1991). The main groups of neurotic disorders include disturbances of mood (dysthymia), anxiety disorders (such as panic, adjustment disorders, agoraphobia, obsessive compulsive disorder, post-traumatic stress disorder, specific phobias and generalized anxiety disorder), dissociative disorders and somatoform disorders (Lindesay 1997).

Epidemiology

As would be expected, neurotic disorders are commoner in community samples compared to hospital populations. As with depression, neurotic symptoms are commoner than a diagnosis of neurotic disorder (Copeland et al. 1987). Symptoms of anxiety scoring below case level were present in 18.5% of men in the community and 16.9% of women compared with diagnosis of anxiety neurosis in 0.2% and 1.7% respectively. The American Epidiemiologic Catchment Area (ECA) study

(Regier et al. 1988, Blazer et al. 1991) reported rates of neurotic disorders in people over the age of 65 – dysthymia (1.8%), phobic disorders (4.8%), panic disorder (0.1%), obsessive compulsive disorder (1.3%), somatisation disorder (0.1%) and generalized anxiety disorder (1.9%). Lindesay and Banerjee (1993) described prevalence rates of 10% for phobic disorders and 3.7% for generalized anxiety.

Aetiology

There are a number of aetiological factors associated with neurotic disorders in elderly people. These include a genetic predisposition, associations with disorders of brain structure and function (post stroke anxiety is well recognised and changes in blood flow have been documented when patients with phobias have been exposed to noxious stimuli). Psychological determinants are similar to those in young people with life events are important precipitants of illness in older people. There is an intricate interplay between physical and neurotic disorders in older people in any combination, i.e. physical illness causing and mimicking neurosis and neurotic disorders causing and mimicking physical illness (Lindesay 1997).

Treatment

Cognitive behavioural treatment has been shown to be of benefit in younger people and some case reports suggest this may also be true for the older population (King and Barrowclough 1991). Drug treatments include benzodiazepines which do have a place in the short term treatment of anxiety in older people. Antidepressants are indicated if there is evidence of depression. Other drugs which can be of use include neuroleptics, β-blockers, antihistamines, buspirone and some patients are still taking barbiturates (Lindesay 1997).

PARAPHRENIA

Clinical features

Late paraphrenia is a heterogenous condition introduced originally to describe elderly people with persecutory delusions and auditory hallucinations with preservation of personality and who are free from affective disorder. From a phenomenological point of view, the syndrome was divided into three (in roughly equal proportions) by Post (1966): a group whose paranoid ideas are circumscribed and directed at neighbours or people close to the individual; a group where the ideas had spread to include others in the locality and often associated with auditory hallucinations; and people whose symptomatology was indistinguishable from schizophrenia. This last group tend to have less evidence of cerebral pathology (Howard et al. 1991).

There is currently debate as to how late paraphrenia is best categorised. Prominent auditory hallucinations are often seen and so they do not satisfy the International

Classification of Disease criteria (ICD-10, WHO, 1992) for persistent delusional disorder. In the American classification (Diagnostic and Statistical Manual, DSM-IV, APA 1994), the disorders would be diagnosed as late onset schizophrenia as the previous arbitrary upper age limit of 45 years for the diagnosis of schizophrenia in DSM-III was removed. From a descriptive point of view persistent persecutory states in the elderly is a useful term but it is likely that many patients in the group are in the early stages of a primary dementia.

Aetiology

The aetiology of a persecutory state in older people is multifactorial. The caricature of an older patient with paraphrenia being female, socially isolated, being deaf and never married is seen fairly regularly in clinical practice. There is usually no past history of note but often pre-existing personality traits (sometimes described as eccentric) can be seen. A significant proportion of patients with late paraphrenia have organic brain pathology (Burns et al. 1989, Holden 1987) including structural brain changes on MRI scan (Howard et al. 1994, 1995).

Management

The mainstay of treatment in an elderly person with paraphrenia is the establishment of a trusting consistent relationship, best effected by a community psychiatric nurse. Antipsychotics can lessen paranoid beliefs, and are usually best given as depot preparations in doses suitably adjusted for the elderly. Rehousing, though often requested, is generally not a useful strategy as persecutory ideas generally reappear (Howard and Levy 1997).

PATIENTS WHO GROW OLD WITH PSYCHIATRIC DISORDERS ('GRADUATES')

Patients of increasing significance to old age psychiatry services are those who have a diagnosis of any chronic psychiatric disorder, predominantly schizophrenia, and who have 'graduated' to their 65th birthday and so come under the relatively arbitrary age range often applied to old age psychiatry. With the closure of long stay mental hospitals and better treatments leading to longer survival, the numbers in this group will increase. There is surprisingly little research specifically into the issue of graduates. There has been recent interest with the closure of the larger mental hospitals, for example the study described by Anderson (1990) on the closure of Friern and Claybury Hospitals in the London area. A number of instruments were devised specifically for that project to assess the effects of discharging patients with chronic mental illness into the community.

Most long stay patients suffer from schizophrenia (Cunningham and Johnstone 1980) and the vast majority of elderly patients in hospital with schizophrenia had been there since before they were 65, with just less than half having been in hospital for over 30 years. Generally, older patients with schizophrenia tend to have fewer positive symptoms (e.g. delusions and hallucinations) and many more negative symptoms (e.g. apathy and cognitive impairment) than younger people (Soni and Mallik 1993). Many patients have associated physical illness and, in addition to those disorders which would be expected in an age matched cohort, these additional disabilities are related to the effects of chronic institutionalization (perhaps predisposing to illnesses resulting from a more sedentary lifestyle), the effects of behavioural disturbance (e.g. conjunctivitis associated with faecal incontinence), the effects of drugs (e.g. extrapyramidal side effects, tardive dyskinesia) and specific associations between illness and schizophrenia (e.g. arteriosclerotic heart disease and myxoedema) (Jablensky, 1988). The association between schizophrenia and dementia has been the subject of several investigations and while it is known that memory deficits do occur in older people with schizophrenia (McKenna et al. 1990, Clare et al. 1993) there is less evidence that a discrete dementia syndrome occurs in people with chronic schizophrenia. This may, at least in part, be due to difficulties in accurate diagnosis. Histologically, patients with schizophrenia do not have Alzheimer's disease (Harrison 1995).

Management

The management of patients with chronic mental illness who grow old is essentially no different to the continued treatment of the primary illness with the obvious caveats that multiple disabilities may occur, cognitive impairment may supervene, and physical ill health may complicate the clinical picture. The side-effects of medication tend to be more severe in older people. This factor and the higher rates of negative symptoms, make the use of atypical antipsychotic drugs particularly appropriate. Older people with a long history of mental illness often become increasingly dependent and may not have developed close relationships to rely on. Consequently, they are often at risk of self-neglect and should be closely supervised by health and social services. It is worth stating that patients with chronic mental illness have the same rights with regard to medical and surgical treatments as anyone else.

ALCOHOL ABUSE

Epidemiology

Alcohol abuse in the elderly is undoubtedly under-recognised and underdiagnosed, possibly in part due to the belief that alcoholics tended to die in middle age or recover spontaneously so that late onset addiction was considered rare (Atkinson 1997). Under-reporting of the problem, even when recognised by clinicians and relatives, may also have a part to play in terms of the embarrassment engendered by such a diagnosis and the therapeutic pessimism generally associated with the condition. Community surveys suggest that 2% of men and 1% of women could be described as being alcoholic but this increases to around 20% when considering admissions to nursing homes or medical wards (e.g. Saunders et al. 1989, Joseph et al. 1995).

Clinical features

Clinical features of alcohol abuse in the elderly are often mild and are very subtle. Non-specific presentations such as mood disorders, behavioural disturbance, weakness, falls, recurrent trauma, incontinence may be present and alcoholic excess is a common cause of dementia and delirium. Elderly people with alcohol problems can be divided into two groups – one consisting of a population who have grown old with their alcohol problem who present primarily with the physical sequelae of alcohol abuse and older people who develop dependence on alcohol later in years. In this latter group, the alcohol dependence syndrome is rarely present and falls, self-neglect and intermittent confusional states are the commonest reason for presentation (Jolley and Hodgson 1985).

Treatment

The treatment for alcohol abuse for those who have grown old with their problem is similar to that of their younger counterpart. Little information is available to guide the clinician about treating the late onset group but common sense dictates that the skill and support service of general alcohol treatment services should be employed along with particular attention to physical and psychiatric complications (Jolley and Hodgson 1985).

DIOGENES SYNDROME

A rare syndrome, Diogenes syndrome is typified by severe self neglect (named after the Greek philosopher who lived in a barrel). Sufferers typically hoard belongings and rubbish, in particular, newspapers and may pose a hazard to neighbours. Frequently they have very poor self care, neglect their diet and are often reclusive. Some are found to be suffering from a frontal lobe dementia or paraphrenia. However, most will have no apparent psychiatric illness, but isolative traits in their personality (Cooney 1997).

DEMENTIA

Introduction

Dementia is not a diagnosis but a syndrome consisting of different signs and symptoms and is defined as an acquired global impairment of intellect, memory and personality without disturbance of consciousness. The syndrome is:

- acquired (which distinguishes it from people with learning disabilities);

- there is global impairment of mental function (as distinct from pure amnesia, as may be seen with chronic alcohol abuse, or pure aphasia which has been described with localised brain pathology);

- there is no impairment of consciousness, emphasising that it is distinct from delirium.

The global nature of the deficits underscores the fact that dementia consists of a wide variety of features and is not merely restricted to disorders of cognitive function, as is often the popular belief. Dementia can be conveniently described as having three main expressions:

- a neuropsychological deficit (characterised predominantly by memory loss, i.e. amnesia but also including aphasia, apraxis and agnosia – see below);

- a neuropsychiatric expression (characterised by psychiatric symptoms and behavioural disturbances);

- difficulties with activities of daily living.

The syndrome of dementia has a number of causes, exhaustive lists of which can be found in many textbooks. It is important to emphasise that dementia is not a diagnosis and is merely a convenient clinical description of a cluster of signs and symptoms. It is as unacceptable to be satisfied with dementia as a diagnosis and do nothing else as it would be for a physician to diagnose jaundice but accept that further investigations were not necessary. In the same way that liver damage is the final pathway to cause jaundice, brain damage is the common pathway to cause dementia. Taking the analogy further, cirrhosis of the liver is one of the causes of jaundice in the same way that Alzheimer's disease is one of the causes of dementia. Cirrhosis has a number of causes in the same way that Alzheimer's disease has many causes.

Clinical features

The syndrome of dementia has common features as described above, irrespective of the cause. Other features include:

- apraxia (an inability to carry out purposeful movement in the presence of normal motor and sensory function);

- aphasia (difficulty with language (two types – receptive, understanding what is being said and expressive, an inability to make oneself understood of which the commonest manifestation is the inability to name objects is impaired);

- agnosia (failure of recognition, especially concerning people).

Neuropsychiatric features are common and include psychiatric symptoms such as depression (which can affect up to 60% of people), delusions (30%), hallucinations

(15–20%), misidentifications (20%) and behavioural problems such as aggression (about 20% of patients affected at some point in their illness, sexual disinhibition, eating disorders and wandering (Burns et al. 1990).

Differential diagnosis of dementia

The main differential diagnoses of dementia include delirium, depression, the effects of drugs and in the early stages of Alzheimer's disease, the differentiation from memory loss associated with normal ageing. The characteristic symptomatology of delirium is described elsewhere in this chapter, and any drug, particularly psychotropic medication, should be suspected of causing the syndrome.

Differentiation from depression can be problematic. Patients with depression usually have an illness whose onset can fairly accurately be dated (as opposed to Alzheimer's disease where the onset cannot be easily dated). Patients complain of a number of symptoms, including depression, which is unusual in dementia. Distress is conveyed by the patient, 'don't know' answers to questions are common and gaps in memory are usually apparent. If there is any doubt, a trial of antidepressants should be given.

Age associated memory impairment is becoming increasingly recognised in particular because patients with memory problems are coming forward worrying they have early Alzheimer's disease. Subjective complaints of poor memory do increase with age and several studies have suggested that complaints of memory loss have more in common with features of depression than impending dementia. Once other disorders have been ruled out, it may be necessary to follow-up the patients over time and assess what changes take place. O'Brien et al. (1992) followed up 68 patients who presented at a hospital memory clinic over 3 years, of whom six developed definite dementia. Reisberg et al. (1986) carried out a 3.6-year follow up and found that 38 out of 40 people with subjective forgetfulness were clinically unchanged.

ALZHEIMER'S DISEASE

This is the commonest cause of dementia in old age accounting for 60–70% of people affected by dementia. It has a characteristic neuropathology and in some cases a strong genetic association. As treatments are now available, the therapeutic nihilism associated with the disorder is now unjustified and inappropriate.

Epidemiology

This is inextricably mixed with the epidemiology of dementia, the proportion of people with Alzheimer's disease varying in different samples of patients. Hofman et al. (1991) described the prevalence of dementia in Europe according to age ranges as detailed in Table 7. 2.

Table 7.2

Age range (years)	Prevalence rates (percentage)
30–59	0.1
60–64	1
65–69	1.4
70–74	4.1
75–79	5.7
80–84	13.0
85–89	21.6
90–94	32.2
95–99	34.7

Women tend to outnumber men from age 75 onwards.

There are many factors which influence significantly the estimates of proportions in people suffering from dementia. Any survey needs to include residents of nursing and residential facilities. Solely concentrating on people living in the community would result in underestimates and diagnostic inaccuracy may occur as a full assessment of patients is not practical for epidemiological studies (Henderson and Kay 1984).

With regard to Alzheimer's disease, cumulative results from European studies have suggested a prevalence rate of 3.2% in people aged 70–79 and 10.8% of people age 80–89 (Rocca et al. 1991). Skoog et al. (1993) showed in a survey of 85 year olds a sweeping 30% were affected by dementia and the prevalence of Alzheimer's disease was just under half, which emphasises the importance of vascular disease as a cause of the clinical syndrome of dementia in elderly people.

Aetiology

There are several risk factors associated with Alzheimer's disease. The three for which the most pressing evidence exists are genetics, age and the presence of Down's syndrome.

Thirty percent of late onset cases of Alzheimer's disease have a positive family history of dementia (Burns and Levy 1992). A number of families have been reported where the disorder is passed as an autosomal dominant gene and in the last ten years, studies of the molecular genetics of these families have demonstrated particular mutations associated with the disease. It has been observed that people with Down's syndrome frequently develop Alzheimer's disease – the majority have the characteristic histological changes of senile plaques and neurofibrillary tangles after the age of 40 and a substantial proportion develop the clinical syndrome of dementia. Within a few months of each other in the late 1980s it was found that a genetic marker was associated with Alzheimer's disease on chromosome 21 and that the gene encoding for amyloid precursor protein (APP, the protein responsible for the smaller amyloid protein, one of the major deposits in Alzheimer's disease) was also on that gene (Clark and Goate 1993). However, in many families (particularly those with late onset disease) no linkage was found between this gene and affected individuals, leading to a search for more genetic markers. Others which had been discovered include changes on chromosome 14 (Harrison 1993, Sherrington et al. 1995) and chromosome 1, the former explaining about three-quarters of genetically inherited early onset Alzheimer's disease. The vast majority of patients suffering from Alzheimer's disease are elderly and an association was found between the presence of a peripheral protein (apolipoprotein E determined by a gene on chromosome 19) and Alzheimer's disease. Everybody has two alleles of the protein E2, E3 or E4 derived from each chromosome, in any combination (i.e. a person can have two of the same or E3/E23, E3/E4, or E2/E4). People with two copies of E4 have an over 90% chance of developing Alzheimer's disease and those with one copy have about a 25% chance of getting the disease. It is important to appreciate that this is not a genetic marker but a very strong biological risk factor for the disease whose main use will be in studies of environmental and genetic risk factors of Alzheimer's disease and not so much in presymptomatic testing (Wrelkin 1996).

In addition to the association with age and Down's syndrome (Holland and Oliver 1995), other risk factors include head injury and depression with suggestions that female sex, increased parental age and a number of other risk factors are implicated (for a review, see Jorm et al. 1987, van Duijn et al. 1991).

Protective factors recently documented include oestrogen (Burns and Murphy 1996) and non-steroidal anti-inflammatory drugs. A number of case control studies of women taking oestrogen have found a protective effect. In one study (Tang et al. 1996) 16% of nearly 1000 women developed Alzheimer's disease who were not taking oestrogen compared with 5.8% of those who were. The protective effect of anti-inflammatory drugs on Alzheimer's disease has been documented and a couple of trials have shown improvement in cognitive function with people taking the drug (Andersen et al. 1995).

Clinical features

In Alzheimer's disease, the onset of dementia is insidious with amnesia usually the first symptom and often manifest predominantly as deficits in short term memory.

Neuropathology of Alzheimer's disease

Alzheimer's disease has a defined biological substrate in terms of gross brain changes (cerebral shrinkage) and protein abnormalities at microscopic level (amyloid deposition and tau protein abnormalities). Neurochemical changes have been consistently described, mainly deficits in the cholinergic neurotransmitter system and this has formed the basis of the neurotransmitter replacement therapies currently available.

VASCULAR (MULTI-INFARCT) DEMENTIA

As cardiovascular and cerebrovascular disease tend to be commoner in men vascular dementia, unlike Alzheimer's disease, is the commonest type of dementia affecting elderly males.

Clinical features

Characteristically, the onset is abrupt and the progression of the illness is step-wise. The clinical features of vascular dementia were enshrined in the Hachinski (ischaemic) score (Hachinski et al. 1975) (table 3).

While the diagnosis of vascular dementia is often clear cut, there are situations in which it can be very difficult to tease out the contribution of Alzheimer's disease and vascular dementia and the concept of 'mixed' dementia is used to denote a suggested combination of the two. Diagnostic criteria for vascular dementia exist (e.g. Roman et al. 1993) which require the presence of dementia, focal neurological signs on either clinical examination or evidence of infarction on brain imaging and a clear relationship between the dementia syndrome and cerebral vascular disease. It is unresolved how patients should be classified who have a disabling stroke (in terms of hemiplegia or aphasia) who develop a cognitive impairment (Erkinjuntti and Hachinski 1993).

- abrupt onset
- fluctuation course
- history of strokes
- associated atherosclerosis
- focal and neurological signs and symptoms
- step-wise deterioration
- nocturnal confusion
- preserved personality
- depression
- somatic complaints
- emotional incontinence (lability)

Table 7.3 – Features suggesting vascular aetiology to dementia (from Hachinski et al. 1975).

LEWY BODY DEMENTIA

In the last 10 years, Lewy body dementia has been increasingly recognised as a cause of the dementia syndrome. It draws its name from the pathological changes consisting of Lewy bodies (an intercellular protein deposit named after the describer) found in the neocortex.

Clinical features

These are fluctuating cognitive impairment affecting memory and higher cognitive functions, visual or auditory hallucinations (usually accompanied by paranoid delusions) spontaneous extrapyramidal features or evidence of extreme sensitivity to antipsychotics and repeated unexplained falls. The fluctuating pattern lasts months rather than weeks (in the case of delirium) and other physical causes (including cerebrovascular disease) have been excluded (McKeith et al. 1992). As with vascular dementia, Lewy body disease can co-exist with Alzheimer's disease (Forstl et al. 1993). The important issue in relation to dementia of Lewy body type is the tendency for patients to be very sensitive to the effects of antipsychotics and injudicious use of these drugs can lead to severe side effects and an increased mortality rate (McKeith et al. 1992).

DEMENTIA OF FRONTAL LOBE TYPE

Dementia of frontal lobe type is characterised by atrophy of the frontal lobe in the absence of Alzheimer type pathology. There seems to be an overlap between this type of dementia and Picks disease (Hodges 1994). Clinical and pathological criteria for fronto-temporal dementia have been published (Lund and Manchester groups 1994). The main features are insidious onset and slow progression. Early loss of personal and social awareness, early signs of disinhibition, hyperorality, stereotyped behaviour, distractibility and emotional changes. Spatial orientation and praxis are relatively preserved.

OTHER DEMENTIAS

Rarer causes of dementia include Huntington's disease, neurosyphilis, normal pressure hydrocephalus, hypothyroidism, vitamin B12 deficiency, head trauma, alcohol related dementias, Jakob-Creutzfelt disease and progressive supranuclear palsy (Burns and Hope 1997).

Treatment of dementia

These are traditionally divided into pharmacological treatments for the neuropsy-chological and neuropsychiatric symptoms and non-pharmacological interventions

(Burns 1995). Current attention is focused mainly on treatments for memory loss in patients with Alzheimer's disease.

Pharmacological treatment of neuropsychological deficits

One of the most consistent findings in neurochemical studies of Alzheimer's disease is loss of the cortical neurotransmitter, acetylcholine. Based on this, a number of strategies have been tried to boost levels of the transmitter: increasing the available precursor using Lethicin or acetylcarnitine (Little et al. 1985, Livingstone et al. 1991); directly stimulating the receptor (using muscarinic agonists, Spiegal et al. 1987) or by inhibiting the enzyme which itself breaks down acetylcholine using anticholinesterases (Thal et al. 1983, Eagger et al. 1991).

It is with this last approach that most success has been achieved. Physostigmine has been used in some studies with demonstrable benefit (Thal et al. 1983) and tacrine was licensed ten years ago in some countries for the treatment of mild to moderate Alzheimer's disease (Summers et al. 1986, Eagger et al. 1991). While the treatment was effective in improving symptoms in patients with Alzheimer's disease, the side effects, notably to the liver, greatly limited the practical use of the drug (Watkins et al. 1994).

The introduction of donepezil hydrochloride (Aricept) has been a significant step forward. The drug is in the UK for the symptomatic treatment of mild to moderately severe Alzheimer's disease. Its mode of action is that of an anticholinesterase but it is extremely well tolerated and has not significant side-effects other than some to be expected from the physiological mode of action of the drug (stomach cramps, nausea, and diarrhoea). Trials have demonstrated improvement in both mental functioning (as measured by standardized cognitive tests) improvements in activities of daily living and improvements in independently rated global assessments of the patient's condition (arguably the most relevant change, Rogers et al. 1996, 1998a, b, Burns et al. 1999).

Rivastigmine (Exelon) was launched one year after donepezil hydrochloride, based on a larger database compared to donepezil. The improvements in cognitive global functioning and activities of daily living are comparable with those published on donepezil. Similar side effects have been noted with Rivastigmine, but the half life is considerably shorter, important if they are troublesome.

Other drugs which may be licensed in the near future include the anticholinesterase galanthamine and propentofylline. There are a host of other treatments available which claim to ameliorate the cognitive deficits of Alzheimer's disease but none, thus far, is as effective as the anticholinesterases. Some trials have demonstrated that the disease progression can be slowed down using selegiline and Vitamin E (Sano et al. 1997). There is some evidence that oestrogen may slow the progression of the disease and further trials are awaited. Anti-inflammatory agents may also be effective (Burns et al. 1999).

Pharmacological treatment of neuropsychiatric symptoms

Depression in dementia is as amenable to treatment as it is in functional psychiatric disorders (Reifler et al. 1989). Theoretically, the anticholinergic effects of tricyclic drugs could worsen the cognitive impairment of Alzheimer's disease and one of the new SSRIs might be more appropriate. Agitation can often be the presenting sign of depression in dementia and a trial of antidepressants may be indicated in this situation. Trazodone is said to be particularly effective against screaming and the commonest reason for prescribing an antipsychotic in dementia is agitation, regardless of its cause (Wilcock et al. 1987). A meta-analysis has shown this to be effective in about 20% of patients (Schneider and Sobin 1994). All antipsychotics are probably equally effective and choice depends on personal experience and preference. Specific psychotic symptoms should be treated with antipsychotics. Particular care should be taken in prescribing these drugs where Lewy body dementia is suspected (McKeith et al. 1992).

Non-pharmacological treatments

A number of therapies have been tried such as memory retraining, validation therapy, reality orientation, and reminiscence therapy. While anecdotally these may be of some benefit, there is a lack of properly conducted double blind randomised controlled trials to support their introduction (Bleathman and Morton 1994).

Social and community support

A patient who suffers from dementia, present with a varying and often complex group of symptoms. For the carer of this person it can be extremely difficult not only to see the changes developing in their loved ones as the disease progresses, but also to deal with the increasing level of dependence, both mental and physical that ensues.

Donaldson et al. (1997) found high levels of psychological distress in carers, which often goes unrecognized and therefore not addressed. Health, social and voluntary services have developed different ways of offering respite to carers, for example, day care, family link, crossroads and regular respite care. Many areas have community nurses specifically to advise carers, and the Alzheimer's Disease Society provides excellent education, advice and support to those who need it. It should be noted that many carers themselves are elderly, and often feel immensely guilty that they are not able to cope with their relatives.

MEDICO-LEGAL ISSUES IN OLD AGE PSYCHIATRY

Various statutory provisions are made under law in England and Wales in relation to people with mental incapacity. Some of these are particularly relevant to older people with dementia or with chronic psychotic illness.

Court of Protection is an office of the Supreme Court that has the function of managing the property and affairs of people with mental disorders who are unable to do so themselves. The Court can take jurisdiction if (a) the person suffers from a mental disorder as defined under the Mental Health Act and (b) if he/she is incompetent to manage their finances (Jacoby 1997). There are no specific criteria laid down but Silberfeld et al. (1995), have suggested that they should include:

- knowledge of income;
- knowledge of expenses;
- an ability to handle everyday financial transactions;
- the ability to delegate financial wishes.

If these are not met and a person has assets exceeding £5000 an application can be made to the Court of Protection (via the Public Trust Office who are responsible for the administration of the Court of Protection) by solicitors, local authority social services or relatives. A medical certificate is also required to support the application (Certificate of Incapacity, Form CP3) to which notes are appended to help the doctor completing the form (usually the patient's general practitioner or a consultant psychiatrist who has examined the patient and, preferably, knows them well). The most important difference is that although the individual has to suffer from a mental disorder within the meaning of the Mental Health Act, the criteria are not the same as for compulsory admission to hospital, i.e. the person can be deemed incapable of managing their own affairs but not necessarily require admission to hospital (Jacoby 1997). A **receiver** is then appointed (this can be a relative or friend, bank manager, solicitor or accountant) to manage the affairs of the individual but the receiver must ask the Court's permission before disposing of capital assets.

An appointee is an individual sanctioned by the Secretary of State to claim social security benefit for an elderly person – in practice this is arranged through the local social security office and is usually a friend or family member of an elderly person who collects their pension. The person has no authority to spend the money without asking the person for whom they are claiming the benefit and receivership supersedes and appointee (Jacoby 1997).

Power of attorney is given by an individual to another to manage his or her financial and property affairs. The drawback is that it becomes invalid when a person becomes mentally incapable. In 1986, Enduring Power of Attorney, which remains valid despite the development of incapacity, was introduced. The crucial difference between this and Court of Protection is that power of attorney is completed before the onset of mental incapacity. Further developments to extend powers to decisions over healthcare are planned.

A further measure is defined under the National Assistance Act of 1948 (Section 47) which allows a person to be removed to a place of safety when they are not suffering from a mental disorder. This usually involves the local officer of public health and only requires the signature of one doctor and the relatives have no power of veto.

Driving in dementia

A recent General Medical Council document (GMC 1995) emphasised that a doctor has a duty of responsibility to society in general which may, in certain circumstances, outweigh the responsibility of confidentiality to the patient. In other words if a doctor knows a patient is driving dangerously and may put the lives of others at risk, he or she has a responsibility to inform the appropriate authorities.

The fundamental issue in relation to driving in dementia is that a doctor is unqualified to make a judgement as to whether an elderly person is able to drive or not. All that a doctor has a responsibility to do is to inform the patient, their relatives (and the authorities if necessary) that the patient has a condition which may impair his or her ability to drive. The responsibility for determining fitness to drive rests with the Driver and Vehicle Licensing Authority and they will usually ask for a report from patient's own doctor. The driver has a legal duty to inform the DVLA if they have a condition which may affect their ability to drive. The situation is usually quite straightforward when a person has moderately severe dementia but it is less obvious when someone is mildly impaired and, indeed, some people may be safe to drive and yet have a diagnosis of dementia. It is reasonable to take the view that driving is a privilege, not a right, and it is important to remember that driving is a complex task involving visuo-spatial skills, vigilant judgement, memory as well as a minimum of physical attributions such as sight and hearing. It is also important to remember that any person has the ability to request a further driving test to clarify whether he or she is fit to drive. Anyone may inform the DVLA of a situation where it is clear someone is unable to drive and medical advisers at the DVLA are extremely helpful and able to discuss particular circumstances with a doctor (Oppenheimer 1997).

References

Abas M, Sahakian BJ, Levy R. Neuropsychological deficits in CT scan changes in elderly depressives. Psychological Medicine 1990; 20: 507–520.

Ames D, Ashby D, Mann A, Graham N. Psychiatric illness in elderly residents of Part 3 homes in one London borough. Age and Ageing 1988; 17: 249–296.

Andersen K, Launer L, Ott A, Hose A, Bereteler N, Hoffman A. Do non-steroidal anti-inflammatory drugs decrease the risk for Alzheimer's disease? Neurology 1995; 45: 1441–1445.

Anderson J. The TAPS project. 1: Previous psychiatric diagnosis and disability of long-stay psychogeriatric patients. British Journal of Psychiatry 1990; 156: 661–666.

Atkinson. Alcohol and drug abuse. In Jacoby R and Oppenheimer C (eds), Psychiatry in the Elderly, 2nd edition, 1997, pp. 661–686.

Baldwin RC. Depressive illness. In Jacoby R and Oppenheimer C (eds), Psychiatry in the Elderly, 2nd edition, 1997, pp. 536–572.

Baldwin R. Late life depression – undertreated? British Medical Journal 1988; 296: 519.

Benbow S. The role of ECT in the treatment of depressive illness in old age. British Journal of Psychiatry 1989; 155: 147–152.

Benbow S, Egan D, Marriot A, Tregay K, Walsh S, Wells J et al. Using the family life cycle with later life families. Journal of Family Therapy 1990; 12: 321–340.

Berrios G. Presbyophrenia: clinical aspects. British Journal of Psychiatry 1985; 147: 76–79.

Blazer D, Williams C. Epidemiology of dysphoria and depression in an elderly population. American Journal of Psychiatry 1980; 137: 439–444.

Blazer D, George L, Hughes D. The epidemiology of anxiety disorders: an age comparison. In Saltzman C, Lebowitz B (eds), Anxiety in the Elderly. New York: Springer, 1991, pp. 17–30.

Bleathlam C, Morton I. Psychological treatments. In Burns A and Levy R. London: Chapman & Hall, 1994.

Bradshaw M. Social work with older persons. In Jacoby R and Oppenheimer C (eds), Psychiatry in the Elderly, 2nd edition. Oxford: Oxford University Press, 1997, pp. 217–231.

British Association for Psychopharmacology. Consensus Committee Guidelines for treating depressive illness with antidepressants. Journal of Psychopharmacology 1993; 7: 19–23.

Burns A, Russell E, Page S. New Drugs for Alzheimer's disease. British Journal of Psychiatry 1999; 174: 476–479.

Burns A et al. A trial of donepezil in Alzheimer's disease: results of a multi-national study. Dementia and Geriatric and Cognitive Disorders 1999: 237–244.

Burns A, Murphy D. Protection against Alzheimer's disease (Editorial). Lancet 1996; 348: 420–421.

Burns A, Hope A. Clinical aspects of the dementias of old age. In Jacoby R, Oppenheimer, C (eds), Psychiatry in the Elderly, 2nd edition. Oxford: Oxford University Press, 1997, pp. 456–493.

Burns A, Jacoby R, Levy R. Psychiatric phenomena in Alzheimer's disease. British Journal of Psychiatry 1990; 157: 72–94.

Burns A, Carrick J, Ames D et al. A cerebral cortical appearance in late paraphrenia. International Journal of Geriatric Psychiatry 1989; 4: 31–34.

Burns A, Levy R. Clinical diversity in late onset Alzheimer's disease. Maudsley Monograph 34, Oxford: Oxford University Press, 1992.

Burns A. Alzheimer's disease: pharmacological developments to the Year 2000. Human Psychopharmacology 1995; 10: s247–s251.

Clare L, McKenna PJ, Mortimer AM, Baddeley AD. Memory in schizophrenia: what is impaired and what is preserved? Neuropsychologica 1993; 1225–1241.

Clarke R, Goate A. Molecular genetics in Alzheimer's disease. Archives of Neurology 1993; 50: 1164–1172.

Cole M. The prognosis of depression in the elderly. Canadian Medical Association Journal 1990; 143: 633–640.

Cooney C. Diogenes syndrome: the role of the psychiatrist. In Homes C, Wrightson HR (eds), Advances in Old Age Psychiatry. Biomedical Publishing, 1997, pp. 246–253.

Copeland J, Dewey M, Wood N, Searle R, Davidson I, McWilliam C. Range of mental illness among the elderly in the community. British Journal of Psychiatry 1987; 150: 815–823.

Cunningham Owens DG, Johnstone EC. The disabilities of chronic schizophrenia. British Journal of Psychiatry 1980; 136: 384–395.

Department of Health. Caring for people: community care in the next decade and beyond, London: HMSO, 1989.

Donaldson C, Tarrier N, Burns A. The impact of the symptoms of dementia on caregivers. British Journal of Psychiatry 1997; 170: 62–68.

Eagger S, Levy R, Sahakian B. Tacrine in Alzheimer's disease. Lancet 1991; 337: 989–992.

Erkinjuntti T, Hachinski V. Rethinking vascular dementia. Cerebrovascular Disease 1993; 3: 3–23.

Evans M. Depression in elderly physically ill inpatients. International Journal of Geriatric Psychiatry 1993; 8: 587–592.

Folstein M, Bassett S, Romanoski A et al. The epidemiology of delirium in the community. International Psychogeriatrics 1991; 3: 169–179.

Forstl H, Burns A, Luthert P, Cairns N, Levy R. The Lewy body variant of Alzheimer's disease. British Journal of Psychiatry 1993; 162: 385–392.

Gerson R. Present status of drug therapy of depression in late life. Journal of Affective Disorders Supplement 1985; 1: S23–S31.

Godber C, Rosenvinge H, Wilkinson D, Smithies J. Depression in old age: prognosis after ETC. International Journal of Geriatric Psychiatry 1987; 2: 19–24.

Gurland B, Copeland J, Kurianskay J, Kelleher N, Sharpe L, Dean L. The mind and mood of ageing. New York: Howarth, 1983.

Gustafson G. Frontal lobe degeneration of the non-Alzheimer type. Archives of Gerontology and Geriatrics 1987; 6: 209–223.

Hachinski V, Illiff L, Zilka E et al. Cerebral blood flow in dementia. Archives of Neurology 1975; 32: 632–637.

Harrison PJ. On the neuropathology of schizophrenia and its dementia: Neurodevelopment, Neurodegenerative or Both? Neurodegeneration 1995, 4: 1–12.

Harrison P. Alzheimer's disease and chromosome 14. British Journal of Psychiatry 1993; 163: 2–5.

Harvey PD, White L, Parrella M, Putnam KM, Kincaid MM et al. The Longitudinal Stability of Cognitive function in schizophrenia. British Journal of Psychiatry 1995; 166: 630–633.

Health Departments of Great Britain. General Practice in the National Health Service: The 1990 Contract. Health Departments of Great Britain, 1989.

Henderson A, Kay D. The epidemiology of mental disorders in old age. In Kay D and Burrows G (eds), Handbook of Studies of Psychiatry in Old Age. Amsterdam: Elsevier, 1984.

Henderson A, Jorm A, Quarton A et al. Environmental risk factors for Alzheimer's disease. Psychological Medicine 1992; 22: 429–436.

Hodges J. Cognitive assessment for clinicians. Oxford: Oxford University Press, 1994.

Hofman R, Rocca W, Brayne C et al. The prevalence of dementia in Europe. International Journal of Epidemiology 1991; 20: 736–748.

Holden N. Late paraphrenia or the paraphrenias. British Journal of Psychiatry 1987; 15: 635–639.

Holland A, Oliver C. Down's syndrome and the links with Alzheimer's disease. JNNP 1995; 59: 111–114.

Hopkinson G. A genetic study of affective illness in patients over 50. British Journal of Psychiatry 1964; 110: 244–254.

Howard R, Almeida O, Levy R et al. Quantitative MRI imaging in delusional disorder and late onset schizophrenia. British Journal of Psychiatry 1994; 165: 474–480.

Howard R, Mellors J, Petty R et al. Magnetic resonance imaging of the temporal and frontal lobes, Hoppocampus, parahippocampal and superior temporal gyri in late paraphrenia. Psychological Medicine 1995; 25: 495–503.

Howard R, Forstl H, Nguib N et al. First rank symptoms in late paraphrenia: cortical structural correlates. British Journal of Psychiatry 1991; 160: 108–109.

Howard R, Levy R. Late onset schizophrenia, lata paraphrenia and paranoid states of late life. In Jacoby R, Oppenheimer C (eds), Psychiatry in the Elderly, 2nd edition. Oxford: Oxford University Press, 1997, pp. 617–631.

Jablensky A. Epidemiology of schizophrenia. In McGuffin P, Bebbington P (eds), Schizophrenia: The Major Issues. Oxford: Heinemann (and the Mental Health Foundation), 1988, pp. 19–35.

Jackson R, Baldwin B. Detecting depression in elderly medically ill patients. Age and Ageing 1993; 22: 349–353.

Jacoby R. Managing the financial affairs of mentally disordered persons in the UK. In Jacoby R, Oppenheimer C (eds), Psychiatry in the Elderly, 2nd edition. Oxford: Oxford University Press, 1997, pp. 765–771.

Jarvik L, Mintz L, Steurer J, Gerner R. Treating geriatric depression: a 26 week interim analysis. Journal of the American Geriatric Association 1982; 30: 713–717.

Johnson P, Falkingham J. Ageing and Economic Welfare. London: Sage, 1992, p. 23.

Jolley D, Hodgson S. Alcoholism and the elderly. In Isaacs B (ed), Recent Advances in Geriatric Medicine 3. Edinburgh: Churchill Livingstone, 1985, pp. 113–122.

Jorm A, Korten A, Henderson A. The prevalence of dementia. Acta Psychiatrica Scandinavica 1987; 76: 465–479.

Joseph C, Ganzini L, Atkinson R. Screening for alcohol use disorders in the nursing home. JAGS 1995; 43: 368–373.

Katona C. The management of depression in old age. In Depression in Old age. Chichester: Wiley, 1994, pp. 93–121.

King P, Barrowclough C. Clinical pilot study of cognitive behaviour therapy for anxiety disorders in the elderly. Behavioural Psychotherapy 1991; 19: 337–345.

Laslett P. A fresh map of life: the emergence of the third age. London: Widenfeld & Nicholson, 1989.

Levkoff S, Clearly P, Pitzin B, Evans D. Epidemiology of delirium. International Psychogeriatrics 1991; 31: 49–67.

Liddle PF, Crow TJ. Age disorientation in chronic schizophrenia is associated with global intellectual impairment. British Journal of Psychiatry 1984; 144: 193–199.

Lindesay J, Banjeree S. Phobic disorders in the elderly: a comparison of 3 diagnostic symptoms. International Jounral of Geriatric Psychiatry 1993; 8: 387–393.

Lindesay J. Neurotic disorders in the elderly. In Jacoby R, Oppenheimer C (eds), Psychiatry in the Elderly, 2nd edition. Oxford: Oxford University Press, 1997.

Lindesay J, MacDonald A, Starke I. Delirium in the elderly. Oxford: Oxford Medical 1990.

Lindesay J. Phobic disorders in the elderly. British Journal of Psychiatry 1991; 159: 531–541.

Lindesay J, Briggs K, Murphy E. The Guy's Age Concern survey. British Journal of Psychiatry 1989; 155: 317–329.

Lipowski Z. Delirium. New York: Oxford University Press, 1990.

Little A, Levy R, Kidd P et al. A double-blind placebo controlled trial on high dose lecithin in Alzheimer's disease. JNNP 1985; 48: 736–742.

Livingstone G, Sax K, McClenahan Z, Blumenthal E, Foley K, Willison J, Mann A, James I. Acetyl L. Carnitine in dementia. International Journal of Geriatric Psychiatry 1991; 6: 853–860.

Lund and Manchester Clinical and neuropathological criteria for fronto-temporal dementia. J Neurol Neurosurg Psychiatry 1993; 57: 416–418.

Mann A. Epidemiology. In Jacoby R, Oppenheimer C (eds), Psychiatry in the Elderly, 2nd edition. Oxford: Oxford University Press, 1996, pp. 63–78.

McKeith I, Fairburn A, Perry R, Thompson P, Perry E. Neuroleptic sensitivity in patients with senile dementia of Lewy body type. British Medical Journal 1992; 305: 673–678.

McKeith I, Perry R, Theoburn A, Jaben S, Perry S. Operational criteria for senile dementia of the Lewy body type. Psychological Medicine 1992; 22: 911–922.

McKenna PJ, Tamlyn D, Lund CE, Mortimer AM, Hamond S, Baddeley AD. Amnesic syndrome in schizophrenia. Psychological Medicine 1990; 20: 967–972.

Murphy E. Social origins of depression in old age. British Journal of Psychiatry 1982; 141: 135–142.

O'Brien J, Beats D, Hill K et al. Do subjective memory complaints precede dementia? International Journal of Geriatric Psychiatry 1992; 7: 481–486.

OADIG. How long should the elderly take antidepressants? A double blind placebo controlled study of continuation/prophylaxis therapy with prothiaden. British Journal of Psychiatry 1993; 162: 175–182.

Ong Y, Martineau F, Lloyd C, Robins I. Support group for the depressed elderly. International Journal of Geriatric Psychiatry 1987; 2: 119–123.

OPCS (Office of Population, Censuses and Surveys). National Population Projections: mid-1989 based OPCS monitor PP291.1. London: HMSO, 1991.

Oppenheimer C. Driving and firearms licences. In Jacoby R, Oppenheimer C (eds), Psychiatry in the Elderly, 2nd edition. Oxford: Oxford University Press, 1997, pp. 772–776.

O'Brien M. Vascular dementia. In Burns A, Levy R (eds), Dementia. London: Chapman & Hall, 1994, pp. 625–640.

Palmore E. Attitudes towards ageing as shown in humour. Gerontologist 1971; 11: 181–186.

Pearlson G, Rabins P, Kim W, Speedie L, Moburg P, Burns A et al. Structural CT changes in cognitive deficits with and without reversible dementia. Psychological Medicine 1989; 19: 573–584.

Post F. Persistent persecutor states of the elderly. Oxford: Pergammon, 1966.

Post F. The clinical psychiatry of late life. Oxford: Pergammon, 1965, pp. 61–105.

Regier D, Boyd J, Burke J, Rae D, Myers J, Krammer M et al. The prevalence of mental disorders in the United States. Archives of General Psychiatry 1988; 45: 977–986.

Reifler B, Teri L, Raskind M et al. Double blind trial of imipramine in Alzheimer's disease with and without depression. American Journal of Psychiatry 1989; 146: 45–49.

Reisberg B, Ferris S, Schulman E et al. Longitudinal course of normal ageing and progressive dementias of the Alzheimer type progress. Neuropsychopharmacology and Biological Psychiatry 1986; 10: 571–578.

Rocca A, Hofman A, Brayne C et al. Frequency and distribution of Alzheimer's disease in Europe. Annals of Neurology 1991; 30: 381–390.

Rogers SL, Friedhoff LT. Long term efficacy and safety of donepezil in the treatment of Alzheimer's disease. European Neuropsychopharmacology 1998; 8: 67–75.

Rogers SL, Farlow M, Doody R et al. A twenty-four double week double blind placebo controlled trial of donepezil in patients with Alzheimer's disease. Neurology 1998; 50: 136–145.

Rogers SL, Friedhoff LT, and the Donepezil Study Group. The efficacy and safety of donepezil in patients with Alzheimer's disease. Dementia 1996; 7: 293–303.

Roman G, Tatemichi T, Erkinjuntti T, Cummings J, Masdeu J and Garcia J. Vascular dementia: diagnostic criteria for research studies. Neurology 1993; 3: 250–260.

Rovner B, Kfonek S, Filipp L. Prevalence of mental illness in a community nursing home. Americal Journal of Psychiatry 1986; 143: 1446–1449.

Royal College of Physicians. Organic mental impairment in the elderly. Journal of the Royal College of Physicians 1981; 15: 141–167.

Sano M, Ernesto C, Thomas RG et al. A controlled trial of selegiline, alpha-tocopherol, or both as treatment for Alzheimer's disease. New England Journal of Medicine 1997; 336: 1216–1247.

Saunders P, Copeland J, Dewey M, Davidson I, McWilliam C, Sharma V et al. Alcohol use and abuse in the elderly. International Journal of Geriatric Psychiatry 1989; 4: 103–108.

Schneider L, Sobin P. Treatments for psychiatric symptoms in behavioural disturbances in dementia. In Burns A, Levy R (eds), Dementia. London: Chapman & Hall, 1994.

Secretaries of State for Health, Social Security, Wales and Scotland. Caring for People: community care in the next decade and beyond. CM849. London: HMSO, 1989.

Sherrington R et al. Cloning of a gene bearing missense mutations in early onset familial Alzheimer's disease. Nature 1995; 375: 754–760.

Shulman K, Tohan M, Setlin A, Mallya G, Kalunian D. Mania compared with unipolar depression in old age. American Journal of Psychiatry 1992; 1493: 41–45.

Silberfeld M, Corber W, Madigan K, Checkland D. Capacity assessment for requests to restore legal competence. International Journal of Geriatric Psychiatry 1995; 10: 191–197.

Skoog I, Nilsson L, Palmartz B et al. A population based study of dementia in 85 year olds. New England Journal of Medicine 1993; 328: 153–158.

Soni SD, Mallik A. The elderly chronic schizophrenic inpatient: a study of psychiatric morbidity in 'elderly graduates'. International Journal of Geriatric Psychiatry 1993; 8: 665–673.

Spiegal R, Azcona A, Wettstein A. First results with RS86, an orally active muscarinic agonist in healthy subjects and in patients with dementia. In Wurtman R, Corkin S, Growden J (eds), Alzheimer's Disease: Advances in Basic Research and Therapy. Cambridge, MA: Centre for Brain Sciences and Metabolism Charitable Trust, 1987; 391–405.

Starkstein S, Fedoroff P, Berthier N, Robinson R. Manic depressive and pure manic states after brain lesions. Biological Psychiatry 1991; 29: 149–158.

Stijnen T, Hofmann A. Risk factors for Alzheimer's disease. International Journal of Epidemiolgoy 1991; 20: 2(supp 2): S4–S12.

Tang MX, Jacobs D, Stern Y et al. The effect of oestrogen during menopause. What risk and age of onset of Alzheimer's disease. Lancet 1996; 348: 429–432.

United Nations 1989. World Population Prospects. United Nations Publications No 106. New York: Department of Economics and Social Affairs, 1988.

Watkins P, Zimmerman H, Knapp N, Gracon S, Lewis K. A hepatotoxic effects of tacrine administration in patients with Alzheimer's disease. Journal of the American Medical Association 1994; 271: 992–998.

Weissman M, Leaf P, Tischler G, Blazer D, Karno M, Livingstone-Bruce M et al. Affective disorders in five United States communities. Psychological Medicine 1988; 18: 141–153.

Whittaker J. Post-operative confusion in the elderly. International Journal of Geriatric Psychiatry 1989; 4: 321–326.

WHO (World Health Organisation) The ICD 10 Classification of Mental and Behavioural Disorders. Geneva: WHO, 1992.

Wilcock G, Stephens J, Perkins A. Trazodone/trytophan for aggressive behaviour. Lancet 1987; 1929–1930.

Wrelkin N. Consensus statement apolopoprotein E genotyping in Alzheimer's disease. Lancet 1996; 347: 1091–1099.

8

PERSONALITY DISORDER – WHAT ROLE FOR THE MENTAL HEALTH SERVICES?

Connor Duggan

INTRODUCTION

Personality disorder is probably unique in this volume as the only disorder in which there is a debate about whether there is a role rather than what kind of role for the mental health services. This raises two questions: why has personality disorder been so neglected and is this neglect justified?

There are many reasons to justify this neglect and negative attitude from mental health professionals. First, personality disorder appears to have little connection with more general theories of personality. Second, it is difficult to separate normal from abnormal personality, particularly if one accepts a dimensional concept so that this appears to make the definition of the disorder an arbitrary process. Third, even though there have been major improvements in defining personality disorder in the past decade, these definitions are still not sufficiently precise to achieve good reliability either over time or with one another (Zimmerman 1994). As a consequence, there has been little good quality research on which to base any argument. Fourth, as shall be argued below, personality disorder is primarily a disorder of interpersonal functioning and, therefore, its presence is likely to evoke a negative response from carers. A core-defining feature of the personality disordered is that they have the capacity 'to get under our skin'. Vaillant (1987) expresses this aversion to those with personality disorder: 'The term personality disorder is reserved for the patients that psychiatry likes least: the deviant, the sinner, and the loathsome'. Fifth, there is a strong association – at least in the public mind – between personality disorder and antisocial behaviour so that the use of the concept may appear to be a medical sanctioning of irresponsible conduct.

Although many of these points contain a grain of truth, I shall argue that over the past decade in particular advances in our understanding of personality disorder have removed much of their potency. In addition, however, one does not need to be especially defensive about justifying an interest in personality disorder. This applies especially to those (and they are in the majority) whose main interest is in Axis I disorders. As Skodol (1997) in a recent review warns 'To ignore personality psychopathology, even in routine assessment, is a serious mistake, however, since the cause of treatment failure or untoward outcome often lies uninvestigated in the "black hole" on Axis II'. This injunction is warranted in that personality disorder is common (Weissman 1993) and its presence increases help seeking behaviour especially in mental health facilities (Norton 1992). It is also a source of considerable marital, interpersonal and occupational disability (Skodol 1997). Finally, personality is the backdrop in which Axis I disorders manifest themselves and personality factors have a considerable influence in the response to treatment and hence the course and outcome of the Axis I disorders (Reich and Vasile 1993).

One of the major problems in this field is not that we lack models to explain personality disorder – rather, it is that we have too many competing models that appear to confuse rather than illuminate. There is now evidence that these are converging and this will be detailed below. Further progress would be made if we were to accept one of these models. As will become apparent, my preference would be for interpersonal theory as the explanatory model. I shall discuss the nature of this theory and its implications as an overarching explanatory principle in what follows, but it may be premature at this stage to force this model on others.

As a valid assessment is critical to coherent treatment planning and service delivery, I shall concentrate in this chapter mainly on the assessment of personality disorder together with the assumptions which underlay this process. I shall also focus on the separation of psychopathic personality from antisocial conduct on the one hand, and from the legal concept of psychopathic disorder on the other, as a failure to make distinctions in this area is a major source of confusion.

DEFINITION

Normal personality

It is important to consider what is meant by normal personality before describing abnormal personality. Indeed, one of the major problems until recently has been that there has been little formal connection between the description of normal personality which has relied largely on factor analytic techniques and the more clinically based descriptions of abnormal personality (and personality disorder) (Strack and Lorr 1997). This is a major conceptual problem for without this connection it is not possible to see personality disorder as an extreme variant of normal traits.

Eysenck (1967) has made an important contribution to a comprehensive description of personality. He believed that there were three major independent dimensions of variation to personality: neuroticism (versus emotional stability), extraversion (versus introversion) and psychoticism (versus fluid and efficient superego functioning). This schema has been extended so that personality is now thought to be described most parsimoniously by the Five Factor Model (FFM) (Costa and McCrae 1995) consisting of the dimensions of neuroticism, extraversion (both of which are in Eysenck's system), consciousness, and agreeableness (perhaps corresponding to psychoticism although these may be broader then the Eysenckian notion) and openness which does not appear to correspond to any of the Eysenckian dimensions (Skodol 1997).

Personality disorder

Categorical approaches DSM-IV and ICD–10

Personality Disorder has progressed from being a residual category resulting from a diagnosis of exclusion (i.e. not organic, psychotic or neurotic) to one requiring the presence of positive features, namely, a pervasive maladjustment that persists over time (Skodol 1997). Additional advances in DSM-III and IV have involved the introduction of a separate axis to ensure that the presence of personality disorder would not be overlooked and to aid diagnosis. The latter in turn have led to the development of structured clinical interviews to improve the reliability of diagnosis. In DSM-IV (APA 1994) there is an explicit relationship between normal personality traits and abnormal personality. Thus, personality traits are defined as 'enduring patterns of perceiving, relating to, and thinking about the environment and oneself that are exhibited in a wide range of social and personal contexts'. It is when these normal personality traits become sufficiently 'inflexible, maladaptive and cause significant functional impairment or subjective distress' that they constitute a personality disorder. In their introduction to the Structural Clinical Interview for DSM-IV Axis II Personality Disorders (SCID-II), the authors emphasize the importance of the three 'P's for personality disorder diagnosis, that is, 'the characteristic has to be *pathological* (i.e. outside the range of normal variation), *persistent* (i.e. frequently present over a period of at last the last five years with onset in early adulthood), and *pervasive* (i.e. apparent in a variety of contexts, such as work or at home, or, in the case of items concerning interpersonal relations, in several different relationships)' (First et al. 1997). ICD–10 (1992) is very similar to DSM-IV. In ICD–10, personality disorder is defined as affecting several areas of functioning (i.e. pervasive), of being enduring (i.e. persistent) and of usually, but not invariably, being associated with significant problems in social or occupational functioning (i.e. pathological). In the ICD–10 definition no mention is made of an age band during which personal distress becomes manifest.

CLASSIFICATION

In DSM-IV, personality disorders are grouped into three clusters. Cluster A, which includes the paranoid, schizoid and schizotypal, is characterized by individuals with odd or eccentric features, whose members are socially isolated, suspicious and distrustful of others. Cluster B includes borderline, narcissistic, antisocial and histrionic personality disorders, and comprises individuals who develop intense relationships, but these are self-serving and manipulative. Cluster C includes the anxious, dependent and obsessive-compulsive personality disorders whose members are fearful, insecure and overcontrolling.

In ICD–10 personality disorders are included in the categories F60, 61 and 62. F60 comprises 10 specific personality disorders which are similar to those in DSM-IV except that in the former schizotypal personality disorder is placed in with schizo-phrenia (F21) and narcissistic PD which is included in F60 but only as one of the other specific personality disorders (F60.8). Each of the 10 major personality disorders are described with several of the traits or behaviour which ought to be present in each and the clinician is advised that at least three of these ought to be present to meet the criteria for inclusion. F61 refers to Mixed and other Personality Disorders where the abnormalities are often troublesome but do not meet the criteria of F60. Finally F62 refers to enduring personality changes which occur either after a catastrophic experience (62.0) or following a severe psychiatric illness (62.1).

Having identified the absence of a connection between normal personality and personality disorder as a problem earlier in this chapter, it is important to mention some recent attempts to integrate the Five Factor Model with DSM-III-R and DSM-IV (Widiger et al. 1994). Here neuroticism is thought to be present in almost any personality disorder with combinations of traits on the other four dimensions determining which type of personality disorder will occur. For instance, Avoidant Personality Disorder is believed to comprise a mixture of high neuroticism and low extraversion (McCrae 1994). Although a dimensional concept is useful, one has to resort to a categorical definition for it to be of clinical value by having a threshold beyond which there is a statistical likelihood of dysfunction. This cut-off on a continuum to define pathology is no different to many other areas of physical medicine (for instance, hypertension, anaemia, renal failure).

Criticism of DSM-IV and ICD–10

Although these classificatory schemes are an advance on their predecessors, they continue to have a number of major problems. One criticism is that while these disorders ought to depend on exaggerated traits, the definitions of items for inclusion in a disorder in some instances depend on behaviours rather than on the underlying traits. For instance, recurrent self-injury is one of the criteria for borderline personality disorder and this is clearly a behaviour rather than an under-lying trait. Similarly, antisocial personality disorder in DSM-IV has been criticized as the criteria overemphasize features associated with criminal behaviour and underemphasize the interpersonal and affective domains (Hare and Hart 1995).

A second problem concerns reliability. Despite the improvements in the criteria, the reliability of un-standardized clinical evaluations (i.e. what a clinician might do using the criteria as specified in the manuals) is only poor to fair (Zimmerman 1994). While it has been shown that structured interviews such as the SCID-II (First et al. 1997) or IPDE (Loranger et al. 1994) have much improved joint-rater reliability, at least when the instruments are used by their developers, the test–re-test coefficients over 6 months are very often low and the diagnostic concordance between different instruments is poor (Perry 1992, Zimmerman 1994). Finally, the use of these structured instruments is excessively cumbersome for a working clinician. Hence, the production of a good method of defining personality disorder that has good clinical reliability remains a problem.

Benjamin (1993) identifies two reasons for these difficulties. First, the symptoms of personality disorder are more difficult to define than the symptoms of an Axis I disorder: 'When trying to diagnose a personality disorder, the interviewer cannot simply ask such questions as "are you vain and demanding" or "are you manipulative or exploitive?" Definition of the symptoms of a personality disorder is largely in the evaluative opinion of the interviewer, whose view is likely to be widely discrepant from that of the interviewee'.

Second, there is the boundary problem as many of the criteria are signs of membership of more than one category. For instance, she points out that anger is listed as a marker for all of the four personality disorders in Cluster B of DSM-IV. This overlap in symptomatology in the definition of specific personality disorders results in the same individual meeting the criteria for more than one personality disorder. As it is logically absurd to have more than one personality (and by extension more than one personality disorder) this is a major criticism. Although it is possible to overcome this criticism by specifying the particular interpersonal context for each symptom (for instance anger in the borderline arises when the caregiver is seen as neglectful and abandoning), this is outside the scope of this chapter although I would encourage interested readers to refer to Benjamin (1993) for further information.

INTERPERSONAL DIAGNOSIS OF PERSONALITY DISORDER

I have already discussed the relationship between the dimensional FFM and the categorical DSM-IV. An alternative approach within the dimensional system that is complementary to the FFM is provided by interpersonal theory. This construes interpersonal behaviour as a function of the two basic motivations: the need for control (power, dominance) and the need for affiliation (love, friendliness). This theory sees individuals as continually negotiating on these two major relationship issues as Kiesler (1996) puts it: 'how friendly or hostile they will be with each other, and how much in charge or control each will be in their encounters'. The interpersonal circle views personality as a circular arrangement (a circumplex) of interpersonal dispositions and styles arranged around these orthogonal dimensions of dominance (or power) versus submission and nurturance (or affiliation) versus hostility (Figure 8.1). An individual with satisfactory adjustment would have a wide range of skills and hence be able to produce behaviour representing all parts of the circle, depending on the situation. The inner circle represents this normal range. However, as the behaviour becomes more pronounced, such a person would then rely less on behaviour from opposite parts of the circle. For instance, an individual who has a pronounced dominant interpersonal style will be unable to act in a submissive manner when it is appropriate to do so. Consequently the behaviour will be rigid, inflexible and maladaptive (i.e. will approximate features of personality disorder). It is possible to relate DSM-IV Personality Disorders to the interpersonal circle so that, for instance, schizoid individual are in the withdrawn quadrant and paranoid in the hostile quadrant, and so on.

An important consequence from interpersonal theory, which increases our understanding of personality disorder, is that in an interpersonal exchange, a particular behaviour 'pulls' a complementary reaction from the other person. Along the dominant/submission axis, this response will be reciprocal so that a dominant style will pull a submissive response; on the hostile/affiliation axis, the response will be congruent so that a hostile action will pull a hostile response, a friendly action will pull a friendly response (Blackburn 1992). This formulation of interpersonal behaviour focusing on the self-fulfilling prophecy nature of the human encounter offers an explanation for why personality disorder persists. What this also does, however, is to use the most important aspect of personality disorder (i.e. its negative reactivity) to a purposeful effect namely, what is evoked from an interactant is what is helpful in understanding an target individual's behaviour.

The Impact Message Inventory of Kiesler (1996) is one measure that has been 'designed to designate the behaviour of target persons by measuring the covert

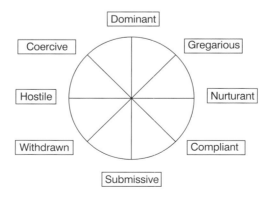

Figure 8.1 – The interpersonal circle

reactions targets induce or evoke in interactants or observers'. Thus a sample item from the Impact Message Inventory that would be indicative of the individual being in the dominant octant would be when the recipient endorsed the item 'When I am with this person, she (he) makes me feel "bossed around"', whereas the response or 'I should tell her to stand up for herself' would indicate that the subject was located in the submissive octant scale. Kiesler (1996) stresses that this interaction is complex and depends on the psychological meaning attributed to others' overt behaviour, not simply from the behaviour itself.

ASSESSMENT

Self-report versus structured interview

Is it possible to obtain accurate information from a personality disordered individual as one might argue that such traits, being egosyntonic, would not be recognized as such by the individual? In addition, even if individuals recognized such traits as being disordered, they might be minimized or denied if they, for instance, infringed social norms as might be the case with antisocial personality disorder. This expectation that individuals underreport their personality abnormalities has not been borne out in practice. For instance, individuals using self-report personality questionnaires are more likely to overestimate rather than underestimate their pathological personality traits (Hyler et al. 1990). Furthermore, under reporting when it does occur is a feature of narcissistic and passive–aggressive rather than antisocial personality disorder (Skodol 1997).

Hunt and Andrews (1992) made a formal comparison of the construct validity of the self-report Personality Diagnostic Questionnaire – Revised (PDQ-R) with the semi-structured interview (The Personality Disorder Examination) in subjects with anxiety neuroses and (in the case of the PDQ-R only) in a group of highly functioning adults. The agreement between the two instruments was poor and while only 7.5% of the patients met criteria for a personality disorder on the PDE, 67.5% of the patients on the PDQ-R met the criteria. Significantly, 12% of the highly functioning adults sampled with the PDQ-R met the criteria for personality disorder and the authors to conclude that the PDQ-R is detecting traits rather than personality disorder and that 'the diagnosis of personality disorder is best made by clinical or structured interview, and not by self-report questionnaires.'

Use of informants

An important question is whether informants should be used to determine whether an individual has a personality disorder. Some interview schedules depend entirely on information from informants (Tyrer et al. 1979, Mann et al. 1981) and while it is always useful to have additional information in any clinical assessment, there are no data to suggest that such informant information is any more or less valid as compared with that from the subject him/herself (Zimmerman 1994). One of the problems here is that with an informant interview, one is depending on the observation and reaction of one subject (with all his or her own personality variables) to the other and it is likely that what ever is reported will be confounded by the observers own response set. This is not to say that such information is not of value but rather that, if informants are used, careful attention to this informant reactivity needs to be made (see above).

Clinical assessment of personality disorder

In addition to the information gathered during a routine clinical interview, the six areas covered in the IPDE provide a useful format whereby personality functioning can be assessed. Attention should, therefore, be given to (1) interpersonal relationships, (2) sense of self, (3) work, (4) affects, (5) impulse control and (6) reality testing.

Personality disorder and criminality

This is an important area that merits discussion especially in the UK where the use of 'Psychopathic Disorder' within the Mental Health Act creates confusion with the pejorative term 'psychopath'. There is also additional confusion with the use of the 'treatability' criterion in order to detain an individual under the Act. The use of the following terms need to be clarified: (1) criminal behaviour (or social deviance), which may be associated with mental disorder (either mental illness, personality disorder or learning disability), antisocial personality, psychopathic personality, and psychopathic disorder (according to the Mental Health Act). The terms include groups who overlap to varying degrees and this has significant implications for the interface between mental health services and the criminal justice system.

First, criminal behaviour and mental disorder are not mutually exclusive so that one can have one or the other or both or neither (Blackburn 1992). Second, even when both occur together, there may or may not be a connection between them. Thus, an individual may have an Axis I or II disorder and be a career criminal and these two conditions could occur independently of one another. In the case of antisocial personality disorder, this can be difficult in practice to disentangle as some of the criteria for ASP are the individual's past criminal behaviour. This overlap between these different domains has been criticized (Hare 1996).

The term 'psychopathic personality' is a much more restrictive concept than the legal term psychopathic disorder. Psychopathic personality, which best approximates what is colloquially known as a 'psychopath', is a cold callous egocentric manipulative individual and is best characterized by high scores from the Hare Psychopathy Checklist PCL (1996). This is a well-validated instrument which, from a semi-structured interview, produces a score from the individual assessed ranging from 0 to 40. It has a two-factor structure with factor 1 items being derived from the Clecklian features of psychopathy such as superficiality, egocentricity, manipulativeness as contrasted with the more antisocial behaviour (factor 2). This distinction has treatment and prognostic implications. For instance, those who load heavily on factor 1 are more likely to (1) engage in instrumental violence (Cornell et al. 1996), (2) re-offend after discharge (Harris et al. 1993) and (3) be less amenable to treatment (Rice et al. 1992), all of which may be a function of the stability of factor 1. Another useful distinction is between primary and secondary sociopaths with the former overlapping with those who score high on the PCL-R (Table 8.1). Primary sociopaths are unable to experience social emotions and exhibit deficits in tasks that typically induce anxiety in others. Secondary sociopaths, have a normal levels of anxiety and responses to punishment but may be especially driven by high reward conditions – they have 'socialized conduct disorder' (Mealey 1995).

The legal designation 'Psychopathic Disorder' has been criticized as empirical research has shown that this is a heterogeneous groups including individuals with multiple Axis II (principally borderline and antisocial personality disorder) and Axis 1 disorders over their lifetime (Coid 1992). Furthermore, Coid found that those with the highest scores on the Hare Psychopathy Checklist (i.e. the most psychopathic) were more likely to be in the criminal justice rather than in the health service. The recent Reed Report recommends that the term Psychopathic Disorder be abandoned and replaced by the appropriate personality disorder (Reed 1994).

Blackburn has illustrated the degree of overlap between these different concepts in a very useful conceptual diagram shown in Figure 8.2. Within this, it is possible for

	PRIMARY PSYCHOPATHS	SECONDARY PSYCHOPATHS
Social Class	Distributed throughout all social classes	Predominate in lower social classes
Importance of genetic/environmental factors	Primarily genetic	Primarily environmental
Capacity to experience normal emotions	Limited	Not impaired
Effect of age on antisocial behaviour	None	Diminishes
Effect of social economic factors and parental rearing on antisocial behaviour	None	Significant
Societal response to reduce antisocial behaviour	High rate of detection and swift retaliation	Specialised parent education and support targeted at high risk groups

Table 8.1 – Two pathway model to sociopathy (After Mealey 1997).

an individual to be convicted of a criminal act and to have a personality disorder. It is also possible for an individual to have both a personality disorder, mental disorder and a history of criminal behaviour or any combinations thereof.

What mental health professionals require at this time is some way of rationally defining a group of personality disordered individuals within the criminal justice system for whom one might offer an intervention. The arbitrariness of this process at the moment (Collins 1991) coupled with the possibility of indefinite incarceration if treatment is unsuccessful (Baker and Crichton 1995) has brought this area into disrepute. How then does the mental health professional make a rational decision so as to provide those with offending behaviour and a personality disorder with the appropriate intervention while at the same time not allow the service to be wrongly used by those who wish to avoid taking responsibility for their actions? The flow diagram in Figure 8.3 is a suggestion as to how this decision-making process could be improved. Here, the mental health professional has to establish (1) the presence of a personality disorder, the criteria for which does not solely include the presence of criminal behaviour. (2) The establishing of some connection between that personality disorder and the criminal behaviour so that it is not simply mere co-occurrence of the two conditions. (3) The determining of treatability by, for instance, only treating those with a low score the PCL-R or those who are secondary psychopaths. Some of these decisions would be difficult in practice but at least this scheme has the merit of being transparent and allows the possibility of challenge at these different stages.

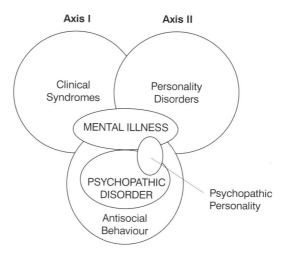

Figure 8.2 – Relationship of the legal categories of mental illness and psychopathic disorder and the concept of psychopathic personality to the domains of clinical syndromes, personality disorders and antisocial behaviour (after Blackburn, personal communication)

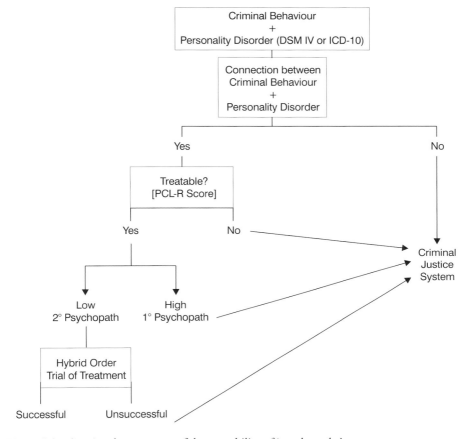

Figure 8.3 – A rational assessment of the treatability of 'psychopaths'

CONTRIBUTIONS OF ORGANIC AND PSYCHOLOGICAL FACTORS TO THE AETIOLOGY OF PERSONALITY DISORDERS

The biopsychosocial model has been used to explain the aetiology of personality disorder as with other Axis I conditions. This implies that many aetiological influences are necessary but that none by themselves are sufficient for the development of a psychiatric disorder (Paris 1993). Within such a model the disorder results from the interactions of multiple risk factors each of which only accounts for a proportion of the variance in pathology. Vaillant (1987) divides personality into the components of temperament and character, the former depending on biology and genetics, the latter on the social environment.

Organic factors

Personality traits arise from the interaction of temperament with social learning (Paris 1993). Temperament is innate and constitutional (Plomin et al. 1990) and personality dimensions have a heritability of 40–50%. There have also been attempts to link these personality dimensions to neurotransmitter systems (Cloninger 1987) (for instance, a link between impulsively and low serotonin; Siever and Davis 1991). Although, there is evidence of the heritability of personality traits, there is less evidence for such heritability for personality disorders (Torgersen 1984).

The use of a dimensional concept for personality is useful in that it allows one to examine whether some aspects of personality have a protective effect. One example of this was provided by Hirschfeld et al. (1983) in a family study of the first-degree relatives of depressed probands. They showed, not surprisingly, that the first-degree relatives recovered from depression had higher scores for introversion, passivity and submission compared with published norms. They also showed that family members without a lifetime history of depression were found to have an extra degree of emotional strength as compared with published norms (i.e. were 'super-normal').

Structural and functional abnormalities in the brain are also of increasing interest especially for antisocial personality disorder. These include impairments in the prefrontal cortex function (Kandal and Freed 1989). Damasio (1994) with his 'somatic marker' hypothesis proposes an alternative explanation suggesting that the absence of emotional markers to representations that contribute to decision making impair that process. Another explanation involves the limbic system that is impaired so that the fear response is not as reliably elicited. Blair (1995) has recently elaborated this explanation proposing that a violence inhibitory mechanism (VIM) which is normally evoked by distress cues and results in withdrawal is not activated in individuals with ASP. Hitherto, there has been a relative absence of attention to brain mechanisms in understanding personality disorder so that these incursions are to be welcomed.

Psychosocial factors

It is clear that while biological factors are important, they are not sufficient in themselves. Psychosocial risk factors are important in converting abnormal traits into disorders. Although several case control studies suggest the link between childhood adversity and subsequent psychopathology, these depend on retrospective accounts and it has been observed that prospective studies are able only to detect much weaker associations. There are reasons for this observation (Rutter and Maughan 1997) but an important one is the base rate effect in which it is usual for the majority who experience the event to escape the consequences (i.e. are resilient). One of the most frequently cited psychosocial associations is that between childhood sexual abuse and borderline personality disorder (Herman et al. 1989). However, this is an association with low specificity as many abused subjects either do not develop a personality disorder at all or a personality disorder other than borderline personality disorder.

Finally, the role of social factors needs to be taken into account although we have little empirical data to judge their impact. Such factors would also interact with temperament and psychological adversity so that, for instance, impulsive individuals might be especially sensitive to the loss of social constraints in a time of social upheaval which might act as a buffer against their impulsive actions (Millon 1993). Conversely, those with psychopathic traits may function very well in times of war or social upheaval.

While this dichotomy between organic and psychosocial influences (or nature versus nurture) is useful heuristically, it is fundamentally false. It is false as it implies that although these factors combine in their effect, they are essentially independent of one another. This, however, is not what happens. For instance, certain inherited temperamental traits are likely to elicit specific responses from the environment which in turn reinforce the pattern of behaviour so that nature to a degree creates its own nurture. Thus, Plomin (1995) speaks of 'the nature of nurture'. This implies more than what the biopsychosocial model suggests and this is of especial importance in the area of personality disorder where such feedback loops are an essential part of the fabric of the disorder.

It is this matching between the individual's temperament and the environment which explains, among other things, why it is that children exposed to the same parents may report very different experiences of parenting. The reason, therefore, that an adult reports poor parenting may have as much to do with his/her difficult temperament as a child (which evoked the poor parenting) as the poor parenting produced the difficult temperament and subsequently the personality disorder. There is a strong continuity from childhood into adulthood so that the child with a difficult temperament may continue as an adult to have a hostile view of the world thereby provoking a negative reaction from significant others which reinforces their world view and so on. Such individuals may even go out and actively seek out others who confirm their view of the world and this explains why personality, despite being disordered, nevertheless continues to persist. Andrews (1991) characterizes this process as follows: 'Personality is stable and enduring, not because it is composed of fixed traits or because it is controlled by external social arrangements, but because it is sustained by the active self via an intricate set of feedback loops with the environment by continuous interaction cycles, shaped partly by the individual, that provide self-confirmation'. For instance, patients with borderline personality disorder have an overwhelming sense of wanting to be nurtured but fear abandonment. The paradox is that they will actively coerce nurturance from the therapist but in a manner that will lead the therapist to 'burn out'. This burn out and abandonment will confirm their fear that they are likely to be abandoned but does nothing to change their own behaviour. Several examples of this phenomenon can be found in descriptions of personality disorder and this process of schema maintenance is well described Young (1990).

IMPACT ON FUNCTIONING

Personality disorder is common and those with personality disorder not only are large consumers of mental health services (Norton 1992, Reich and Vasile 1993), but also are generally dissatisfied with what they are given. Although it is claimed that 10% of the population suffer from personality disorder (Weissman 1993), others regard this as an overestimate because 'Clinicians who do not specialise in these disorders frequently underestimate the severity of the disturbance required before the DSM-III criteria are satisfied' (Andrews 1991).

Severe personality disorder, in this sense, has about the same prevalence as severe mental disorder (i.e. between 2 and 3%) (Bond et al. 1994). Even with this lower estimate, personality disordered individuals have a significant impact on services. They appear to have little tolerance of psychological pain, use primitive defence mechanisms (Bond et al. 1994) and, therefore, engage in a number of self-defeating strategies such as drug taking, alcohol dependence and self-harm. An important area to consider is the interaction between Axis I and II together with their co-occurrence.

Co-morbidity with other Axis I disorders

In an important early review of the relationship between personality and affective disorders, Akiskal et al. (1983) identified four different ways in which these Axis I and II might interact. First, personality traits might be pathogenic so that its presence might increase the likelihood of developing an Axis I condition. Second, personality traits might exert a pathoplastic effect altering the natural course of the disorder, response to treatment, etc. Third, personality traits (or disorder) may themselves be a consequence of an Axis I disorder as, for example, depressive personality emerging after a severe major depression. Fourth, they proposed that personality traits (and disorders) may be attenuated forms of an Axis I condition. There is good evidence particularly for the pathoplastic effect of personality (Akiskal et al. 1983, Reich and Vasile 1993). As this conceptualization focuses more on personality traits rather than on personality disorder, I will not consider it further here; but the importance of co-morbidity of Axis I and II requires that this be considered further.

The co-occurrence of depression with borderline personality disorder is the one which has received the greatest attention. The co-occurrence is common and in the five studies that examined the prevalence of major affective disorder in a follow-up of BPD subjects, the mean prevalence estimate was 42% (Perry 1993). In Perry's own follow-along study, he showed that BPD subjects had a mean of 1.7 episodes of major depression per year of follow-up (Perry 1988). Another important co-occurrence is between antisocial personality disorder with alcohol and drug abuse. Guze (1976) found that 54% of his incarcerated male felons (79% with ASP) had alcoholism at intake and after 8–9-year follow-up, 38% had remained alcoholic. Martin et al. (1982) in their 6-year follow-up of incarcerated female felons (65% with ASP) found that 47% had alcohol and 26% had drug problems at intake. After 6 years, 30% of the sample had alcoholism and 9% had drug abuse.

From a clinical perspective, a common problem is that an individual with a long-standing personality disorder may come in contact with services only when he/she develops an Axis I condition. There are two hazards associated with this presentation: (1) that treatment for the Axis I disorder is withheld because the Axis I condition is not recognized within the context of a long-standing personality disorder or (2) the response to treatment of the Axis I condition is diminished by the presence of the personality disorder.

The following example illustrates the significance of this combination. A 30-year-old woman had a long-standing borderline personality disorder but had minimal contact with any mental health service and significantly she was without any criminal history. She was always fractious, difficult to live with and had long-standing relationship difficulties including the relationship with her current partner. She had an unplanned pregnancy but decided to keep the baby. Within weeks of the birth, she developed a significant depressive illness took an overdose and was admitted to hospital. The severity of her depressive episode was not recognized and she was discharged. While social services were in the process of finding an alternative placement for her baby, she killed the child. The two clinical lessons to be learnt from this tragic story are (1) that it is the combination an Axis I together with an Axis 2 disorder that made this a noxious state and (2) that individuals are probably less likely to get treatment of their treatable condition (in this case the depressive episode) in the context of an already existing personality disorder.

COURSE/PROGNOSIS

This area has been well reviewed by Stone (1991) and Perry (1993) and I will focus only on the main points. The general picture is that individuals with personality disorder show a gradual improvement over the long-term so that the pessimism associated with this disorder is not justified. However, this conclusion is subject to two caveats. First, most of the studies are restricted to specialized populations and usually having a borderline or antisocial personality disorder diagnosis. Hence, we do not have any systematic long-term follow-up data for the vast majority of patients with milder character pathology (Stone 1993). Second, even though personality disordered individuals generally have a more favourable outcome compared with, say, a severe enduring mental illness such as schizo-phrenia, studies show that the majority of subjects with personality disorder had significant impairment at follow-up irrespective of its length which further supports the notion that 'Axis II disorders have a serious social impact' (Perry 1993).

Borderline personality disorder

The best comparative follow-up data comes from borderline personality disorder and schizophrenia. Several well-conducted follow-up studies (McGlashan 1986, Stone 1990) have concluded that provided the follow-up is long-term (15 years plus), the outcome of the borderline patients is generally favourable and superior to that of schizophrenia. That is to say, those with a borderline diagnosis were read-mitted less frequently (one-third as likely as schizophrenia in Stone's series) and significantly more likely to obtain employment. Perry (1993) has summarized this gradual improvement of borderline pathology as follows: reviewing five follow-up studies, he reported that the percentage meeting the criteria for BPD were 57, 52 and 33% after 8.7, 10 and 15 years respectively.

Another important outcome measure in this group is suicide. The mean percentage of deaths by suicide in BPD across nine studies was 6.1% (range 3–9%) over a mean follow-up of 7.2 years (Perry 1993). The reported lifetime prevalence figure for suicide in personality disorder of 10% is the same as for schizophrenia but this conceals an important point namely, that suicide in personality disorder tends to occur at an early age (i.e. between 20 and 30 years of age) unlike as in schizophrenia where it can occur throughout the lifecycle. Hence, there is an especial need to be vigilant in the immediate period after hospitalization as this is when the likelihood of suicide is greatest (Perry 1993). The data from the P1–500 follow-up (Stone 1990) also illustrate the importance of the impact of co-morbidity in predicting the occurrence of suicide in those women with BPD, in that women with major affective disorder and alcoholism in addition to BPD had a 38% increased chance of committing suicide compared with a 10% level for the BPD alone.

Antisocial personality disorder

There is general agreement that many with antisocial lifestyle outgrow their wildness by 30–40 years of age and not surprisingly most follow-up studies in this group focus on criminal behaviour even though this is strictly not a personality trait. Epidemiological (Weissman 1993) and follow-up (Robins 1966) data provide evidence that the number meeting criteria for antisocial personality disorder diminishes with age. West and Farrington conducted the important prospective longitudinal survey in a community sample by following up a sample of boys from a working class area of South London (Farrington 1995). Their ascertainment rate was high (e.g. 94% at 32 years of age) and they were able to obtain information from multiple sources. Over the period of follow-up, one-third of the boys (37%) were convicted of criminal offences. In most offenders offending began at 17 years of age, lasted 6 years and ended at 23 years of age. A small group of chronic offenders (6%) committed a disproportionate number of offences (about 50%) and went on committing them longer. They found that delinquency was just one element of a larger syndrome of antisocial behaviour.

Those with antisocial personality disorder do not appear to do as well compared with borderline personality disorder (Perry 1993). In the Robins (1966) follow-up, while delinquent children stopped their antisocial conduct in adulthood, a significant continuity remained between childhood conduct disorder and adult antisocial behaviour. For instance, she showed in her 30-year follow-up that arrests for rape and murder only occurred in those adults who had a history of conduct disorder in childhood. Likewise, prostitution in women occurred only in those with a history of conduct disorder in childhood. In addition, while many with antisocial personality cease their offending, this does not mean that such individuals turn out to be agreeable individuals (Hare 1996). Again the subdivision into high and low scorers on the PCL-R is of particular interest for long-term course prediction in that it has been shown that while factor 2 features (i.e. antisocial behaviour) attenuates over time, factor 1 features (i.e. the affective and interpersonal domains) do not (Hare 1996).

One of the factors that may protect against further re-offending is social integration. This inverse relationship between social integration and further re-offending among those with antisocial or psychopathic tendencies was shown by Reiss et al. (1996) in a study of young men who were legally detained under the Mental Health Act's category of psychopathic disorder. Steels et al. (1998), in comparing the long-term course of individuals discharged from maximum security showed that those with the legal category PD fared much better for psychosocial functioning but worse for subsequent re-offending compared with those with mental illness (i.e. predominantly with schizophrenia). Black et al. (1995) in comparing the long-term course of antisocial personality disorder with schizophrenia, found that the former had better social functioning but no difference in employment compared with the latter.

In antisocial personality disorder, the rates of suicide are lower than that of BPD. In the Robins (1966) sample, only 10% of her follow-up ever attempted suicide in most cases to avoid incarceration or to obtain a hospital transfer. Guze (1976) found that three of a series of 223 male felons with ASP had met with a violent death over an 8–9-year follow-up. Martin et al. (1982) found that only one female with ASD died of an overdose over a 6-year follow-up. However, for those with personality disorder admitted to hospital, both Black et al. (1995) and Steels et al. (1998) found an increased standardized mortality ratio with suicide being common.

Schizotypal personality disorder

The outcome of this group is generally poor being closer to that of schizophrenia than that of BPD so that they continue to have problems with under performing at work together with social isolation. In the Chestnut Lodge follow-up, a number developed schizophrenia during the follow-up (Fenton and McGlashan 1989).

Narcissistic personality disorder

There is little systematic follow-up information on this group. Plakun (1989) compared the outcome of NP with BPD and showed that the outcome of the latter was superior. Owing to the core psychopathology, one might expect that individuals with NP would be especially prone to commit suicide and thus has been partially borne out in follow-up studies although the series are too small to permit anything other than tentative conclusions (Stone 1993).

Predictors of prognosis

There are few data on predictors of outcome in personality disorder and our capacity to predict long-term course and outcome in psychiatric illnesses in general is limited. For instance, Stassen (1990) has the sobering suggestion that one-sixth is the maximum amount of the variance in long-term outcome which can be predicted using all the known predictors. Using 14 predictors in Stone's own series of borderline patients, could only account for 11.65% of the outcome variance of which parental brutality was the most important (7%) of the outcome variance.

SUMMARY

Despite the vicissitudes associated with personality disorder (and these are many), there is no doubt that this is an important area for mental health workers and for the services they provide. It is important not only because personality disorder is common and the source of morbidity in its own right, but also, perhaps more importantly, it is the cause of very significant problems for the evaluation and management of Axis I problems with which it often co-occurs. The assessment of personality disorder remains a problematic area but there are encouraging signs that several different systems are converging with one another and within the next decade it is likely that a less complicated system will develop. In addition, I believe that developments in interpersonal theory will make a major contribution to the understanding of the problems in this area. Associated with these developments are some new more targeted treatments that challenge the pessimism associated with these disorders hitherto. These are not discussed here but useful reviews are to be found in Gabbard (1997) and Soloff (1998). Within the next decade it is to be hoped that personality disorder will assume the same status for mental health workers and services as other Axis I disorders.

References

Akiskal HS, Hirschfeld RMA, Yerevanian BI. The relationship of personality to affective disorders. Archives in General Psychiatry 1983; 40: 801–810.

American Psychiatric Association. Diagnostic and Statistical Manual of Mental Disorders, 4th edn. Washington, DC: American Psychiatric Association, 1994.

Andrews G. Treatment outlines for borderline, narcissistic and histrionic personality disorders. Australian and New Zealand Journal of Psychiatry 1991; 25: 392–403.

Andrews JDW. The Active Self in Psychotherapy: An Integration of Therapeutic Styles. New York: Gardner, 1991.

Baker E, Crichton J. Ex parte a: psychopathy treatability and the law. Journal of Forensic Psychiatry 1995; 6: 101–119.

Benjamin LS. Interpersonal Diagnosis and Treatment of Personality Disorders. New York: Guildford, 1993.

Black DW, Baumgard CH, Bell SE. The long-term outcome of antisocial personality disorder compared with depression, schizophrenia and surgical conditions. Bulletin of the American Academy of Psychiatry and Law 1995; 23: 143–52.

Blackburn R. Criminal Behaviour Personality Disorder, and mental illness: the origins of confusion. Criminal Behaviour and Mental Health 1992; 2: 66–77.

Blair RJ. A cognitive developmental approach to morality: investigating the psychopath. Cognition 1995; 57: 1–29.

Bond M, Paris J, Zoreng-Frank H. Defense styles and borderline personality disorder. Journal of Personality Disorders 1994; 8: 28–31.

Cloninger CR. A systematic method for clinical description and classification of personality variants. Archives of General Psychiatry 1987; 44: 579–588.

Coid JW. DSM-III diagnosis in criminal psychopaths. Criminal Behaviour and Mental Health 1992; 2: 78–94.

Collins P. The treatability of psychopaths. Journal of Forensic Psychiatry 1991; 2: 103–110.

Cornell DG, Warren J, Hawk G, Stafford E, Oram G, Pine B. Psychopathy in instrumental and reactive violent offenders. Journal of Consulting and Clinical Psychology 1996; 64: 783–790.

Costa PT JR, McCrae RR. Primary traits of Eysenck's P-E-N system: three and five factor solutions. Journal of Personal and Social Psychology 1995; 69: 308–317.

Damasio AR. Descartes' Error: Emotion, Rationality and the Human Brain. New York: Putnam, 1994.

Eysenck HJ. The Biological Basis of Personality. Springfield: CC Thomas, 1967.

Farrington DP. The Twelfth Jack Tizard Memorial Lecture. The development of offending and antisocial behaviour from childhood: key findings from the Cambridge Study into Delinquent Development. Journal of Child Psychology 1995; 36: 929–964.

Fenton WS, McGlashan TH. Risk of schizophrenia in character disordered patients. American Journal of Psychiatry 1989; 146: 1280–1284.

First MB, Gibbon M, Spitzer RL, Williams JBW, Benjamin LB. User's Guide for the Structured Clinical Interview for DSM-IV Axis 1 Personality Disorders. SCID-II. Washington, DC: American Psychiatric Press, 1997.

Gabbard GO. Psychotherapy of personality disorders. Journal of Practical Psychiatry and Behavioral Health 1997; 3: 327–333.

Guze SB. Criminality and Psychiatric Disorders. New York: Oxford University Press, 1976.

Hare RD. Psychopathy: a clinical construct whose time has come. Criminal Justice and Behavior 1996; 23: 25–54.

Hare RD, Hart S. Commentary on antisocial personality disorder: the DSM-IV field trial. In Livesley WJ (ed.), The DSM-IV Personality Disorders. New York: Guildford, 1995, pp. 127–134.

Harris GT, Rice ME, Quinsey VL. Violent recidivism of mentally disordered offenders: The development of a statistical prediction instrument. Criminal Justice and Behaviour 1993; 20: 315–335.

Herman JL, Perry C, van der Kolk BA., Childhood trauma in borderline personality disorders. American Journal of Psychiatry 1989; 146: 490–495.

Hirschfeld RMA, Klerman GL, Clayton, Keller MB. Personality and depression. Archives in General Psychiatry 1983; 40: 993–998.

Hunt C, Andrews G. Measuring personality disorder: the use of self-report questionnaires. Journal of Personality Disorders 1992; 6: 125–133.

Hyler SE, Skodol AE, Oldham JM, Kellman HD, Doidge N. Validity of the Personality Diagnostic Questionnaire-Revised (PDQ-R): a replication in an outpatient sample. Comprehensive Psychiatry 1990; 33: 73–77.

ICD–10. The ICD–10 Classification of Mental and Behavioural Disorders: Clinical Descriptions and Diagnostic Guidelines. Geneva: WHO, 1992.

Kandal E, Freed D. Frontal lobe dysfunction and antisocial behaviour: a review. Journal of Clinical Psychology 1989; 45: 404–413.

Kiesler DJ. Contemporary Interpersonal Theory and Research: Personality, Psychopathy and Psychotherapy. New York: Wiley, 1996.

Loranger AW, Sartorius N, Andreoli A, Berger P, Buchheim P, Channabasavanna SM. The International Personality Disorder Examination. Archives in General Psychiatry 1994; 51: 215–224.

Mann AH, Jenkins R, Cutting JC, Cowen PJ. The development and use of a standardised assessment of abnormal personality. Psychological Medicine 1981; 11: 839–847.

Martin RL, Cloninger CR, Guze SB. The natural history of somatization and substance abuse in women criminals: a six year follow-up. Comprehensive Psychiatry 1982; 23: 528–537.

McCrae RR. A reformulation of Axis II: personality and personality related problems. In Costa PT Jr, Widiger TA (eds), Personality Disorders and the Five-Factor Model of Personality. Washington, DC: American Psychological Association, 1994.

McGlashan TH. The Chestnut Lodge follow-up study: III. Long-term outcome of borderline personalities. Archives of General Psychiatry 1986; 43: 20–30.

Mealey L. The sociobiology of sociopathy: an integrated evolutionary model. Behavioral and Brain Sciences 1995; 18: 523–541.

Millon TH. Borderline personality disorder: a psychosocial epidemic. In Paris J (ed.), Borderline Personality Disorder: Etiology and Treatment. Washington, DC: American Psychiatric Press, 1993.

Norton KRW. 'The Health of the Nation': the impact of Personality Disorder on 'Key areas'. Postgraduate Medical Journal 1992; 68: 350–354.

Paris J. Personality disorders: a biopsychosocial model. Journal of Personality Disorders 1993; 7: 255–264.

Perry JC. A prospective study of life stress, defenses, psychotic symptoms and depression in borderline and antisocial personality disorder. Journal of Personality Disorders 1988; 2: 49–59.

Perry JC. Longitudinal studies of personality disorders. Journal of Personality Disorders 1993; vol?: 63–85.

Perry JC. Problems and considerations in the valid assessment of personality disorders. American Journal of Psychiatry 1992; 149: 1645–1653.

Plakun EM. Narcissistic personality disorders: a validity study and comparison to borderline personality disorder. Psychiatric Clinics of North America 1989; 12: 603–620.

Plomin R. Beyond nature versus nurture. International Journal of Methods in Psychiatric Research 1995; 5: 161.

Plomin R, DeFries JC, McClearn GE. Behavioural Genetics: A Primer. New York: Freeman, 1990.

Reed J. Department of Health and Home Office Working Group on Psychopathic Disorders. London: Department of Health, 1994.

Reich JH, Green AI. Effect of personality disorders in a community sample. Journal of Nervous and Mental Diseases 1991; 179: 74–82.

Reich JH, Vasile RG. Effect of personality disorders on the treatment outcome of Axis I conditions: an update. Journal of Nervous Mental Disease 1993; 181: 475–484.

Reiss D, Grubin D, Meux C. Young 'psychopaths' in special hospital: treatment and outcome. British Journal Psychiatry 1996; 168: 99–104.

Rice ME, Harris GT, Cormier CA. An evaluation of a maximum security therapeutic community for psychopaths and other mentally disordered offenders. Law and Human Behaviour 1992; 16: 399–412.

Robins LH. Deviant Children Grown Up: A Sociological and Psychiatric Study of Sociopathic Personality. Baltimore: Williams & Wilkins, 1966.

Rutter M, Maughan B. Psychosocial adversities in childhood and adult psychopathy. Journal of Personality Disorders 1997; 11: 4–18.

Siever LJ, Davis L. A psychobiological perspective on the personality disorders. American Journal of Psychiatry 1991; 148: 1647–1658.

Skodol AE. Classification assessment and differential diagnosis of personality disorders. Journal of Practical Psychiatry and Behavioural Mental Health 1997; 3: 261–274.

Soloff PH. Symptom-oriented psychopharmacology for personality disorders. Journal of Practical Psychiatry and Behavioral Health 1998; 4: 3–11.

Steels M, Roney G, Larkin E, Jones P, Croudace T, Duggan C. Discharged from hospital: a comparison of the fates of psychopaths and the mentally ill. Criminal Behaviour and Mental Health 1998; 8: 37–53.

Stone MH. Long-term outcome in personality disorders. British Journal Psychiatry 1993; 162: 299–313.

Stone MH. The Fate of Borderline Patients. New York: Guildford, 1990.

Strack S, Lorr M. Invited Essay: The challenge of differentiating normal and disordered personality. Journal of Personality Disorders 1997; 11: 105–122.

Torgersen S. Genetic and nosological aspects of schizotypal and borderline personality disorders: a twin study. Archives of General Psychiatry 1984; 41: 546–554.

Tyrer P, Alexander MS, Cicchetti D, Cohen MS, Remington M. Reliability of a schedule for rating personality disorders. British Journal Psychiatry 1979; 135: 168–174.

Vaillant GE. A developmental view of old and new perspectives of personality disorders. Journal of Personality Disorders 1987; 1: 146–156.

Weissman MM. The epidemiology of personality disorders: A 1990 update. Journal Personality Disorders 1993; 7 (suppl.): 44–62.

Widiger TA, Trull TJ, Clarkin JF, Sanderson C, Costa PT Jr. A description of the DSM-III-R and DSM-IV personality disorders with the five-factor model of personality. In Costa PT Jr, Widiger TA (eds), Personality Disorders and the Five-Factor Model of Personality. Washington, DC: American Psychological Association, 1994, pp. 41–56.

Young JE. Schema Therapy for Personality Disorders: A Schema-focused Approach. Florida: Professional Resources Press, 1990.

Zimmerman M. Diagnosing Personality Disorders. Archives General Psychiatry 1994; 51: 225–245.

9

UNDERSTANDING THE NEED

Graham Thornicroft, Sonia Johnson, Michael Phelan and Mike Slade

INTRODUCTION

Defining Needs

Despite the ubiquitous current clamour to base services upon assessed needs, there remains at present no consensus on how needs should be defined (Holloway 1994), and who should define them (Ellis 1993, Slade 1994, Corrigan et al. 1996) Individual needs, for example, may be defined at the levels of impairment, disability or in terms of interventions. The fact that a need is defined does not mean that it can be met. For example, some needs may remain unmet because other problems take priority, because an effective method is not available locally, because the person in need refuses treatment or because there is no known way to meet the need.

A need may exist, as defined by a professional, even if a patient refuses the intervention. Further, a needs assessment is not intended to endorse the status quo. It is important to define need in terms of the care/agent/setting required, not those already in place. At the same time, a proper needs assessment process should not lead to the imposition of expert solutions on patients. A professionally defined need may remain unmet, and have to be replaced by one acceptable to the patients. Health economists have suggested another approach to defining need. Their contributions include first the proposal that need refers both to the capacity to benefit from an intervention and the amount of expenditure required to reduce the capacity to benefit to zero – it is, therefore, a product of benefit and cost-effectiveness (Culyer and Wagstaff 1992) and, second, that empirical data should guide operational needs definitions (Beecham et al. 1993).

The specification of particular interventions, if accepted by the service user can lead to the key worker providing a care package (Mangen and Brewin 1991). In addition, it is important to distinguish need from demand care package provision (Figure 9.1) (Stevens and Gabbay 1991).

Demand

A demand for care exists when an individual expresses a wish to receive it. Some demands are expressed in an unsophisticated form, e.g. 'something needs to be done'. The user should be involved in a negotiation about what interventions should be provided for what problems. This will include an explanation of the options. Experts or professionals should not purely direct the process.

Provision

Provision includes interventions, agents and settings, whether or not used. Care coordination entails providing such a pattern of service after initial evaluation and then updating the review regularly to assess outcomes and to modify the care if needs remain unmet. Over-provision is provision without need. Under-provision is need without provision (unmet need).

Utilization

Utilization occurs when an individual actually receives care, for example, an inpatient admission. Need may not be expressed as demand; demand is not necessarily followed by provision or, if it is, by utilization; and there can be demand, provision and utilization without real underlying need for the particular service used.

NEEDS ASSESSMENT AT THE INDIVIDUAL LEVEL

In an ideal planning framework, a comprehensive needs assessment would be undertaken on all patients and the aggregated data would be used to plan the overall service. In practice this is seldom possible, but systematic assessment, review and evaluation over months and years of contact should allow services to work with

Need	= what people benefit from
Demand	= what people ask for
Supply	= what is provided

Figure 9.1 – Definition of needs, demand and supply

their users to evolve services more appropriate to their needs (Brewin et al. 1987). Patients who suffer from severe mental illness have a range of needs that goes far beyond the purely medical, such as those described in the US National Institute of Mental Health's document 'Toward a Model Plan for a Comprehensive Community-Based Mental Health System' (1987).

The issue of how best to make an individual assessment of need has taxed both researchers and clinicians, not least because their requirements differ. An ideal assessment tool for use in a routine clinical setting would be one which is brief, easily learned, takes little time to administer, does not require the use of personnel additional to the usual clinical team, is valid and reliable in different settings and, above all, which can be used as an integral part of routine clinical work. Macdonald (1991) suggests that in addition such a scale should be sensitive to change, the potential inter- and test-rater reliability should be high, and it should logically inform clinical management. The decision about which scale to use will depend on whether the approach is to focus on particular diagnostic or care groups, and on the balance to be struck between economy of time and inclusiveness of the ratings, and should include a range of areas of clinical and social functioning.

The Camberwell Assessment of Need

A clinically orientated and relatively brief instrument is the CAN (Camberwell Assessment of Need; Table 9.1), published by the PRiSM team at the Institute of Psychiatry. It is intended for both research and clinical use, especially in relation to the requirements of the NHS and Community Care Act (1990) to undertake needs assessments of people with severe mental health problems, and it includes both patient and staff views, considers a comprehensive range of health and social needs, and assesses need separately from interventions. Thornicroft (1994) describes the areas assessed by the CAN (Slade et al. 1999).

The principles that have guided the development of the CAN are that needs are universal, that many psychiatric patients have multiple needs, that need assessment should be an integral part of clinical practice, and that this should allow ratings by both staff and by patients. In the construction of the scale we attempted to establish that it had adequate psychometric properties, could be completed within 30 min, was comprehensive, was usable by wide range of staff, could record help from informal carers and staff, and would be suitable for both research and clinical use.

The areas of assessment included refer to basic needs (accommodation, food, occupation), health needs (physical health, psychotic and neurotic symptoms, drugs and alcohol, safety to self and others), social needs (company, intimate relationship, sexual expression), everyday functioning (household skills, self-care and childcare, basic education, budgeting), and service receipt (information, telephone, transport, welfare benefits).

- Accommodation
- Occupation
- Specific psychotic symptoms
- Psychological distress
- Information about condition and treatment
- Non-prescribed drugs
- Food and meals
- Household skills
- Self care and presentation
- Safety to self
- Safety to others
- Money
- Childcare
- Physical health
- Alcohol
- Basic education
- Company
- Telephone
- Public transport
- Welfare benefits

Table 9.1 – Areas of potential need included in the CAN (Camberwell Assessment of Need).

The psychometric properties of the scale have now been established both in terms of validity (face, consensual, content, criterion and construct) and reliability (Phelan et al. 1994/1995) and the results are acceptable (Table 9.2). It was striking that in a survey of severely disabled psychiatric patients in south London, the mean number of problems identified by staff was 7.5 (95% CI, 6.7–8.4), and by patients was 7.9 (6.8–8.9). When examined in detail, however, the degree of agreement by staff and patients for individual items was rather poor, rejecting the hypothesis that staff and patients would rate problems similarly (Slade 1994). The CAN is now being introduced to field trials in routine clinical settings, is being translated into 12 European languages, and is being published in an electronic PC version (called PELiCAN).

The MRC Needs for Care Schedule

The MRC Needs for Care schedule (Brewin 1992) is based on the following formal definition of need for care: (1) a need is present when (a) a patient's

		R	SIGNIFICANCE LEVEL
Inter-rater	Staff	0.99	p<.001
	Patient	0.98	p<.001
Test – re-test	Staff	0.78	p<.001
	Patient	0.71	p<.001

Table 9.2 – Camberwell Assessment of Needs: summary of reliability scores.

functioning (social disablement) falls below or threatens to fall below some minimum specified level, and (b) this is due to a remediable, or potentially remediable, cause; (2) a need (as defined above) is met when it has attracted some at least partly effective item of care, and when no other items of care of greater potential effectiveness exist; and (3) a need is unmet when it has attracted only partly effective or no item of care and when other items of care of greater potential effectiveness exist.

In this schedule 'needs for care' have been defined as requirements for specific activities or interventions that have the potential to ameliorate disabling symptoms or reactions. In contrast, 'needs for services' reflect institutional requirements and are defined as needs for specific agents or agencies to deliver those interventions (Brewin et al. 1987). Mangen and Brewin (1991) outline a procedure for deriving estimates of needs for services from individuals' needs for specific items of care. Substantial data have now been presented on individual needs assessments using this instrument (Brewin et al. 1988, 1990, McCarthy et al. 1988, Lesage et al. 1991, Pryce et al. 1993, van Haaster et al. 1994) along with a detailed critique of this approach (Hogg and Marshall 1992, Brewin and Wing 1993).

Cardinal Needs Schedule

A third formal approach to individual needs assessment is that of Marshall (1994) who is developing the Cardinal Needs Schedule. This is a modification of the MRC Needs for Care approach, and identifies cardinal problems as those which satisfy one of three criteria:

- 'Cooperation criterion' (the patient is willing to accept help for the problem).

- 'Carer stress criterion' (the problem causes considerable anxiety, frustration or inconvenience to people caring for the patient).

- 'Severity criterion' (the problem endangers the health or safety of the patient, or the safety of other people).

To rate this schedule, data are collected using the Manchester Scale for mental state assessment, the REHAB scale and a specially developed additional information questionnaire. A computerized version (Autoneed) has also been developed. Patients' views are rated using the Client Opinion Interview and the Carer Stress Interview which includes carers ratings, and the author is undertaking both inter-rater and test–re-test reliability studies

POPULATION LEVEL NEEDS ASSESSMENT

The rational approach to planning services that are fully appropriate for the local population, and which are consistent across a wider area, is the systematic assessment of the needs of all individuals identified as mentally ill within each catchment area. This should also include those who have severe mental health problems but are not currently in contact with services. A local case register should then be used to aggregate the needs detected in all these individuals, and services developed to fit them (Wing 1989). However, planners in many districts do not currently have access to the extensive information this approach requires. A more pragmatic approach, therefore, has to be taken to assessment of local needs for services by interpreting the incomplete mosaic of data that is to hand.

Widely available demographic and service use data may be used to assess current local service needs and provision. The methods outlined here should not be regarded as more than approximations, which can be used as proxies for more detailed local needs assessment. However, they do provide a means of beginning to plan services in a way which is informed by some of the characteristics of the local population, without having to undertake further local research. As well as using the methods outlined here, service planners may take into account any available reports on local services from bodies such as the Health Advisory Service, or other epidemiological or service-related research which has been carried out locally.

The demographic indicators discussed here are for the most part readily available in Office of Population Censuses and Surveys (OPCS) data, and in the Health Service Indicators (HSI) published by the NHS Executive. The data on local service provision which are referred to are also usually readily available. However, health purchasers and providers sometimes have surprisingly little access to accurate information about voluntary sector and social services provision. A key initial step in assessing local services will often be collating information already available from disparate sources about current levels of residential and daycare provision.

Here, this pragmatic process of assessing local services on the basis of a group of demographic and service use characteristics will be illustrated using the example of an imaginary health district, here called Planchester. Tables 9.3 and 9.4 show the main characteristics of Planchester, which are referred to in the examples that follow:

DEMOGRAPHIC INDICATOR	FIGURE FOR PLANCHESTER
Population	250 000
Location	inner-city
Jarman index	39th most deprived of 400 districts
Ethnic mix	70% white, 15% Asian, 12% black Caribbean, 2% black African
Homeless known to local authority	1500 households
Street homeless	175 individuals
Unemployment	17% economically active population unemployed
Suicide rate	16.2 per 100 000 per year
Age structure	slight over-representation of 25–44-year-olds compared with national age structure

Table 9.3 – Basic information required for population-based estimation of service needs: demographic characteristics of Planchester.

SERVICE	PLANCHESTER LEVEL OF PROVISION
Number of people admitted at least once to hospital	1900 (1400 general adult service)
Admissions per annum (including re-admissions)	2820 (2110 general adult service)
Number of outpatient attendances	6500
Acute psychiatric beds	170 general adult service
Day centre placements – all functional mental illness	150
Sheltered work placements	100
Community psychiatric nurses for general adult service – maximum total caseload	200 clients
Places in 24-h staffed hostels (18–65 years of age, mental illness)	30 residents
Places in day staffed hostels	90 residents
Group homes	25 residents
Intensive care unit beds	3
Patients in Regional Secure Unit or Special Hospitals	14

Table 9.4 – Mental Health Service provision in Planchester.

The data in Table 9.2 illustrate an issue, which it is important to remember in comparing local data with national figures. There are no standard classifications for collection of service information, and there will often be inconsistencies between data sets in the age ranges and diagnostic categories included. Care is, therefore, needed to ensure that like is compared with like.

Simple information of the types illustrated in Tables 9. 3 and 9.4 may be used to assess current local services by four main methods, each with some limitations:

- 1 – Local need may be estimated on the basis of epidemiological studies, which give figures for the national prevalence of psychiatric disorders.

- 2 – Levels of service provision, which would be expected locally, may be calculated from national and international patterns of service use and service provision.

- 3 – Current local services may be compared with expert views on desirable levels of service provision.

- 4 – The validity of estimates derived from Method 3 may be increased by using a deprivation-weighted approach. Estimates of service need may be adjusted on the basis of current knowledge about the relationships of mental health disorders to age, sex, ethnic group, marital status, economic status and other social variables.

Finally, the degree of fit between current service provision and the population's needs should be assessed from a geographical perspective as well as in terms of numbers of individuals who can be provided for. In particular, those demographic variations within catchment areas that may produce especially high levels of need in certain areas need to be considered. Here, each of the above methods is explained and illustrated using the example of Planchester.

Method 1 – Using epidemiological studies of the prevalence of psychiatric disorder

An estimate of local morbidity may be derived from community studies of levels of psychiatric morbidity carried out elsewhere in the UK. Table 9.5 shows the expected numbers of people with psychiatric disorders in our fictional district, Planchester, based on the figures for expected morbidity summarized in the 'Health of the Nation':

Survey and case identification data from inner-city London suggests that about 0.7% of the population at risk suffers from some form of psychotic disorder (Campbell et al. 1990). This would suggest an expected prevalence for Planchester of some form of psychotic disorder of 1750, compatible with the ranges in table 3.

Epidemiological data provide an overall estimate of needs in the community. It does not indicate which forms of service are needed; most people with depression or

	ESTIMATED PREVALENCE/500 000	ESTIMATED PREVALENCE FOR PLANCHESTER (POPULATION 250 000)
Schizophrenia	1000–2500	500–1250
Affective psychosis	500–2500	250–1250
Depression	10 000–25 000	5000–12 500
Anxiety	8000–30 000	4000–15 000
Data are based on Department of Health (1993).		

Table 9.5 – Estimates of psychiatric morbidity in Planchester based on national prevalence data.

anxiety do not need referral to specialist services. However, for schizophrenia and other psychoses these data are more useful, as it may be assumed that most patients with these severe mental illnesses will need some form of long-term contact with psychiatric services. Returning to our fictional district, Planchester's community services accommodate 200 people on Community Psychiatric Nurses' caseloads, 150 people in day centres and 100 people in sheltered work placements This might cause concern when considered in relation to epidemiological data. If the estimate that there are 1750 people with psychotic illnesses in the district is accurate, local community services do not currently have the capacity to provide for more than a small minority of these people.

The local suicide rate is another important epidemiological indicator. Suicide rates have a dual function in service assessment. They may be seen both as an indicator of psychiatric morbidity, and as a marker of service outcome. Suicide rates for each district and national rankings for males and females are available in the Health Service Indicators. Table 9.6 shows suicide rates for Planchester and for the country as a whole for 1991/92.

Thus, Planchester has a relatively high suicide rate, particularly among women. This cannot be unambiguously interpreted without access to other data. However, it suggests that needs for development of mental health services may be great compared with other areas, either because it indicates high levels of morbidity, or because it reflects ineffective services.

	MALES	FEMALES	PERSONS
Planchester	20.1	14.1	16.2
England and Wales	16.9	5.7	11.2

Table 9.6 – Rates of suicide/100 000 per year.

In deciding what form of intervention may reduce local suicide risks, it is important to consider which groups are particularly at risk. For example, Planchester has a large Asian community, and it is important to investigate the possibility that its high rates for women are due to suicide among young Asian women, known to be elevated nationally (Soni-Raleigh and Balarajan 1992).

Method 2 – Estimating service need on the basis of national patterns of service use

The work of Goldberg and Huxley (1980, 1992) may be used to compare local service use with national and international data on service utilization. Table 9.7 shows the expected Planchester levels of morbidity and of service use, based on Goldberg and Huxley's calculations of the proportion of the population using services at various levels. These figures include the elderly as well as younger adults.

LEVEL OF SERVICE	ONE YEAR PREVALENCE FOR POPULATION AT RISK (%)	EXPECTED LEVELS FOR PLANCHESTER (POPULATION 250 000)
Adults suffering from mental illness/distress	26–31.5	65 000–78 750
Consulting primary care	23	57 500
Identified by doctors as having mental illness/distress	10.2	25 500
Seen by specialist mental health services	2.4	6000
Admitted to psychiatric hospital	0.6	1500
Data are based on Goldberg and Huxley (1992).		

Table 9.7 – National and Planchester expected morbidity and service use.

Referring to the figures for Planchester, the number of people admitted at least once to a psychiatric hospital (1900) is high compared with these estimates of service use. However, the information considered so far gives no grounds for choosing between various possible explanations, including higher than average levels of need, greater than usual willingness to admit, and shortage of services providing alternatives to admission.

Wing (1992) gives the following national figures for patients with mental disorder in contact with services per 250 000 in 1990/91 (Table 9.8). These figures include people with dementia. Again expected levels of provision for the population of Planchester may be derived:

TYPE OF CONTACT	NATIONAL FIGURES FOR 1990/91 PER 250 000 POPULATION	EXPECTED FOR PLANCHESTER
No. of patients attending GP per annum	64 250	64 250
No. of patients attending outpatients per annum	2858	2858
Total no. of outpatient attendances per annum	8586	8586
No. of inpatients on 1 day, stay < 1 year	135	135
No. of acute admissions per annum	1095	1095
No. of inpatients on 1 day, stay 1–5 years	93	93
No. of inpatients on 1 day, stay < 5 years	70	70
No. in local authority residential care on 1 day	18	18
No. in Local Authority long-term day place on 1 day	63	63

Data are from Wing (1992).

Table 9.8 – National figures for service use and expected Planchester figures.

Planchester again has large numbers of acute admissions compared with rates predicted from national figures (2820 actual admissions compared with 1095 predicted). The number of outpatient contacts, on the other hand, is smaller than expected (6500 actual attendances compared with 8586 predicted). This pattern could be explained in various ways. One important possibility is that the outpatient service might currently be under-resourced, leading to an inability to respond swiftly to referrals. Alternatively, patients may find the outpatient service geographically inaccessible or psychologically unwelcoming, or local professionals may have limited awareness of how to make referrals to it. If such difficulties exist, the ability of the outpatient service to avert inpatient admissions may be compromised.

Wing (1992) quotes other national figures for service use on the basis of the Local Authority Profile of Social Services for 1989/90. Again, these may be extrapolated to give expected figures for Planchester, assumed to be an inner-city borough (Table 9.9).

Comparing these figures with the actual provision figures, it appears that Planchester has low levels of day centre provision compared with current national levels (150 actual places compared with 200 predicted from national levels). Looking at residential placements, on the other hand, suggests greater provision than is available nationally (145 actual places compared with 85 predicted from national levels).

An important disadvantage of national service use data is that they are often based on incomplete or inaccurate returns, especially where they refer to community

	LOCAL AUTHORITY RESIDENTIAL	OTHER RESIDENTIAL	DAY CENTRE
England	0.4/10 000 population	0.3/10 000	4/ 10 000
Shire Counties	0.2/10 000	0.2/10 000	3/10 000
Outer London	0.5/10 000	0.9/10 000	4/10 000
Inner London	1.2/10 000	2.2/10 000	8/10 000
Planchester	30	55	200

Table 9.9 – Use of local authority services: predicted service levels in Planchester based on national data.

services (Glover 1991). A good alternative may be use of data from studies in areas such as Salford where detailed case registers recording all service contacts have been kept (Fryers and Wooff 1989, Wing 1989).

Service utilization data do not, of course, allow for a normative assessment of the services that the health authority **should** have. However, planners may find it helpful to use them to get some idea whether numbers of contacts for particular components of their local services are relatively large or small compared with services elsewhere.

Method 3 – What are desirable levels of service provision?

The disadvantage of comparing local services with national data is that national average service use cannot be assumed to represent ideal levels of service provision. It is also unwise to assume that the current balance between service components such as acute beds, residential services outside hospital, daycare services and community services is the best possible. The development of ways of determining optimal levels of service provision is still in its infancy, but a number of writers have contributed to the debate. For a discussion of service models and their components, see Chapter 10.

The 1975 British White Paper suggests targets of 50 District General Hospital beds per 100 000 of the population, together with 35 for the elderly severely mentally infirm and 17 for the 'new' long-stay patients. More recently, the House of Commons Social Services Committee report on Community Care (1985) noted that 'a smaller number of in-patients beds is now thought necessary for general psychiatric services', and a Royal College of Psychiatrists working party has specified this as 44 acute beds for a population of 100 000 (Hirsch 1988).

Strathdee and Thornicroft (1992) have set out targets for service provision based on a 'Delphi' method of summarizing expert opinion in the UK and on likely prevalences of mental illness nationally. These targets assume that services should as far as possible be community based, with community residential places and daycare taking the place of institutional care. Naturally, none of these suggested levels of provision should be taken in isolation – if one component of the mental health services is underdeveloped, this is likely to lead to a higher demand on the other elements in the system (Audit Commission 1994). Wing (1992) has made similar estimates of targets for general adult residential services. These two sets of estimates are shown in Table 9.10.

Wing (1992) also provides some figures for targets for day provision by mental health services and for total numbers in contact with any mental health services, again taking account of the prevalence of severe mental illness in the community. These figures appear to include elderly people who have functional mental

TYPE OF ACCOMMODATION	MIDPOINT NUMBER OF PLACES	RANGE	MIDPOINT NUMBER OF PLACES	RANGE
	Wing		Strathdee and Thornicroft	
Staff awake at night				
Acute and crisis care	100	50–150	95	50–150
Intensive care unit	10	5–15	8	5–10
Regional Secure Unit and Special Hospital	4	1–10	5	1–10
Hostel wards	50	25–75		
Other staffed housing				
High-staffed hostel	75	40–110	95	40–150
Day-staffed hostel	50	25–75	75	30–120
Group homes (visited)	45	20–70	64	48–80
Respite facilities			3	0–5
No specialist staff				
Supported bed-sits			30	–
Direct access			30	–
Adult placement schemes			8	0–15
Total per 250 000	394	226–565	357	174–540

Data are from Wing (1992) and Strathdee and Thornicroft (1992).

Table 9.10 – Estimated need for general adult residential provision per 250 000 population.

illnesses. Figures based on his calculations for the full range of provision for the mental health service are shown in Table 9.11.

Method 4 – The deprivation-weighted population approach to needs assessment

The above calculations of expected levels of morbidity and of service utilization in Planchester have not taken into account its particular population characteristics. This is unsatisfactory, as there is strong evidence that social and demographic factors are closely associated with rates of psychiatric disorder.

The association between psychiatric disorders and social class (particularly for schizophrenia and depression) is one of the most consistent findings in psychiatric epidemiology. The Jarman combined index of social deprivation has been shown to be highly correlated with psychiatric admission rates for health districts in the South-East Thames Region (Jarman 1983, 1984, Hirsch 1988, Thornicroft 1991, Jarman and Hirsch 1992).

It thus seems reasonable to use Jarman scores to make deprivation-weighted assessments of likely local needs for services. Weightings based on Jarman scores may be used to estimate where each district should fall within the national ranges for desirable levels of service provision which are shown in Tables 9.10 and 9.11. For example, if Planchester has a Jarman score 10% below the top of the national range, a useful approximation of numbers of places needed can be obtained by assuming that the district should have service levels about 10% below the upper end of the national range. Table 9.12 shows the estimated requirements for Planchester, calculated on this basis from Strathdee and Thornicroft's estimates of ideal levels of national service provision reproduced in Table 9.10.

FORM OF PROVISION	PLACES PER 250 000
Total in contact with specialist services	572–1716
NHS specialist residential care with night staff	82–246
Other residential	115–345
Specialist daycare (4+ half days a week)	183–548*
Other active contact with specialist team (excluding those in above categories)	250–750

*Including people in non-NHS residential care, of whom half are assumed also to require daycare. Data are from Wing (1992).

Table 9.11. Estimated numbers of day and residential places needed for 250 000 population.

TYPE OF PROVISION	ESTIMATED REQUIREMENTS IN PLANCHESTER
24-h staffed residences	139
Day staffed residences	111
Acute psychiatric care	140
Unstaffed group homes	77
Adult placement schemes	14
Local secure places	10
Respite facilities	5
Regional secure unit	9

Table 9.12 – Estimated residential service requirements in Planchester – calculated on basis of deprivation scores.

The same approximation may be applied to Wing's (1992) figures given in Table 9.11 (Table 9.13).

Fit between current services and deprivation-weighted estimates of requirements

Returning to Table 9.4, which shows current levels of service provision in Planchester, some of the actual levels of provision may now be compared with the deprivation-weighted estimates of requirements (Table 9.14).

FORM OF PROVISION	ESTIMATED REQUIREMENT FOR PLANCHESTER, BASED ON JARMAN SCORE
Total in contact with specialist services	1602
NHS specialist residential care with night staff	230
Other residential	322
Specialist daycare (4+ half days a week)	512*
Other active contact with specialist team (excluding those in above categories)	700

*Including people in non-NHS residential care, of whom half are assumed also to require daycare). Data are based from those of Wing (1992).

Table 9.13 – Deprivation weighted estimates of required day and residential services in Planchester.

SERVICE	ACTUAL LEVEL OF SERVICE	ESTIMATED NUMBER REQUIRED	GAP BETWEEN ACTUAL AND REQUIRED
Acute psychiatric beds expected requirement)	170	140	+ 30 (21% above
Day centre or sheltered work placements – all functional mental illness	250	512	−262 (49% of expected requirement)
Places in 24-h staffed residences (18–65 years of age, mental illness)	30 residents	139 residents	−130 residents (22% of expected requirement)
Places in day staffed hostels	90 residents	111 residents	−21 residents (81% of expected requirement)
Group homes	25 residents	77 residents	−52 residents (32% of expected requirements
Local intensive care beds	3	10	−7 (30% of expected requirements)
Patients in Regional Secure Unit or Special Hospitals	14 patients	9 patients	+5 patients (56% above expected requirement)

Table 9.14 – Actual levels of services and estimated requirements in Planchester.

Thus, this simple exercise allows us to begin to evaluate the overall pattern of service provision in Planchester, which seems to be a relatively high level of inpatient service provision, but levels of day service and community residential services which are lower than estimates of what is required. Again it must be noted that it is crucial to look at all the elements in local services together. If the acute bed provision were considered in isolation, it might be judged to be unnecessarily high. However, if considered in relation to the low levels of community provision, it becomes apparent that reliance on inpatient beds and high admission rates may well be a consequence of undeveloped community facilities. It thus seems unlikely that numbers of acute beds could reasonably be reduced without considerable further development of community services.

An example of the deprivation weighted approach is the Mental Illness Needs Index (MINI) developed by Glover (1996). The MINI has been used as a means of comparing the actual levels of residential and inpatient provision found with those that would be predicted for London boroughs from their demographic conditions. Since the NHS reforms of 1991, there has been a trend for purchaser health authorities to amalgamate into larger units with a population base of three-to-four times the size of the old district health authorities, which tended to be about

200 000. Within the territory of each of these large purchasing authorities, several separate mental health units commonly provide care for geographically defined catchment areas (often reflecting former district boundaries). Service delivery within these provider units increasingly tends to be shared between several separate clinical teams, often on the basis of geographically defined catchment areas. These arrangements produce resource allocation problems at two levels: how should the purchaser assign mental healthcare resources between the provider units and how should the provider units allocate between clinical teams?

Epidemiological studies shed some light on these problems. Thornicroft's (1991) exploratory study of prediction of district level admission rates in the South-East Thames Region began by reviewing this literature. He identified a range of social variables (lower social class, male gender, single marital status, some aspects of domicile such as living alone, in overcrowded accommodation or in highly transitory neighbourhoods, high residential mobility, living in inner cities, population density and poverty) with established relation to psychiatric morbidity. By a principal components analysis he identified components of general deprivation and social isolation and permanent sickness which were effective predictors of district admission rate.

The problem for resource allocators is to determine the quantitative weight such issues should be assigned. Two groups (Jarman et al. 1992) have undertaken work to produce methods of predicting resource requirements on a reasonably wide scale (i.e. wider than a single district) on the basis of independent statistical indicators. Neither study solves theses problems altogether satisfactorily. At a practical level using the conclusions below the district level is difficult as the model incorporate data elements not routinely published at lower levels. From a theoretical perspective both studies develop models which make use of data about population ethnicity categorizing black Caribbeans and individuals with roots in the Indian Subcontinent as a single group, despite evidence that the former show a high rate of mental health services use while evidence for the latter is conflicting, but they may show a low rate (Harrison et al. 1988, Glover 1991). In the experience of the author of the MINI, this confusion has caused considerable argument about relative needs in at least one London health district.

The index is widely available for use within the NHS and local government in the form of a computer program that calculates values of the index for any area which can be geographically defined in terms of electoral wards. In addition to calculating the MINI, the program shows the population structure and, based on calibrations from the North-East Thames Region HES for 1991, predicts the age standardized psychiatric admission prevalence for adults of 15–64 years of age. This rate is translated into a predicted number of adults likely to be admitted by reference to the relevant population figures.

The program goes on to make estimates of the numbers of hospital, residential and daycare facilities likely to be required. These estimates are based on the two major recent studies of the range in requirements for elements of a comprehensive mental health service. Wing (1992) based his estimates on an extensive review of the research literature; Thornicroft and Strathdee (1992) undertook a modified Delphi study. In each case, for each type of facility (acute beds, 24-h staffed residential accommodation, etc.), the authors suggest the range of provision (places per unit total population) likely to be required from the least to the most needy district.

The MINI program suggests for each type of facility, where within the suggested range the chosen area is likely to fall. This estimate is produced as a rate per unit population and, based on the population figures, as a number of places. The location of each place within the suggested range is based on its place within the range of predicted admission prevalence figures

The relevance of this work for district purchasers is that it provides a simple method for obtaining a first estimate of how a rational apportionment would distribute whatever is the level of resources available to them. While helpful, this type of method still has many problems, some of them particularly important to the present task of predicting expected levels of provision for London (Johnson et al. 1997). Local factors, such as resettlement of patients in clusters or the existence of extreme local idiosyncratic geography, may determine the distribution of need in ways the model could not anticipate. The model is based only on predicting the numbers of people likely to have an admission, not the associated costs. If patients in deprived areas present more complex problems and possibly enjoy less informal support, then in addition to being more numerous in relation to the population, the care of each may be more expensive. Finally, and for the present purposes crucially, the early part of the study demonstrated that the distribution of morbidity within inner-city catchment areas is not so easily modelled as that within suburban or rural areas. In at least one district, Hackney, no satisfactory model for the distribution of morbidity within the catchment area could be derived using any apparently relevant population characteristics. This may result from poorer quality census or hospital admission data, more uniform deprivation scores, a greater ability of the council to re-house mentally ill people in any part of the borough (thus dispersing the problem), or idiosyncratic behaviour by staff caring for one or more clinical sectors. However, the observation indicates that this type of analysis should be viewed with particular caution in inner-city areas.

Specific local modifying factors

Weighting according to overall deprivation levels is a helpful beginning in planning epidemiologically based services. However, various other local demographic factors should also be considered in tailoring the overall approach to local conditions. These will be outlined below.

Ethnicity

Ethnicity has a major influence on service utilization and on the types of services needed. Black Caribbeans are an important group, as several studies have indicated a higher risk than their white neighbours of being admitted to psychiatric hospital (Moodley and Thornicroft 1988) or of being diagnosed as suffering from schizophrenia (Harrison et al. 1988, King et al. 1994).

It has not been very clearly established that Asians have an elevated rate of admission for psychosis (Thomas et al. 1993), although King et al. (1994) argue that elevated rates of psychosis may be general among immigrant groups. However, it has also been found that, despite identical rates of consultation in general practice, Asians are less likely than the white population to be referred to the psychiatric services, and that psychological disorders in this group may be more likely to go unrecognized (Brewin 1980), perhaps reflecting linguistic and cultural barriers to service delivery. Refugee communities also have important specific needs. High levels of deprivation and possibly of post-traumatic stress disorders are likely to be found among the various communities of recently arrived refugees in the UK.

Planchester has substantial Asian and black Caribbean populations, and this will need to be taken into account at all stages of service planning. The presence of the black Caribbean population may create greater needs for services for the severely mentally ill. For each group, great attention will need to be paid to making services culturally and linguistically appropriate. There may be greater barriers to early access to mental health care than for the white population, so that particular attention will need to be paid to outreach and making services accessible. Distrust of psychiatric services may also be greater than among the white population, so that consultations with members of these communities and effective advocacy services are important.

Homelessness

Recent research in the UK suggests that the homeless in hostels and night shelters and on the street probably have a rate of mental illness of between 30 and 50%, and that psychoses predominate (Marshall 1989, Timms and Fry 1989, Scott 1993). Conventional psychiatric services often fail to contact or engage the homeless mentally ill, so that specific services are needed. For example, clinics may be provided in places where the homeless tend to congregate or assertive outreach work carried out on the streets.

The extent and location of the local homeless population thus needs to be known in order to plan comprehensive services for the long-term mentally ill. Unfortunately, it is often very difficult to obtain an accurate enumeration of local numbers of homeless people, particularly the street homeless. Any 'official' figures should be treated with caution, and enquiries made about the methods used for data collection. It is helpful to ask national and local agencies concerned with homelessness how accurate they think any figures obtained are likely to be, and whether they know of any counts carried out locally. If there have been no thorough local enumerations, this should be a priority.

Unemployment

Another characteristic of Planchester with specific significance for mental health service provision is the high unemployment rate. High levels of unemployment and suicide rates have been found to be correlated in several Western countries (Platt et al. 1992, Pritchard 1992), and becoming unemployed has been associated with a general decline in mental health (Warr et al. 1988). Thus, this demographic characteristic again may suggest an increased need for mental health services.

Age structure

The age structure of the population may also serve as a pointer for service needs. Over-representation in the 20–29-year age range may indicate a greater population at risk of developing psychotic disorders. Thus, there may be a slightly greater need than nationally for general adult services, and a slightly lower one for services for the elderly mentally ill.

Service needs from a geographical perspective

To meet needs across the catchment area, services should not only provide adequate numbers of places in a range of forms of care, but also should locate these services so that they are accessible to their users. The geography of the catchment area thus needs to be considered as well as its overall characteristics. Two principles are important: sectorization, and the development of services which are highly accessible to parts of the catchment area where particularly high levels of need are likely to be found.

The term sector generally refers to a delineated geographic area, with a defined catchment population. Sectorization, with services for each sector located centrally within it, is likely to be an important principle in ensuring that services are reasonably accessible to people throughout the catchment area. To ensure that services match population needs, it is helpful to examine in detail local maps which include public transport routes to check that local bases are accessible without too much time and effort from every part of the catchment area they serve. This can present considerable problems in rural areas with dispersed populations and poor public transport.

It is also important to consider on an epidemiological basis which parts of the catchment area should be particularly targeted. Attention needs to be paid to providing accessible and well-resourced services with good facilities for outreach work in those areas where levels of overall deprivation are high or where there are large numbers of homeless people or unemployed people. Demographic indicators such as Jarman scores, ethnic mix and levels of unemployment are available for individual electoral wards. It is worth marking on local maps those areas where higher levels of need would be expected, and considering where service bases are located in relation to these areas. In dividing the catchment areas into sectors, variations in deprivation within the area need to be considered – in the more deprived parts of the catchment area, sector populations should be smaller than elsewhere, or else be served by more staff. Information on deprivation in rural areas and the effects of rurality on service need and delivery are still largely lacking in the UK (Gregoire and Thornicroft 1998).

CONCLUSION

This central theme of this chapter is that it is feasible to use currently available information for each local area as the basis for a rational approach to planning mental health services. There is evidence that current mental health services throughout England and Wales are often not distributed in relation to need, however estimated (Audit Commission 1994). It is thus important to develop and apply simple pragmatic approaches to assessment of local population needs. However, more fine-tuned planning of services in each local area will require investment in an information infrastructure that can monitor service performance and continue to provide relevant information to underpin future planning cycles.

References

Audit Commission. Finding a Place: A Review of Mental Health Services for Adults. London: HMSO, 1994.

Brewin, C. Explaining the lower rates of psychiatric treatment among Asian immigrants to the United Kingdom. Social Psychiatry 1980; 15: 17–19.

Brewin C. Measuring individual needs for care and services. In Thornicroft G, Brewin CR, Wing J (eds), Measuring Mental Health Needs. London: Gaskell and Royal College of Psychiatrists, 1992.

Brewin C, Veltro F, Wing J et al. The assessment of psychiatric disability in the community: a comparison of clinical, staff, and family interviews. British Journal of Psychiatry 1990; 157: 671–674.

Brewin C, Wing J, Mangen S et al. Needs for care among the long-term mentally ill: a report from the Camberwell High Contact Survey. Psychological Medicine 1988; 18: 457–468.

Brewin C, Wing JK, Mangen SP, Brugha TS, MacCarthy B. Principles and practice of measuring needs in the long-term mentally ill: the MRC Needs for Care Assessment. Psychological Medicine 1987; 17: 971–982.

Brewin C, Wing J. The MRC Needs for Care Assessment: progress and controversies. Psychological Medicine 1993; 23: 837–841.

Campbell PG, Taylor J, Pantelis C, Harvey C. Studies of schizophrenia in a large mental hospital proposed for closure, and in two halves of an inner London borough served by the hospital. In Weller M. (ed.), International Perspectives in Schizophrenia. London: John Libbey, 1990.

Corrigan P, Buican B, McCracken S. Can severely mentally ill adults reliably report their needs? Journal of Nervous and Mental Disease 1996; 184: 523–529.

Department of Health. The Health of the Nation. London: HMSO, 1993.

Ellis K. Squaring the Circle: User and Carer Participation in Needs Assessment. York: Joseph Rowntree Foundation, 1993.

Fryers T, Wooff K. A decade of mental health care in an English urban community. Patterns and trends in Salford 1976–1987. In Wing JK (ed.), Contributions to Health Services Planning and Research. London: Gaskell, 1989.

Glover G. The official data available on mental health. In Jenkins R, Griffiths S (eds), Indicators for Mental Health in the Population. London: HMSO, 1991.

Goldberg D, Huxley P. Mental Illness in the Community. London: Tavistock, 1980.

Goldberg D, Huxley P. Common Mental Disorders. A Bio-Social Model. London: Routledge, 1992.

Gregoire A, Thornicroft G. Rural Mental Health. Psychiatric Bulletin 1998; 22: 273–277.

Harrison G, Owens D, Holton A, Neilson D, Boot D. A prospective study of severe mental disorder in Afro-Caribbean patients. Psychological Medicine 1988; 18: 643–657.

Hirsch S. Psychiatric Beds and Resources :Factors Influencing Bed Use and Service Planning. London: Gaskell and Royal College of Psychiatrists, 1988.

Hogg L, Marshall M. Can we measure need in the homeless mentally ill? Using the MRC Needs for Care Assessment in hostels for the homeless. Psychological Medicine 1992; 22: 1027–1034.

Holloway F. Need in community psychiatry: a consensus is required. Psychiatric Bulletin 1994; 18: 321–323.

House of Commons. Second Report from the Social Services Committee, Session 1984–85, Community Care. London: HMSO, 1985.

House of Commons. The National Health Service and Community Care Act. London: HMSO, 1990.

Jarman B. Identification of underprivileged areas. British Medical Journal 1983; 286: 1705–1709.

Jarman B. Underprivileged areas: validation and distribution of scores. British Medical Journal 1984; 289: 1587–1592.

Jarman B, Hirsch S. Statistical models to predict district psychiatric morbidity. In Thornicroft G, Brewin C, Wing JK (eds), Measuring Mental Health Needs. London: Gaskell and Royal College of Psychiatrists, 1992, Chapter 4.

Johnson S, Ramsay R, Thornicroft G, Brooks L, Lelliot P, Peck P, Smith H, Chisholm D, Audini D, Knapp M, Goldberg D. London's Mental Health. London: Kings Fund, 1997.

King M, Coker E, Leavey G, Hoare A, Johnson-Sabine E. Incidence of psychotic illness in London: comparison of ethnic groups. British Medical Journal 1994; 304: 1115–1119.

Lesage AD, Mignolli G, Faccincani C et al. Standardised assessment of the needs for care in a cohort of patients with schizophrenic psychoses. In Tansella M. (ed.), Community-based Psychiatry: Long-term Patterns of Care in South-Verona. Psychological Medicine Monograph Supplement 19, 1991, pp. 27–33.

Liss P. Health Care Need: Meaning and Measurement. Linkoping: Studies in Arts and Science, 1990.

Mallman CA, Marcus S. Logical clarifications in the study of needs. In Lederer K. (ed.), Human Needs. Cambridge, MA: Oelgeschlager, Gunn & Hain, 1980, pp. 163–185.

Mangen S, Brewin CR. The measurement of need. In Bebbington PE (ed.), Social Psychiatry: Theory, Methodology and Practice. Transaction (in press).

Marshall M. Collected and neglected: are Oxford hostels filling up with disabled psychiatric patients. British Medical Journal 1989; 299: 706–709.

Marshall M. How should we measure need? Philosophy, Psychiatry and Psychology 1994; 1: 27–36.

Marshall M, Reed A. Psychiatric morbidity in homeless women. British Journal of Psychiatry 1992; 160: 761–768.

Moodley P, Thornicroft G. Ethnic group and the compulsory admission of psychiatric patients. Medicine, Science and the Law 1988; 28: 324–328.

Phelan M, Slade M, Thornicroft G, Dunn D, Holloway F, Wyles T, Strathdee G, Loftus L, McCrone P, Hayward P. The Camberwell Assessment of Need (CAN): the validity and reliability of an instrument to assess the needs of people with severe mental illness. British Journal of Psychiatry 1994/95; 167: 589–595.

Platt S, Micciolo R, Tansella M. Suicide and unemployment in Italy: description, analysis and interpretation of recent trends. Social Science and Medicine 1992; 34: 1191–1201.

Pritchard C. Is there a link between suicide in young men and unemployment: a comparison of the UK with other European Community countries. British Journal of Psychiatry 1992; 160: 750–756

Pryce I, Griffiths R, Gentry R, Hughes I, Montaguss L, Watkins S, Champney-Smith J, McLackland B. How important is the assessment of social skills in a long-stay psychiatric inpatients? British Journal of Psychiatry 1993; 163: 498–502.

Scott, J. Homelessness and mental illness. British Journal of Psychiatry 1993; 162: 314–324.

Slade M. Needs assessment: who needs to assess? British Journal of Psychiatry 1994; 165: 287–292.

Slade M, Thornicroft G, Loftus L, Phelan M, Wyles T (1999). The Camberwell Assessment of Need (CAN). London: Gaskell and Royal College of Psychiatry.

Snee K, Church E. Hotchkiss J, Marchbank A. The assessment of mental health need and its translation into policy and practice. In Gilman E, Munday S, Somervaille L, Strachan R (eds), Resource Allocation and Health Needs: From Research to Policy. London: HMSO, 1994.

Soni-Raleigh V, Balarajan R. Suicide and self-burning among Indians and West Indians in England and Wales. British Journal of Psychiatry 1992; 161: 365–368

Strathdee G., Thornicroft G. Community Sectors for Needs-Led Mental Health Services. In Thornicroft G, Brewin C, Wing JK (eds), Measuring Mental Health Needs. London: Gaskell and Royal College of Psychiatrists, 1992.

Stevens A, Gabbay J. The purchases information requirements on Mental Health needs and controlling for Mental Health Services. In Thornicroft G, Brewin C, Wing JK (eds), Measuring Mental Health Needs. London: Gaskell and Royal College of Psychiatrists, 1992.

Stevens A, Raftery J (eds). Introduction. In Health Care Needs Assessment. Oxford: Radcliffe Medical, 1994, pp 11–30.

Stevens A, Gabbay J. Needs assessment, needs assessment. Health Trends 1991; 23: 20–23.

Thomas CS, Stone K, Osborn M, Thomas PF, Fisher M. Psychiatric morbidity and compulsory admission among UK born Europeans, Afro-Caribbeans and Asians in central Manchester. British Journal of Psychiatry 1993; 163: 91–99

Thornicroft G. Social deprivation and rates of treated mental disorder: developing statistical models to predict psychiatric service utilisation. British Journal of Psychiatry 1991; 158: 475–484.

Thornicroft G. The NHS and Community Care Act, 1990. Psychiatric Bulletin 1994, 18: 13–17.

Thornicroft G, Brewin C, Wing J. Measuring Mental Health Needs. London: Royal College of Psychiatrists, 1992.

Timms P, Fry A. Homelessness and mental illness. Health Trends 1989; 21: 70–71.

Van Haaster I, Lesage A, Cyr M, Toupin J. Problems and needs for care of patients suffering from severe mental illness. Social Psychiatry and Psychiatric Epidemiology 1994; 29: 141–148.

Warr P, Jackson P, Banks MH. Unemployment and mental health: some British studies. Journal of Social Issues 1988; 44: 47–68

Wing JK (ed.), Health Services Planning and Research: Contributions from Psychiatric Case Registers. London: Gaskell, 1989.

Wing JK. Epidemiologically based Needs Assessment: Mental Illness. London: NHSME, 1992a.

Wing JK. Epidemiologically based Needs Assessments: Review of Research on Psychiatric Disorders. London: Department of Health, 1992b.

10

MODELS OF CARE FOR SEVERE MENTAL ILLNESS

Richard Ford and Matt Muijen

BACKGROUND

De-institutionalization

The past 40 years have seen a dramatic change in the ideology, structure and delivery of mental health services. In 1955 inpatient services dominated specialist mental healthcare with a peak of 150 000 beds in England, but in the second half of the 20th century there has been a dramatic decline of inpatient bed numbers to 37 000 in 1997/98 (Health and Personal Social Services Statistics, England 1998). The speed of bed closure has accelerated over the past decade with a 55% reduction. Although more difficult to track, there is evidence that many of these beds have been replaced by nursing and residential home places (Davidge et al. 1993).

In the past, many people with severe mental illness (SMI) would have become long stay patients. Although this may have guaranteed a basic level of care, this model of service provision was increasingly seen as inappropriate, based on among others the work of Goffman (1961) who described institutionalization. Furthermore, institutional care was seen by some authors as the cause of additional mental illness. For example, Barton (1959) described 'institutional neurosis'.

The run-down of hospital beds has led to a gap in care services for people with SMI. Particularly at risk are people with predominantly psychotic disorders, who need long-term care and have difficulties with functioning in society, and may consequently present for repeated short admissions.

Community care

With the run-down of mental hospitals, only people suffering from the most intractable problems remained in hospital. Community care developments, however, have not gone hand-in-hand with bed closures, partly as the result of systematic underfunding, in particular of local authorities.

As a consequence, many people with SMI are admitted for short periods of inpatient care but may be discharged to low levels of aftercare. In a one-year follow-up study of people with schizophrenia being discharged from hospital, Melzer et al. (1991) found that 55% of people continued to experience psychotic symptoms and 22% were functioning socially at very poor or severely maladjusted levels. Although 94% had contact over the last 3 months with a health professional, only 16% were in residential care and 23% using day services. Further follow-up of this cohort by Conway et al. (1994) over 4 years found that 65% had been readmitted at least once. Both Melzer et al.'s and Conway et al.'s work, therefore, raised serious questions about the quality of life for people with SMI living in the community. The non-institutionalization of people with SMI had not, in itself, provided them with a reasonable quality of life.

In addition to inadequate levels of service provision, problems in access to services for this client group have also arisen out of poor care coordination. People with SMI need to access multiple services, varying over time, to optimize their quality of life, and coordination and continuity become essential (Bachrach 1981, Clifford et al. 1988). In the past the care given by the mental hospital may not have been appropriate but coordination was simpler, care being under one roof with clear lines of authority, responsibility and accountability. Now, multiple statutory and non-statutory agencies provide care, while health, social services and housing authorities each have a complex commissioning role.

Community-based services have proved acceptable to people with less SMI who would not have been referred, or would have accepted referral, for hospital care. For example Goldberg and Gater (1991) have demonstrated how community services increased by threefold the prevalence of people with less SMI in contact with mental health services.

In the face of such a massive increase in demand mental health services have had difficulty in continuing to provide adequate care to people with SMI. For example, the Audit Commission (1994), in a multi-site study, has found that community mental health nurses (CMHN) were not providing any more intensive care to people with the most severe illness than they were to the rest of their case load. Ford and Sathyamoorthy (1996) found that a community mental health team (CMHT), comprised of mainly CMHN and no social workers, was receiving so many new referrals from general practitioners (GP) that it was unable to prioritize people with the most serious problems. In this study there was little relationship between need and resources; indeed, there was evidence that people with the greatest needs were seriously under-provided with care. Butterworth (1994) summarizes the lack of attention given to people with SMI in the review of mental health nursing and extrapolates that only 20% of people with schizophrenia have contact with a CMHN.

Challenges to community services

Safety

Much of the criticism levelled at mental health services is concerned with public safety, as opposed to improving the quality of life for people with SMI. Best known is the Clunis Inquiry (Ritchie et al. 1994), called after the killing of Jonathan Zito at the hands of Christopher Clunis. Clunis's care had been a series of uncoordinated transfers of care over 5.5 years, involving 30 psychiatrists, 10 inpatient stays and three remands to prison or police custody. He also lived in a bail hostel, two rehabilitation hostels, two hostels for the homeless and six separate bed-and-breakfast accommodations. At the time of the homicide Clunis was out of contact with services and not receiving treatment for his paranoid schizophrenia.

Following concerns about the amount of contact that SMI people have with the police and courts, most areas of the UK are now covered by court diversion schemes seeking to prevent the criminalization of the mentally ill. Joseph and Potter (1993) reported on a scheme that had over 200 referrals from two inner London courts over 18 months. Of these referrals, 60% suffered from a psychotic disorder, 29% having been in hospital in the previous 6 months. Incarceration of the mentally ill still occurs and diversion from prison schemes have also been set up. Robertson et al. (1994) estimated that 15% of all receptions had a psychotic illness. Gunn et al. (1991) established that most people with a psychotic disorder do get diverted to mental healthcare before or soon after sentencing. The latter study of the prevalence of mental illness among sentenced prisoners found only 2% with a psychotic illness. The potential for prisons to take over as the new institutions for people with SMI has been demonstrated in the USA where it has been estimated, e.g. by Torrey et al. (1992), that there are 50 000 schizophrenics in jails and prisons, and that generally 6–8% of prisoners suffer from a psychosis.

On the issue of safety, Lehman et al. (1986) showed how people with SMI were more likely to be the victims rather than the perpetrators of crime, with 5% of community residents reporting having been assaulted during the past year. The situation was far worse for inpatients, with 27% reporting assaults, including two rapes by a fellow inpatient. Such fears for the safety of women patients have also arisen in the UK, and many organizations, such as MIND (The National Association for Mental Health), now call for women-only wards. However, a recent National Visit by the Mental Health Act Commission of 47% of acute admission wards in England and Wales found that only one-quarter of women had access to self-contained bedroom, bathing and toilet facilities (Ford et al. 1997).

Homelessness

Homelessness for those with SMI has also received attention as a more visible problem. Craig and Timms (1992) estimated that half of all residents of hostels for the homeless had a mental illness, one-third having a diagnosis of schizophrenia. Craig et al. (1995) went on to undertake a detailed study of the homeless mentally ill in contact with specialist teams in London. They found that former long-stay patients were rare among the homeless mentally ill, but that de-institutionalization had, in a broader sense, led to an increase in the number of the homeless mentally ill. Failure in community care provision was more common for those with the most severe illness. Of the 159 homeless people with schizophrenia, 77% had lost contact with psychiatric services, 96% with primary healthcare, 100% with social services and 38% were evicted from their housing. The researchers attributed half of these lost contacts to service failures. Craig et al. were particularly damning of the care given to the 25% of people whose latest period of homelessness followed a council housing tenancy: 'services were unable to prevent their homelessness and at times encouraged it, through rejection and misguided attempts to regulate behaviour through eviction, due to the lack of alternative, more supportive interventions'.

Needs

The highly publicized public worries about homicides, other criminal behaviour and homelessness have received much attention, but deficiencies in the quality of life, which affect very many people with SMI, go relatively unnoticed. For example, a recent survey of all those with SMI resident in one relatively affluent outer-London borough found that 13% of people had problems of aggressive or disruptive behaviour, mostly minor, but that more people (17%) were at risk of deliberate self-injury (Ford and Warner 1996). However, the most prevalent problems were not safety concerns, but unemployment (88%), poor social relationships (49%), no useful way to keep occupied (39%) and inappropriate or inadequate housing (22%).

Only 19% of Harvey's (1996) sample of all those with schizophrenia within one location were in open employment. This was probably an optimistic finding given that all levels of disability were included in this broad epidemiological study. Despite the inclusive nature of the study, 45% of people had no daytime occupation. The lack of meaningful occupation has been reported in journalistic pieces: 'You can see some of them going back and forward across the road counting their steps. They've nothing else to do. It's so sad' (Wallace 1993a); and 'Peter is a familiar figure to his neighbours, as he wanders up and down the road, clad in numerous layers of thick, dirty clothing, even in the height of summer. His distinctive appearance and the slow shuffling walk caused by his medication mark him out. Bobby, Peter's younger brother spends up to 20 hours a day alone in his room, chain smoking and staring at the walls' (Wallace 1993b).

An inevitable correlate of unemployment is low income. Goldie (1988) argues that poverty is at the root of much of the poor living conditions of people with SMI that he observed. He documented people's dependence on benefits and the effect this has on their living conditions, appearance and cleanliness, paucity of possessions and lack of involvement in meaningful activities. He cites a typical example: 'I can afford 50 pence a day for the gas fire. When that runs out I have no more heating for the rest of the day'.

Social relationships are particularly effected by SMI, in particular schizophrenia. Harvey (1996) reported that 24% of her sample had no contact with their family and that 35% had no contact with friends. Goldie (1988) gave qualitative detail of what this meant to one person: 'I have no friends – except maybe Paul who comes around here sometimes – I met him in hospital. He sometimes comes around with another ex-Claybury patient'.

The lack of social contact can lead to intolerable loneliness. Wallace (1993), for a piece in *The Times*, quoted from the diary of a young man with schizophrenia who had recently committed suicide: 'February 5', he wrote in his diary, 'Very depressed. I do not understand the circumstances of my illness. I am at a loss to know which is the right direction. I don't understand why I feel so alone or appear to be so alone. This loneliness is the thing that will KILL me in the end'.

It is not just homelessness that is a difficulty in the housing domain for people with SMI. Weller (1993) dramatically points out that next to losing a close relative a housing move is the most stressful life event and yet he gives an example of one of his patients who, after waiting a year on an acute ward, then had to move three times in 2 weeks. Wallace (1993), again in *The Times*, has also documented the poor living standards in some residential care homes: 'These places are so filthy and lonely. Last weekend I took a meal to an elderly mentally ill woman. She didn't have a piece of cutlery to eat it with. I had to borrow from next door. The people in charge don't want to hear these stories'. However, despite all the difficulties of living in the community, people with SMI do not want to live in hospital: 'I can't believe this is all mine. I keep thinking it's a dream and one day I will wake up and it will be gone and I will be back in Claybury' (Goldie 1988).

Stigma

People with SMI do not just have to contend with some of the worst material conditions in society, they also, as Warner (1994) poignantly describes, have become a pariah group. The effects of labelling and stigma compound their poor quality of life, leading to social isolation and alienation. Lehman et al. (1982) have shown how those with SMI perceive their quality of life to be worse than the general population of the USA in terms of their living situation, family situation, social relations, finances, personal safety and life in general. Further analysis revealed that those with SMI felt worse about their lives than other socially disadvantaged groups, being under substantial psychological, domestic and financial stress. Interestingly, of the mentally ill in employment, only 15% of the total were as happy as the general population with their work.

Rose (1996), who quotes two service users, has also documented this process of alienation within the British context: 'The media make people afraid of us. One person is violent and it's all over the press and then people think it applies to everyone who's been in hospital. If you're a big man like me, it's worse. People cross the street to avoid me'; and 'A man from the local mental hospital came into the shop and everyone talked about him once he'd gone. They said he shouldn't be allowed out and shouldn't be allowed in the shop. I felt so embarrassed and worried they'd find out about me'.

Warner (1994) argues that de-institutionalization may have eliminated some institutional neurosis (Barton 1959), although he documents that much of this process only moved people in the USA from hospitals to other institutions, such as prisons, where care may be even more inhumane. Warner (1994), having considered what Wing and Morris (1981) referred to as impairments, social disadvantages and adverse personal reactions, concludes that institutional neurosis has been replaced by 'existential neurosis' and poor outcome: 'Now public policy has created the poverty, unemployment and squalid conditions in which the mentally ill live in much of the Western world and, indirectly has inflamed the pessimism and alienation that are to blame for the malignant course of schizophrenia in our society'.

De-institutionalization, originally based on public concerns about the quality of life of those with SMI living in long-stay hospitals, has proceeded apace. However, people with SMI living outside of the institutions have not been able to access adequate care to optimize their quality of life, either because it is unavailable, unsuitable because it was designed for people with less severe illness, or poorly coordinated. The result has been public concern, not about the quality of life for people with SMI, but about public safety, which has in turn exacerbated poor material circumstances and increased alienation.

THE POLICY RESPONSE

1990's Legislation and guidance

De-institutionalization commenced in the 1950s, but it was not until the early 1990s that extensive legislation and policy guidance was introduced in the UK. Policy has consistently been influenced by concerns about the safety of the public, particularly inquiries into major incidents. Conclusions invariably addressed poor coordination and interagency working resulting in both poor care for users and risk to the public. In the UK, as in the USA, forms of case management have been at the core of policy, placing considerable emphasis on engagement through assertive outreach, followed by comprehensive assessment of client need, developing a negotiated package of care, direct care provision, care coordination, monitoring and review (Ryan et al. 1991). Intagliata (1982) defines case management as that which 'involves having a single person, or to the extent possible, a team of persons responsible for maintaining a long-term supportive relationship with the client, regardless of where the client is and regardless of the number of agencies involved. The Case Manager is a helper, service broker and advocate for the client'.

In the UK, both the Care Programme Approach (CPA) (DoH 1990), with the appointment of keyworkers, and care management (DoH/SSI 1990) have their roots in case management systems. Under the CPA all people in contact with specialist mental health services must have a keyworker who assesses the client's needs and coordinates the inputs of all agencies involved in care provision. The guidance is non-prescriptive on how this should happen. In practice, the professional who delivers most care is the keyworker, usually a health professional. Other agencies retain responsibility for their own care delivery. The keyworker coordinates the overall response, without the authority to direct other agencies.

Guidance on care management is more prescriptive. It is clearly the duty of local authority social services departments (LASSD) to assess each client's needs, decide on their eligibility for services against set criteria and, if eligible, commission a package of community care. Usually this role is carried out by social workers or occasionally health staff authorized by the LASSD. Care managers can thus directly coordinate and monitor the package of care delivered through the contracts they set up with the other agencies providing care.

The twin developments of the CPA and care management have led to a set of incompatible care processes. Local arrangements for combining the CPA and care management, as recommended in the Building Bridges (DoH 1995) guidance, and for the joint commissioning of care may overcome these incompatibilities (Muijen and Ford 1996). These, however, remain the exception rather than the rule (Handcock and Villaneau 1997).

Even if the CPA and care management were operating effectively, there would still be difficulties. Both are administrative systems, relying on the availability of a wide range of high-quality services. Neither care management nor CPA keyworking necessarily offer assertive outreach to link clients with services and maintain long-term contact. Nor does either approach specify low caseloads or access to adequate resources.

The development of other specific mental health policies and legislation in the UK has been reactive, prompted by the rising tide of critical public opinion over perceived failings of community care. As a result of these criticisms the then Health Secretary announced a 10-point plan for developing successful and safe community care (DoH 1993). This plan reinforced the government's support for community care while seeking to make the health and safety of patients, and the public, the paramount priority. In addition to amendments to the 1983 Mental Health Act to allow for supervised discharge, the 10-point plan placed considerable emphasis on ensuring that community care limited risk. The measures included fresh guidance on hospital discharge and continuing care in the community, training for keyworkers in their duties under the CPA and special supervision registers for patients most at risk and in need of most support.

The late 1990s, with a new UK government, has seen a continued policy emphasis on mental health. The direction of policy has though seen little change. The *Modernising Mental Health Services – Safe, Sound and Supportive* (DoH 1998) government strategy again placed the emphasis on public safety, having concluded that community care had failed under the previous government.

Positive steps

On a more positive note, the new strategy (DoH 1998), in keeping with the previous one (DoH 1996), goes on to promote a system of mental healthcare that has the potential to meet both society's safety concerns and the individual needs of service users. Essentially, a model of mental healthcare that is comprehensive, integrated and focused is required. Comprehensive in that all the necessary elements of a service are present; integrated so that mental health services function as one system through which users can receive coordinated multiple inputs that change over time; and focused so that the level and type of response from the mental health system is appropriate to the level and type of presenting need.

Such service developments have been encouraged in the UK by the provision of Challenge Funds to the NHS and Mental Illness Specific Grants (MISG) to social services. These were made available to providers who put in bids for innovative services addressing the needs of people with SMI. Although limited, they made an impact, if only by focusing thinking of providers across agencies on this group and their needs. It is hoped that further improvements in resources for both NHS and Personal Social Services (DoH 1999) will extend the impact of earlier funding by inducing whole system change.

PRINCIPLES BEHIND EFFECTIVE MODELS OF ADULT MENTAL HEALTHCARE

The main challenge for mental health services is to offer a vision of care that can be operationalized, reconciling the many contradictory demands such as being sensitive to users and offering choice, integration into the community, avoiding risk, cost efficiency and evidence based. Community care is undoubtedly vision based, which should be made explicit (Figure 10.1).

Over the past decades many research projects have offered evidence of effective components of mental health services. In particular, there is considerable evidence for assertive community treatment approaches, as reviewed by Muijen (1994), Scott and Dixon (1995a) and Marshall et al. (1997). There is also a long-standing

1. Care should be built around the individual needs of users and carers.

2. A range of services that function as a system should be available.

3. Service users should be involved in the delivery of their own care and the planning of services.

4. Mental health services should be sensitive to local needs, resources and culture.

Figure 10.1 – Community care should have explicitly stated vision

body of evidence for the use of psychotropic medication (Dixon et al. 1995) and novel drugs that are more effective for treatment-resistant schizophrenia have recently been introduced (Buchanan 1995). A growing body of evidence supports specific psychosocial interventions, such as interventions for people with schizophrenia and their families (Scott and Dixon 1995b) (see also Chapter 15). However, despite the evidence, many of these innovative service elements and interventions have not become common practice.

It is worth noting the contrasting experiences of introducing new antipsychotics, and community-based care. The introduction of novel antipsychotic drugs, such as clozapine, was not unduly problematic, although the high cost of such drugs has led to some controls on their availability. The traditional hospital-orientated system provided a favourable environment, since psychiatrists were in the lead and could prescribe, and a system to undertake blood tests to monitor for catastrophic side-effects could fit in easily with inpatient care and standard outpatient care. Setting up systems to allow people with schizophrenia to start on such drugs without being admitted to hospital has been far more difficult.

In comparison, assertive community treatment services have been difficult to establish and sustain (Audini et al. 1994). Often demonstration community research projects such as the Daily Living Programme found it hard to integrate with a hospital-orientated system. The tension of having a community and a hospital-orientated system running in parallel is not sustainable because individuals with SMI need to access a whole system, not parts of two systems. For specific interventions to become standard practice, it is first necessary to have a system of mental healthcare within which they can operate.

Services should be established around the needs of individual service users and their carers, mostly relatives (Figure 10.2). Services built up in this way will be community orientated as this is where the vast majority of service users live. Service users will access most mental healthcare via their GP and the primary healthcare team. The next level of access should be home-orientated services acting as the gatekeeper to all other specialist mental health services, including hospital care. It is essential that services act as a system – the second principle – so that individual users can rapidly access the services they require while the system ensures that care remains coordinated over the longer term.

A system of care needs to consist of vertically and horizontally integrated services. Users need to move from level to level in a seamless fashion. For example, referring from primary care to the CMHT (levels 1 to 2), or from the CMHT to a forensic unit (levels 2 to 3), should not be hindered by complex and time-consuming bureaucracy. Equally, referral from daycare to a work unit, both at similar levels, should be smooth. This requires the responsibility of an individual professional, whether they be called a keyworker, a case manager or a care manager. The care system should fit in with such an individual approach, rather than keyworkers having to adapt to the existing system, i.e. a shift from supply- to demand-driven care. The consequence is that the building block of service should be a locality or sector with a population between 40 000 and 100 000 people, allowing planning at an individual need level, rather than at district level, traditionally the unit of planning for a hospital. This will be discussed in more detail below.

The third principle concerns user access and acceptability. This can lead to a paradox, since the more community orientated the service, the more accessible and acceptable it becomes. However, as Goldberg and Gater (1991) have shown, it is mainly those with less severe illness who become the new users of such mental health services, potentially marginalizing people with SMI. Mental health professionals visiting at home or at a local GP surgery, offering counselling and other forms of non-specific care, is a far cry from a long journey to a large and frightening institution. As mental health services become more popular for a larger number of

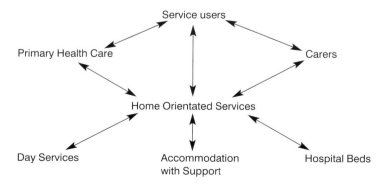

Figure 10.2 – Mental Health Services

people with less severe illness, many of those with the most severe illness find that such services are less relevant to their needs. When mental health services were predominantly provided in institutions, such people became institutionalized and continued to receive services. They may quickly lose contact with community services they are poorly motivated to use.

The unwillingness to engage with mental health services becomes doubly apparent with users from social groups who feel alienated from mainstream society, such as those from many ethnic minorities. Culturally sensitive approaches that take the service out to people on their terms, such as the Tulip Outreach Service in East Haringey, London, can successfully engage with 95% of users (Gauntlett et al. 1996). For today's mental health services user involvement at all levels of service development and provision has become a necessity.

Fourth, it has to be accepted that there is no one model of mental healthcare that can be bought off the shelf and plugged in. The model developed in each locality has to be based on local need with an appreciation of local financial and human resources, and a sensitivity to local culture. For example, in one locality it may make sense to pool resources and have one CMHT that meets all needs at all times of day and night, in another locality it might be better to set up an out-of-hours team in addition to the CMHT. What is clear is that there are functions that home-orientated services must fulfil, but that these can be fulfilled by varying structural configurations. These functions will be considered below within a service framework.

THE NECESSARY ELEMENTS

CMHT and uni- versus multi-disciplinary working

There is a considerable body of research evidence to support the formation of locality based multi-disciplinary CMHT as the principal access point for mental health services (Onyett and Ford 1996). This is not to say that CMHT should attempt to undertake multi-disciplinary work under all circumstances. Where users have a lower level of need, uni-disciplinary working should rightly continue. Many people who come into contact with specialist mental health services do not need input from more than one person and a team approach then risks becoming inefficient. It is still vital that professionals work together so that individual people receive appropriate services with effective overall coordination of services. The most common uni-professional services are psychiatrist, psychologist and psychotherapy outpatient clinics. In common with specialist teams there should be clear protocols for how these clinics relate to other mental health services, in particular CMHT. The review of psychotherapy services (NHS Executive 1996a) has in particular promoted the idea of psychologists and psychotherapists providing specialist training and supervisory inputs for generic CMHT. The review also states that there should be clear protocols for whom these clinics should work with, what they will offer to these clients and how they will monitor and report outcomes.

Services have to prioritize the needs of people with SMI who will usually require, and benefit from, multi-disciplinary interventions. Teamwork is indicated for people with such needs. Furthermore, there is evidence for the effectiveness of multi-disciplinary teams (Marks et al. 1994) but less research support for uni-disciplinary working (Muijen et al. 1994).

It is important to have a clear single route of referral to mental health services to ensure that referrals are allocated to the most appropriate service, whether uni- or multi-disciplinary, within such services to the most appropriate member of staff, and to monitor the focus of the service. If not, it will be difficult to prioritize the needs of people with SMI and to link needs with supply. With multiple access points to mental health services for each and every profession, no systematic control is available, and a shift towards care for people with less severe or urgent conditions can be hard to avoid.

CMHT: specialist or generic?

CMHT are expected to provide a wide range of functions, such as speedy assessments and a rapid response to crisis for new and existing users of mental health services, short-term interventions for people with less severe problems, and assertive outreach and continuing care for people with long-term and severe mental health problems (DoH 1999). Both commissioners and providers around the country are taxed with the question of how best to organize such services in practice.

The two main options are to set up a number of separate teams in a locality, each offering a specialist function, or to combine several functions within one generic team.

Evaluation findings and experiences of the eight sites in England and Wales funded by the Sainsbury Mental Health Initiative to implement state-of-the-art community care indicate some lessons for the development of service models (Minghella and Ford 1997a). Two major principles have become apparent: decisions should be based on an understanding of the local culture of services and service development, and on a local assessment of needs and resources.

The CMHT described in Figure 10.3 was set up to provide a number of functions within the one team. However, in its first year, the team found it difficult to achieve most of its objectives. First, targeting was ineffective: fewer than half of its clients had a diagnosis of a psychotic disorder. Second, many people were discharged from hospital without the subsequent involvement of the CMHT, implying poor integration between hospital and community services. For example, between April 1995 and March 1996, of 73 people discharged from hospital, 38 (52%) were not on the CMHT caseload in May 1996. Third, the formal GP liaison scheme has not been implemented. Finally, the team has not extended its hours, partly because there was a new development of a district wide out-of-hours on call service to which local community psychiatric nurses (CPN) contribute, and partly because some out-of-hours services are provided through daycare facilities locally.

The team charged with integrating a wide range of functions experienced major problems in implementation. But the problems may not be due to the nature of an integrated team *per se*, but, rather, to the required shift from one set of values and practices to another. Originally, there were separate teams dealing with all-comers and offering interventions such as counselling to people with less severe mental health problems. The newly configured multi-disciplinary team targeting the severely mentally ill meant a radical shake up for the existing staff, having skills and attitudes more suited to the former type of service. For example, while a number of staff have diplomas in counselling, none received training in skills known to be effective with SMI, such as psychosocial interventions. The staff also lacked clarity about the team's role and their own professional roles and responsibilities within it.

Stein (1992) indicated the difficulties of innovating against the tide when he was involved in developing the first assertive community treatment teams for people with SMI in Madison, WI, USA. He faced strong resistance from staff based in the

Principal plans for CMHT under Sainsbury Mental Health Initiative:	Reconfigure existing community mental health services to set up new CMHT for people with most severe and enduring problems from 8am to 8pm. Plus primary care liaison.
Location:	Suburban
Main agencies involved:	Health & Social Services
Staffed by:	CPNs, SWs, OT, Community Support Workers. Team Leaders – 1 CPN, 1 SW
Relevant functions for CMHT (aims):	Target SMI
	Integrate community service through central focus of the CMHT
	Extend hours
	Primary health care liaison

Figure 10.3 – Case history 1: providing all statutory community mental health care through one Community Mental Health Team (CMHT)

mental health centre. Staff who did change only changed *where* they worked (e.g. working in clients' homes) not **what** they did. When they were given the choice of either leaving their job or working in the new team, most resigned. On the other hand, new workers who were appointed specifically for the new teams were keen and able to work effectively. It may be that appointing new staff to novel teams is a way of driving service development initially, although this is hardly possible on a large scale. More feasible is the option to introduce change agents into teams, preferably in leadership roles.

This multi-disciplinary team (Figure 10.4) was set up to work with people in crisis with the aim of avoiding unnecessary hospitalization. Responding to a clear need, it had over 370 referrals in its first year; of these 210 were accepted as clients. It was well targeted and referrals were generally of those who were at risk of hospitalization, rather than the feared over-representation of people in temporary emotional crisis who can easily overwhelm similar services (Ford and Kwakwa 1996). For example, the vast majority had psychotic disorders or was considered suicidal on referral (66%). The team achieved this by taking most of its referrals from the generic CMHT, which acted as a filter (only 20% of referrals were from a GP). The rapid response team acted as gatekeeper to hospital beds. This was only possible with a community consultant psychiatrist working as part of the team. He had the assessment skills, power and authority to ensure that admission was used only as a last resort, and had access to beds as necessary.

Despite the fact that this was a 24-h service, most face-to-face client contacts took place within reasonable working hours. Of a month's 360 face-to-face client contacts, only 18 (5%) took place between 20:00 and 09:00 hours, with just eight (2%) after midnight. These figures are not insignificant – they account for between four and five contacts a week – but it may be that a separate team is not necessary to provide this level of cover for such a relatively small number of contacts, and better service coordination could involve existing emergency provision.

Coordination is a major potential problem when separate teams combine to provide 24-h cover or target particular groups. While in this service there were good alliances with the CMHT, integration with the inpatient wards was not so strong. Very few referrals came from inpatient units for facilitating early discharge (about 6%), resulting in a weak link in the coordination of care for people leaving hospital.

In this area separate teams for GP liaison, continuing care and assertive outreach are being developed. This could lead to gaps, overlap and confusion between agencies about which teams provide which sorts of service for which clients. A profusion of teams may result both in inefficient duplication and in people 'falling through the net'. Some service users may find it difficult to receive coordinated input from two or more agencies or teams when they need it. Other groups may be excluded by the various entry criteria that operate for the different teams.

Principal plans for crisis team under Sainsbury Mental Health Initiative:	Set up a new emergency team to act as gatekeepers to the in-patient beds, assess people in crisis and treat in the community where possible.
Location:	Inner city
Main agencies involved:	Health & Social Services
Staffed by:	CPNs, SWs, Consultant Psychiatrist, Community Support Workers. Team Leaders – CPN
Relevant functions for crisis teams (aims):	Assess all people at risk of admission
	Maintain people at home where possible
	Control hospital admissions and length of stay
	Facilitate early discharge
	Be available 24 hours a day

Figure 10.4 – Case history 2: setting up a separate rapid response team

Addressing problems of coordination, in another Sainsbury Mental Health Initiative team, a CPN manager and a social work manager share management of a specialist team providing intensive care to the most-in-need. Each manager has other additional responsibilities across health and social services. The advantage is that the managers have knowledge, understanding and responsibility about the rest of the community services, which should promote good integration with existing services. However, managers re-deploy staff from the specialist team to provide cover for staff in the generic CMHT when necessary. Since the CMHT is under-resourced and works under stressful conditions, along with high sickness rates, this happens frequently, leading to a diluted and reduced service by the specialist team.

Problems of service coordination can be exacerbated by inequity of resource distribution across services. When new, separate teams are set up they tend to receive an injection of resources – financial, planning, training. Meanwhile, existing services remain pressured, resulting in envy and friction. A lack of resources has been identified as a major source of pressure for CMHT (Onyett et al. 1995).

Furthermore, while separate designated teams may be more responsive and target effectively, clear thinking around targeting and resourcing is still required. The seriously mentally ill are not a homogenous group. There are at least two groups with different needs: those with acute and possibly recurring mental health problems, and those with stable, long-standing disabilities. One specialist team has targeted the latter group and has a caseload of about 95% people with SMI. But this group constitutes only about 40% of local people with psychotic diagnoses. Moreover, the team is only looking after about half of those with a psychotic diagnosis **who have had a recent hospital admission**. So, many seriously mentally ill people with acute problems and needs receive care from a more pressured and less targeted service than those with serious and enduring, but relatively stable, conditions. The conclusion is that the target group should be defined across a range of dimensions, including their history of using services.

Other yet more highly specialized teams may be warranted if there is sufficient local need. A balance needs to be reached between needs and resources, and many of such services are provided for a larger area than the locality based CMHT. For example, many drug and alcohol, forensic, perinatal and eating disorder teams have a district wide or broader responsibility. It should be clear what the precise responsibility of such teams are, and how such tertiary teams relate to other mental health services, both at the inter-agency and at the individual service user levels. This is particularly important for people with 'dual diagnoses', i.e. a combination of SMI and drug or alcohol misuse. Some areas will also find sufficient need for other specialist teams such as for homeless people or people with SMI who have come into contact with the criminal justice system. The emphasis should always be specialist services working to the local team and not the local team thinking that they are subordinate to specialist services.

Minghella and Ford's (1997a) conclusions are summarized in Figure 10.5.

- Implementing change requires consideration of the history and culture in which that change is to take place, the local service context and the needs of priority groups locally. These multi-faceted elements influence how effectively new services can work with those most in need and whether services will be properly integrated.

- When considering how to implement new service structures, the attitudes and skills of staff need to be addressed. This requires an acceptance of the radical nature of the changes expected at the level of service delivery.

- Separate teams can work well and target effectively. For crisis response, they need to access most referrals from secondary sources and act as gate-keepers to hospital beds, which requires a psychiatrist to be part of the team.

- However, if services are to be responsive to a wider range of needs through the use of several separate teams, there could be a confusing proliferation of teams and poor service co-ordination. It may be more useful to view separate teams as a lever for change.

- Setting up separate teams can lead to inequity of resource allocation, which in turn may affect targeting and service co-ordination. If resources are directed primarily to the specialist teams, other services will be hard-pressed and there may be a temptation to dilute the specialist service in order to address under-resourcing elsewhere.

- Separate teams for the SMI may mean service gaps or overlap, unless a local assessment of the needs of identified client groups has been carried out. Such an assessment must recognize the diversity of needs, including service use. If not, planning, financial and training resources may be misplaced.

Figure 10.5 – Summary of Minghella and Ford's findings

CMHT and primary care

CMHT of all types have to work with staff in primary healthcare teams, especially the GP. It has been estimated that 20% of the population has a psychological problem at some point during any one year and that one-third of those visiting their GP has a definable mental illness (Goldberg and Bridges 1988). In a traditional mental health service only the most severely ill would have been accepted. Although a community-oriented service significantly increases the number of people accepted by the specialist services, this still leaves the majority to be cared for by the primary healthcare team (Goldberg and Huxley 1991, Jackson et al. 1993). Referral should not mean comprehensive transfer of responsibility. People with the most severe illness have also been reported to have high levels of physical ill-health (Allebeck 1989) and care, therefore, needs to be shared between specialist mental health staff and primary healthcare teams.

Specialist mental health teams and primary healthcare teams have often found working together problematic (Durcan 1997). Typically, primary care professionals have argued that specialist mental health services are unclear about how they should be contacted in the first place, are poor at communication and are unwilling to offer services to people who do not meet their overly restrictive definitions of SMI. Furthermore, specialist mental health services' definitions of SMI are not always relevant in a primary setting. On the other hand, mental health professionals claim that few primary healthcare staff have any training or interest in mental health. Therefore, they seem to make vast numbers of referrals for people with non-severe illness who could be treated by primary care staff in the same way that they care for non-severe general medical conditions.

Considering the large number of GPs as compared with general psychiatrists, respectively covering populations of about 2500 and 40 000 each, perspectives are bound to differ. However, each is tremendously pressured, and increasingly so. The GP is experiencing an increase in visits and, disproportionately, of people with mental illness. About one-third of attenders suffers from a mental illness, mostly neuroses. Nevertheless, 95% of those with a mental health problem are cared for exclusively by the primary care team, including 40% of those with schizophrenia (Nazarath and King 1992). People attending with mental health problems visit more often, and visits are of longer duration. In combination, the burden on primary care is considerable.

So, how should mental health and primary care services work together? Several models have been suggested such as liaison or attachments (Strathdee and Sutherby 1996). Another model is to maintain the CMHT but to have separate mental health link workers working with primary healthcare teams. Such link workers should be responsible for setting up care coordination systems, including the identification of all people with SMI on the lists of each primary healthcare team followed by the application of the CPA to the practice. Such systems work best when the mental health link worker is also the main provider of care for patients with SMI attending the practice, but not requiring multi-disciplinary input.

Day opportunities

Peripatetic home-oriented staff cannot provide all the necessary elements of care. They need to access other services, such as day opportunities, while sustaining their overall care coordination role. Day opportunities is a complex area of provision as funding may come from health, social service, education, employment and, indeed, other sources such as the European Community and the UK National Lottery. In addition, there is a wide variety of statutory and non-statutory providers. This complexity is not helped by the almost total lack of rigorous research evidence!

The one exception is the provision of acute day hospital care, funded by health authorities, as an alternative or compliment to acute inpatient care. Creed et al. (1990) established in well-conducted studies that day hospitals that provide this function are cost effective. However, this model is not widely implemented and many day hospitals provide on-going support to people with long-term needs or short-term psychotherapy to the less severely ill.

Beyond day hospital care there is no research evidence to go on. However, there is a growing consensus among all agencies, as well as among users and carers, that a range of options, available in the least stigmatizing locations, is required. In particular, work schemes are highly valued by users (Pozner et al. 1996). Again, a range of provision will be required as schemes should be small in scale and no one project can meet all needs resulting from very different levels of disability. Shneider and Hallam (1996) have shown that work schemes are usually less expensive than standard day settings. Drop-ins run by service users are also well supported.

Traditional day centres run by statutory agencies are not generally well supported by service users. In particular, they dislike the forced structure and group activities. Day services are usually more popular when provided by the voluntary or user-led sectors who can provide dynamic schemes in flexible ways, at hours that people want them and in locations that users prefer. The role of the statutory sector is probably best left to day hospital care and then to support non-statutory organizations in establishing and maintaining small-scale, local, innovative day opportunities.

Residential supports

Having somewhere to live, somewhere to call home, is vital for us all. For people with SMI the need is greater as their mental health problems may affect the opportunities they have to obtain secure housing and, once obtained, their ability to keep hold of their home. In turn, not having housing may adversely affect peoples' mental health problems. The importance of housing, with adequate support, is emphasized in dramatic terms by inquiries into tragic events (Ritchie et al. 1994). But, difficulties with obtaining appropriate housing are common place, with, for example, 25% of London acute mental health beds occupied by those in need of move-on accommodation. Yet more common are those who have housing that may be insecure or inappropriate to their needs.

Responsibilities for providing housing have changed over the past decade. Health authorities originally provided much accommodation for people with the most serious mental illness within large hospitals. Those with less serious difficulties were, by and large, expected to make provision for themselves, with the help of their families. As hospital beds have declined, responsibilities have shifted. Provision for the mentally ill in the UK has now become the responsibility of the local authority social services departments, housing departments, housing associations, and other voluntary and private sector bodies. It is seldom seen as the health authority's responsibility to provide accommodation, although they may provide the staff support that people need.

Financial systems and access to housing systems have been affected by the introduction of assessment and care management under the NHS and Community Care Act 1990. Before 1 April 1993 large amounts of funding for accommodation with attached care was obtained from the Social Security, where there was no budget cap and anyone who was eligible could receive funding. Now, social services departments have to allocate funding for accommodation, with care on the basis of need, from a fixed budget. The Act has also promoted the growth of the independent sector, in particular housing associations and other voluntary sector providers, as local authorities become 'enablers' as opposed to direct providers.

The burden of decreased NHS provision has also fallen on local authority housing departments who have decreasing stocks, through council house sales, to meet housing needs. The local authority's role in housing is also seen increasingly as 'enabler', not provider, and there has been a similar growth in the role of housing associations for the provision of affordable ordinary housing.

As with day opportunities a range of specialist accommodation provision is required. At the most intensive this will be '24-h nursed care' where residents have the legal status of inpatients and can be detained under provisions of the mental health act (NHS Executive 1996b). There is evidence that users prefer this type of care to either an acute ward or a long stay ward and that the clinical outcomes are superior (Hyde et al. 1987). However, users would still prefer their own self-contained homes (Rose and Muijen 1998).

Bearing in mind user preference, most models now try to separate out accommodation from support (Carling 1993). In this way, those with SMI can have self-contained and stable accommodation while receiving variable levels of support. One model that has sustained over many years is dispersed intensively supported housing (DISH) schemes. In DISH schemes, users not only have their own tenancies, but also receive intensive support from a peripatetic team. Support workers can spend 24 h a day with someone, for a few days if necessary. These schemes are often run in conjunction with local authority housing departments or housing associations that own the dwellings. It is often a requirement of the tenancy agreement that support be provided.

Some people's social disabilities are so great that they require support in communal living situations and others may prefer the social contact that goes with group living. As with day opportunities the most sensitive, flexible and non-stigmatized models are those provided by the voluntary sector. The role of statutory staff will likewise be as supporters, rather than direct providers of residential care. For commissioners of care there will need to be monitoring of standards to avoid a repeat of the scandals that occurred in the Victorian institutions. The National Housing Federation and the Mental Health Foundation (1996) have developed a useful good practice guide. This has further been developed by Warner et al. (1997).

Inpatient care

The number of inpatient beds may have fallen quite dramatically over the second half of the 20th century. However, they are still an essential element of community-focused mental health services. To be effective, inpatient care must be fully integrated with the rest of the system of mental healthcare. Contemporary models of mental healthcare do not see admission as the start of care or discharge as the end. Rather, there is continuous contact with mental health services for as long as is required that may, from time to time, require that the individual spends time in a hospital. Therefore, inpatient care must relate to the core of the system, the community team, as well as to the other elements of day opportunities and accommodation with support.

In a recent study of the pathway through care for 100 consecutive discharges Minghella and Ford (1997b) found that relationships between the inpatient service and the rest of the mental health system were not fully effective. Community staff, such as CPN and social workers, were not doing 'in-reach' work to assist with achieving timely planned discharge. In part this appeared to be not only because of their heavy workload, but also because they felt that they had transferred some of their responsibilities once someone was admitted to hospital. Day hospitals, which can function as an alternative to admission or allow for early discharge (Strathdee and Sutherby 1996), were not functioning as acute treatment centres. They had evolved as continuing care centres and, therefore, had long waiting lists making them difficult to access for the acutely ill. Suitable accommodation with support was also not available and 10% of the discharges, 26% of occupied bed days, had been delayed for this reason. The difficulty in the area under study was that accommodation with integrated support had been developed for former long-stay patients. New long-term users of services were reluctant to be placed in communal living circumstances such as these and require more self-contained options, with a high level of support.

Of equal concern to the integration of inpatient care with the broader system of mental healthcare is the quality of care provided on the wards. In the UK, morale has been reported as low (Carson et al. 1995); and patients also have little contact with nursing staff. For example, the Mental Health Act Commission (Ford et al. 1997a), under their statutory powers to visit wards, found that there were no staff in contact with patients on 25% of the wards they visited. The commission visited 47% of wards in the UK on one day for this report, and also found that only one-third of women had access to women-only facilities where men had no access.

It is clear that inpatient ward staff must be given the right leadership, management and training. In leadership terms they must be convinced that their work is as worthwhile and as important as that of community staff. Too many staff have been affected by the philosophy of community 'good'–hospital 'bad'. To feel part of an integrated system of care inpatient wards need to be part of the same management unit as the other components of the system. They should not be managed as a separate inpatient unit. Staff also need to acquire contemporary skills to work with a more severely ill group of patients. The level of severity of problems that inpatients have has risen dramatically as the number of beds has fallen. One-third of patients (Ford et al. 1997a) are detained against their will and two-thirds have a psychotic disorder (Shepherd et al. 1997). Counselling for people with neurosis is now of only limited value in these environments. Cognitive–behavioural therapies for people with considerable thought disorder have been shown to be effective and should be in more general use (Drury et al. 1996) (see Chapter 15).

Finally, as with all the other elements of the system of care, there will be a need for a range of services. This should include general acute inpatient care, intensive care for people with acute safety needs, and medium and high secure care for those with significant offending histories. There may also be advantages to 'step-down' units that provide a lower level of, usually nurse-led, care to people close to discharge or awaiting suitable long-term placement. In addition, issues of gender must be considered so that a safe environment can be provided.

INTEGRATION: THE MANAGEMENT AND ORGANIZATION OF CARE

Management and organizational processes are required that integrate services and support their long-term sustainable development. It is most helpful to think about these processes from the perspective of the individual user upwards, through team and locality levels, to health and local authorities and, indeed, to the level of government policy.

Integrating care for individual users

Some form of 'case management' process is necessary to ensure that care is both coordinated and continuous. However, it should be remembered that the research evidence for case management indicates that this approach only brings about benefits when utilized for people with the most severe illness (Ford et al. 1997b, c) and when it is linked to a therapeutic process as an integral part of assertive community treatment (Marshall et al. 1997). The English CPA, if implemented in keeping with the more recent guidance which recommends a 'tiered approach' (DoH 1995), provides a useful framework. Following this guidance case management should prioritize people with the most SMI who meet criteria for the top tier of the three-tiered CPA. For those receiving this level of intensive organization and follow-up of their care, there should be a clearly identified keyworker responsible for the coordination, provision and monitoring of all elements of care. The care plan has to be negotiated with other agencies and the service user following an assessment of need. Care plans should be copied to the service user. The CPA keyworker should take responsibility for the provision of home-oriented services including the provision of assertive follow-up to ensure that the user does not lose contact with services. Clearly this is a time-consuming role and keyworkers should have reasonable caseloads. There is some research evidence that caseloads should be a maximum of 15 top-tier clients per keyworker (Bond et al. 1995).

For people on the lower tiers of the CPA, there should be a less intensive form of case management that may be as simple as the user knowing who to contact in the first instance if problems occur concerning their mental health.

The co-existence of a requirement for local authority social services department to undertake a needs assessment and appoint a care manager for all people who may require some form of social care does create additional organizational difficulties. Typically, there is a low degree of overlap between people who have a local authority care manager and those who have been identified for the top tier of the CPA (Figure 10.6) (Ford and Rose 1997). There are examples of further integration of health and social care in England. In Waltham Forest, Essex, all social workers, most of whom function as both care managers and approved social workers under the Mental Health Act, have been fully seconded to the local NHS Trust under the terms of a service agreement. The management of day and residential services was retained in-house by the local authority, although these services can be purchased by care managers. Local authorities can also put out for tender all of its social care provision to other local providers. In the London Borough of Westminster, the city council has contracted out its day and residential provider services, but not care management or approved social work services, to Riverside NHS Trust, which already provided healthcare in the south of the borough. This has unintentionally created a natural experiment about the

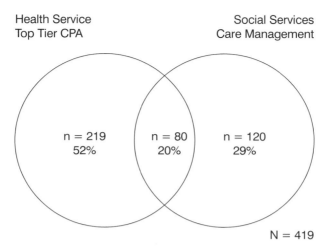

Figure 10.6 – Clients in receipt of CPA and care management (from Ford & Rose 1997)

effectiveness of a single or separate provider model. Health and social care are provided by one agency (Riverside) in the south and by two agencies (Riverside for social care; a different NHS Trust for healthcare) in the north. Early results from an evaluation of this service have revealed greater levels of communication between health and social care staff in the south when compared with the north (Figure 10.7) (Warner and Ford 1996).

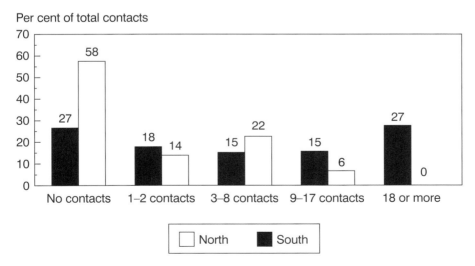

Figure 10.7 – Frequency of communication contacts in North and South Westminster (health and social care provided by one agency in the south)

Integrating care for localities

Although it is necessary to separate the different elements of mental healthcare to describe them and discuss their internal functioning, it is equally necessary to consider how they operate together as one system. The system is usually intended to function at a locality level.

The size of a locality will vary according to the level of need, density of population and naturally occurring size of communities. Generally a UK locality will have a total population of about 100 000 people. Within the locality there will usually be one or more CMHT and a range of day, residential and inpatient services. Often these services will be dedicated to only the one locality, but not always so. For example, an NHS Trust may provide a CMHT, a ward and several residential settings within a locality. Some NHS services such as rehabilitation and forensic teams will have a wider responsibility. However, other complementary or even overlapping local services, including residential services and daycare are likely to be purchased by social services, although often run by the independent sector. This can cause considerable perverse incentives and bureaucracy, both within and especially across agencies (Muijen and Ford 1996).

This raises two issues: the organizational scale of health services and the split across the range of agencies responsible for aspects of mental healthcare. The care provided by the NHS is likely to be managed by one organization across several localities. Typically a population of 200 000–500 000 will be covered, although this is rising. Again, there is no blueprint for the ideal size of management organization. The local context of service development, resource availability and identified need should be the prime drivers for decisions on the over-arching management of services. A recent review of the evidence for the shift towards larger general hospitals concluded that ideal cost economies of scale were reached at a relatively small level and that the benefits of larger scale operations had to be justified in terms of quality (Sheldon 1997). For mental health services it is important to consider whether the organization is large enough to contain a critical mass of highly skilled clinicians sufficient to offer stimulation and support across the whole structure. Another critical mass of 'change agents' is necessary to bring about long-term sustainable improvements in services.

Integrated commissioning of services at the locality level will be vital in creating shared responsibility for services across the range of providers, all accountable to a single agent. A locality-commissioning group can act as the gel between a variety of local providers. In this way the advantages of having a number of local providers offering a broad range of flexible services can be obtained without all the disadvantages of a fragmented system. The present situation is not facilitating this. Although the NHS is likely to be the largest provider, local authorities and the independent sector are also important contributors to the overall system of mental healthcare. For example, CMHT cannot operate as teams if they are receiving three different sets of priorities from health authorities, social services and GPs. For integrated commissioning to happen in the UK context, the health authority, local authority and GPs need to agree a unified local strategy for mental health, and this needs to be followed through by combining budgets. Although this is currently illegal, there are many examples of creative systems that by-pass this, and the UK government is keen to support such initiatives.

Although the most important level of organization is the locality, there is also a need to have a broad strategic framework at the local and health authority levels. In particular, there are the many services that have to be commissioned at this supra-locality level. Authorities will need to ensure they work together to a clear strategy and implementation plan, and focus on locality level and community needs. Handcock and Villaneau (1997) identified that a minority of authorities has joint strategies. To move forward the guidance shown in Figure 10.8 may be helpful.

CONCLUSIONS

Development of comprehensive community services for people with SMI between 16 and 64 years of age is tremendously complex, involving a wide range of decisions about priorities and pay-offs, especially considering the tight budgets available. This has not been helped by unrealistic expectations: high in terms of therapeutic benefit, low when considering cost.

- jointly agreed between each health authority and all local authorities within catchment area

- active involvement of key providers from NHS Trusts and social services

- representation of other relevant agencies – voluntary sector, user/care organizations and housing

- representation on the strategy group of people with organizational backing and the ability to commit resources

- health and social services to have formal agreement for the involvement of GPs

- joint strategic timescales congruent with other organizational time scales

- public acknowledgement of achievements and failures against previous years measurable objectives

- transparency of financial statement

- chairs of health authority, social services and Trust(s) to sign off

- public acknowledgement of each agency's political, economic and social priorities

---

Figure 10.8 – Criteria for developing joint strategies (after Handcok and Villaneu 1997)

It has become clear that community care is not a simple alternative to institutional care. The number of people in contact with mental health services has trebled and the range of services available is far broader, with different skills required for staff (Duggan et al. 1997). Nevertheless, despite many obstacles, there has been considerable progress with the development of comprehensive and locally available services across the Western world. The challenge now is to integrate these services into a coherent system of mental healthcare that prioritizes care of the most severely ill and achieves a match between needs and resources. Research into comprehensive and integrated models of mental healthcare shows the way forward. In particular, there is now considerable evidence for assertive outreach systems of care (Sainsbury Centre for Mental Health 1998). With these models the twin demands of achieving an optimal quality of life for service users and meeting public confidence can be met.

References

Allebeck P. Schizophrenia: a life-shortening illness. Schizophrenia Bulletin 1989; 15: 81–89.

Audini B, Marks I, Lawrence R, Connolly J, Watts V. Home-based versus outpatient/inpatient care for people with serious mental illness. British Journal of Psychiatry 1994; 165: 204–210.

Audit Commission. Finding A Place: A Review of Mental Health Services For Adults. London: HMSO, 1994.

Bachrach L. Continuity of care for chronic mental patients: a conceptual analysis. American Journal of Psychiatry 1981; 138: 1449–1456.

Barton W. Institutional Neurosis. Bristol: Wright, 1959.

British Journal of Psychiatry paper on ward in a house.

Bond G, McGrew J, Fekete D. Assertive outreach for frequent users of psychiatric hospitals: a meta-analysis. Journal of Mental Health Administration 1995; 22: 4–16.

Buchanan R. Clozapine: Effically and safety. Schizophrenia Bulletin 1995; 21: 579–591.

Butterworth A. Working in Partnership. London: HMSO, 1994.

Carling PJ. Housing and supports for persons with mental illness: emerging approaches to research and practice. Hospital and Community Psychiatry 1993; 44: 439–449.

Carson J, Fagin L, Ritter S. (eds) Stress and Coping in Mental Health Nursing. London: Chapman & Hall, 1995.

Clifford P, Craig T, Sayce E. Towards Coordinated Care. London: Sainsbury Centre for Mental Health, 1988.

Conway A, Melzer D, Hale A. The outcome of targeting community mental health services: evidence from the West Lambeth schizophrenia cohort. British Medical Journal 1994; 308: 627–630.

Craig T, Bayliss E, Klein O, Manning O, Reader L. The Homeless Mentally Ill Initiative: An Evaluation of Four Clinical Teams. London: Department of Health and Mental Health Foundation, 1995.

Craig T, Timms P. Out of the wards and onto the streets? De-institutionalization and home-lessness in Britain. Journal of Mental Health 1992; 1: 265–275.

Creed F, Black D, Anthony P, Osborn M, Thomas P, Tomenson B. Randomised controlled trial of day patient versus inpatient psychiatric treatment. British Medical Journal 1990; 300: 1033–1037.

Davidge M, Elias S, Jayes B, Wood K, Yates J. Survey of English Mental Illness Hospitals. Birmingham: Health Services Management Centre, 1993.

Department of Health. Building Bridges: A Guide to Arrangements for Inter-agency Working for the Care and Protection of Severely Mentally Ill People. Wetherby: Department of Health, 1995.

Department of Health. Legislation Planned to Provide for Supervised Discharge of Psychiatric Patients. Press release H93/908. London: DoH, 1993.

Department of Health. Modernising Mental Health Services: NHS Modernisation Fund for Mental Health Services and Mental Health Grant 1999/2002 (HSC 1999/038: LAC(99)8). London: DoH, 1999.

Department of Health. Modernising Mental Health Services: Safe, Sound and Supportive. London: DoH, 1998.

Department of Health. The Care Programme Approach for People with a Mental Illness Referred to the Specialist Psychiatric Services. (HC(90)23). London: Department of Health, 1990.

Department of Health. The Spectrum of Care: Local Services for People with Severe Mental Health Problems. Leeds: DoH, 1996.

Department of Health/SSI. Caring for People: Community Care in the Next Decade and Beyond, Policy Guidance. London: HMSO, 1990.

Dixon L, Lehman A, Levine J. Conventional antipsychotic medications for schizophrenia. Schizophrenia Bulletin 1995; 21: 567–577.

Drury V, Birchwood M, Cochrane R, MacMillan F. Cognitive therapy and recovery from acute psychosis: a controlled trial I. Impact on psychotic symptoms. British Journal of Psychiatry 1996; 169: 593–601.

Duggan M, Ford R, Hill R, Holmshaw J, McCulloch A, Warner L, Muijen M, Raftery J, Strong S, Wood H. Pulling Together: The Future Roles and Training of Mental Health Staff. London: Sainsbury Centre for Mental Health, 1997.

Durcan G. Evaluation of Mental Health Nurse Attachments to Primary Care. London: Sainsbury Centre for Mental Health, 1997.

Ford R, Durcan G, Warner L, Hardy P. The National Visit: A One-day Visit to 309 Acute Psychiatric Wards by the Mental Health Act Commission in Collaboration with the Sainsbury Centre for Mental Health. London: Sainsbury Centre for Mental Health, 1997a.

Ford R, Kwakwa K. Rapid reaction, speedy recovery. Health Service Journal 1996; 18 April: 30–31.

Ford R, Raftery J, Ryan P, Beadsmoore A, Craig T, Muijen M. Intensive case management for people with serious mental illness: II. Site 2. Cost-effectiveness. Journal of Mental Health 1997c; 6: 191–199.

Ford R, Rose D. Into the wilderness? Community Care (Inside) 1997; 28 August: 2–4.

Ford R, Ryan P, Beadsmoore A, Craig T, Muijen M. Intensive case management for people with serious mental illness: I Site 2. Clinical and social outcome. Journal of Mental Health 1997b; 6: 181–190.

Ford R, Sathyamoorthy G. Team Games. Health Service Journal 1996; 27 June: 32–33.

Ford R, Warner L. Reasoning the Need. Health Service Journal 1996; 30 May: 24–25.

Gauntlett N, Ford R, Muijen M. Teamwork: Models of Outreach in an Urban Multi-cultural Setting. London: Sainsbury Centre for Mental Health, 1996.

Goffman, E. Asylums. New York: Doubleday, 1961.

Goldberg D, Bridges K. Somatic presentation of psychiatric illness in primary care settings. Journal of Psychosomatic Research 1988; 32: 137–144.

Goldberg D, Gater R. Estimates of need. Psychiatric Bulletin 1991; 15: 593–595.

Goldberg D, Huxley P. Common Mental Disorders – A Biosocial Model. London: Routledge, 1991.

Goldie N. 'I hated it there, but I miss the people'. London: North London Polytechnic, 1988.

Gunn J, Maden A, Swinton, M. Treatment needs of prisoners with psychiatric disorders. British Medical Journal 1991; 303: 338–341.

Handcock M, Villaneau L. Effective Partnerships: Developing Key Indicators for Joint Working in Mental Health. London: Sainsbury Centre for Mental Health, 1997.

Harvey C. The Camden Schizophrenia Surveys I. The psychiatric, behavioural and social characteristics of the severely mentally ill in an inner London health district. British Journal of Psychiatry 1996; 168: 410–417.

Health and Personal Social Services Statistics, England, 1998 Edition. London: HMSO, 1999.

Hyde C, Bridges K, Goldberg D, Lowson K, Sterling C, Faragher B. The Evaluation of a Hostel Ward. British Journal of Psychiatry 1987; 151: 805–812.

Intagliata J. Improving the quality of community care for the chronically mentally disabled: the role of case management. Schizophrenia Bulletin 1982; 8: 655–674.

Jackson G, Gater R, Goldberg, D, Tantum D, Loftus L, Taylor H. A new community mental health team based in primary care: a description of the service and its effect on service use in the first year. British Journal of Psychiatry 1993; 162: 375–384.

Joseph P, Potter M. Diversion from custody: I. Psychiatric assessment at the magistrates court. British Journal of Psychiatry 1993; 162: 325–330.

Lehman A, Possidente S, Hawker F. The quality of life of chronic patients in a state hospital and in community residences. Hospital and Community Psychiatry 1986; 37: 901–907.

Lehman A, Ward N, Linn S. Chronic mental patients: the quality of life issue. American Journal of Psychiatry 1982; 139: 1271–1276.

Marks I, Connolly J, Muijen M, Audini B, McNamee G, Lawrence R. Home-based versus hospital-based care for people with serious mental illness. British Journal of Psychiatry 1994; 165: 179–194.

Marshall M, Gary A, Lockwood A, Green R. Case management for severe mental disorders. In Adams CE, Duggan L, de Jesus Mari J, White P (eds), Schizophrenia Module of the Cochrane Database of Systematic Reviews. Oxford: Cochrance Collaboration [updated 1 September 1997].

Melzer D, Hale A, Malik J, Hogman G, Wood, S. Community care for patients with schizophrenia one year after hospital discharge. British Medical Journal 1991; 303: 1023–1026.

Minghella E, Ford R. All for one or one for all? Health Service Journal 1997a; 13 March: 30–31.

Minghella E. Ford R. Focal Points. Health Service Journal 1997b; 11 December: 26–27.

Muijen, M. Rehabilitation and care of the mentally ill. Current Opinion in Psychiatry 1994; 7: 202–206.

Muijen M, Cooney M, Strathdee G, Bell R, Hudson A. Community psychiatric nurse teams: intensive support versus generic care. British Journal of Psychiatry 1994; 165: 211–217.

Muijen M, Ford R. The market and mental health: intentional and unintentional incentives. Journal of Interprofessional Care 1996; 10: 13–22.

National Housing Federation/Mental Health Foundation. Housing, Care and Support Code. London: Mental Health Foundation, 1996.

Nazarath I, King M. Controlled evaluation of the management of schizophrenia in one general practice: a pilot study. Family Practitioner 1992; 9: 171–172.

NHS Executive. 24 Hour Nursed Care for People with Severe and Enduring Mental Illness. Leeds: NHS Executive, 1996b.

NHS Executive. NHS Psychotherapy Services in England. Leeds: NHS Executive, 1996a.

Onyett, S. and Ford, R. Multidisciplinary community teams: where is the wreckage? Journal of Mental Health 1996; 5: 47–55.

Onyett S, Pilinger T, Muijen M. Making Community Mental Health Teams Work. London: Sainsbury Centre for Mental Health, 1995.

Pozner A, Ng M, Shepherd G. Working It Out. Brighton: Pavilion and Sainsbury Centre for Mental Health, 1996.

Ritchie J, Dick D, Lingham R. Report of the Christopher Clunis Enquiry. London: HMSO and North East/South East Thames Regional Health Authorities, 1994.

Robertson G, Dell S, James K, Grounds A. Psychotic men remanded in custody to Brixton Prison. British Journal of Psychiatry 1994; 164: 55–61.

Rose, D. Living in the Community. London: Sainsbury Centre for Mental Health, 1996.

Rose D, Muijen M. 24 hr nursed care: user views. Journal of Mental Health, 1998; 7(6): 603–610.

Ryan, Ford R, Clifford P. Case Management and Community Care. London: Sainsbury Centre for Mental Health, 1991.

Sainsbury Centre for Mental Health. Keys to Engagement. London: Sainsbury Centre for Mental Health, 1998.

Scott J, Dixon L. Assertive community treatment and case management for schizophrenia. Schizophrenia Bulletin 1995a; 21: 657–668.

Scott J. Dixon L. Psychological interventions for schizophrenia. Schizophrenia Bulletin 1995b; 21: 621–630.

Sheldon T. Concentration and Choice in the Provision of Hospital Services. CRD Report 8. York: University of York, 1997.

Shepherd G, Beadsmoore A, Moore C, Hardy P, Muijen M. Relation between bed use, social deprivation, and overall bed availability in acute adult psychiatric units, and alternative residential options: a cross sectional survey, one day census, and staff interviews. British Medical Journal 1997; 314: 262–266.

Shneider J, Hallam A. Specialist Work Schemes and Mental Health. Canterbury: University of Kent Personal Social Services Research Unit, 1996.

Simpson C, Hyde C, Faragher E. The chronically mentally ill in community facilities: a study of quality of life. British Journal of Psychiatry.

Stein L. Innovating against the current. New Directions for Mental Health Services 1992; 56: 5–22.

Strathdee G, Sutherby K. Liaison psychiatry and primary health care settings. In Watkins M, Hervey N, Carson J, Ritter S. (eds), Collaborative Community Mental Health Care. London: Arnold, 1996.

Torrey F, Steiber J, Ezekiel J. et al. Criminalizing the Seriously Mentally Ill: The Abuse of Jails as Mental Hospitals. Washington, DC: Public Citizens Health Research Group and National Alliance for the Mentally Ill, 1992.

Wallace M. The Forgotten Illness I. London: SANE, 1993a.

Wallace M. The Forgotten Illness II. London: SANE, 1993b.

Warner L, Bennett S, Ford R, Thompson K. Good Practice in the Provision of Supported Housing to People with Mental Health Problems. London: Sainsbury Centre for Mental Health, 1997.

Warner L, Ford R. Sathyamoorthy, G. Divisions and revisions. Health Service Journal 1996; 5 September: 26–27.

Warner, R. Recovery From Schizophrenia: Psychiatry and Political Economy. London: Routledge, 1994.

Weller, M. Where we come from: recent history of community provision. In Weller M, Muijen M.(eds), Dimensions of Community Mental Health Care. London: Saunders, 1993.

Wing J, Morris B. Clinical basis of rehabilitation. In Wing, J, Morris B. (eds), Handbook of Psychiatric Rehabilitation Practice. Oxford: Oxford University Press, 1981.

11

POLICY DEVELOPMENT FOR SEVERE MENTAL ILLNESS: THE UK EXPERIENCE

Amanda Reynolds, Jonathan Bindman and Graham Thornicroft

INTRODUCTION

This chapter presents a brief overview of the many recent and important policy and legal changes for mental health services in the UK (Table 11.1). As policies have been introduced rapidly and in large numbers, many clinicians and managers are not always fully aware of their contents. Some policies are not always fully operational in all areas, and as Peck et al. write in the Kings Fund London Commission Mental Health Report, 'It is reasonable to assume that implementation of particular policy requirements will take longer than policy makers may wish' (Peck et al. 1997: 347). Knowing the details of these policies will help: (1) to make decisions which are consistent with national policy, (2) provide a common language for the various agencies involved, (3) achieve realistic expectations of the roles of other agencies and (4) meet the demands set by contracts, recommendations from mental health enquiry reports and from central government.

In this chapter we shall summarize the main components of current policy on services for adults who suffer from mental illnesses, which include: (1) the 1990 NHS and Community Care Act, (2) the 1990 Care Programme Approach, (3) the 1992 Health of the Nation, (4) the 1994 Ritchie Report into case of Christopher Clunis, (5) the House of Commons Health Select Committee Report, (6) the 1994 Supervision Register, (7) the 1996 Mental Health (Patients in the Community) Act, which introduced Supervised Discharge Orders, (8) the Spectrum of Care, (9) the 1996 report on 24-h nursed care and (10) the National Service Framework.

1988	Report by Sir Roy Griffiths. Community Care: Agenda for Action	
1990	National Health Service and Community Care Act	
1990	Department of Health Guidance 'Care Programme Approach'	
1992	Department of Health 'Health of the Nation'. Mental Health a Key Area	
1994	Introduction of Supervision Registers	
1995	Zito Trust Report, 'Learning the Lessons'	
1995	Mental Health (Patients in the Community) Act	
1996	Spectrum of Care	
1999	National Service Framework	

Table 11.1 – Key components in the development of community care policy.

THE NHS AND COMMUNITY CARE ACT (1990)

The NHS and Community Care Act was introduced in 1990 to bring greater coordination to the provision of community care by the health and social services. In essence it brought in the following important changes: a clear distinction between purchasing and providing functions, the requirement for local community care plans, the creation of provider trusts and fund-holding general practices, care management, the transfer of funds for residential care from the Department of Social Security to the social services. The objectives of the Act are summarized in Table 11.2.

A **community care plan** is an annual report to the NHS Executive with details of the mental health service for the following year and beyond. It needs to be agreed by chief officers of the local health and social service provider agencies and formally

- To promote the development of domiciliary, day and respite services to enable people to live in their own homes wherever feasible and sensible

- To promote the development of a flourishing independent sector alongside good quality public services

- To coordination of social care by the 'care manager'

- To make proper assessment of need

- To provide services on the basis of needs assessments to clarify the responsibilities of agencies and so make it easier to hold them to account for their performance

- To secure better value for taxpayers' money by introducing a new funding structure for social care. To ensure that service providers make practical support for carers a high priority

Table 11.2 – Key objectives of the NHS and Community Care Act (1990).

endorsed by the local Health Authority and elected members of the Social Services Committee. This plan sets the framework within which more detailed local plans are developed and funded. At the local level, joint Health and Social Services (called Joint Planning Teams or Joint Community Care Planning Groups) were established whose functions include writing an annual Community Care Plan and bidding for Mental Illness Specific Grants. These are strategic forums that oversee inter-agency initiatives, and which play a part in prioritizing local projects for funding.

A key role that has been defined in the Act is that of the **care manager**. The term 'care management' was introduced in 1991 to describe the role of qualified social workers who assess the needs of clients and who then purchase direct care services from other providers. It is different from the role of health service 'key workers' who assess needs and who then also provide direct care. The Act makes the following statutory requirements of care managers: 'where it appears to a local authority that any person for whom they may provide or arrange for the provision of community care services may be in need of any such services, the authority (a) shall carry out an assessment of his needs for those services and (b) having regard to the results of that assessment, shall then decide whether his needs call for the provision by them of any such services'.

A central part of the act concerns **needs assessment**. Needs can be defined on a population or individual basis, and from the perspectives of politicians, clinicians, carers and patients; clearly these will differ. A working definition of need in the sense in which it is used in the CPA is that a need exists where the patient 'is able in some way to benefit from care', where this care is medical or social. The needs are not limited to the care that happens to be available; a broader definition of need may suggest services that should be developed (see Chapter 9).

THE CARE PROGRAMME APPROACH

The Care Programme Approach (CPA) is an administrative measure which the government instructed mental health and social services to introduce in 1991. It aims to guide good clinical practice and to prevent patients from 'slipping through the net' of follow-up. The CPA is a central part of the government's mental health policy, and was brought in following concern that, after discharge, many patients did not have a named member of staff to contact, nor was there a defined care plan. The CPA consists of four parts, as outlined below:

Assessment of health and social care needs

The systematic assessment of needs begins with a good clinical and social history which covers both the needs for diagnosis and treatment, and needs for social care. Most patients with severe mental illnesses will have a wide range of needs, and a full assessment will involve information from informants: family, friends, professional and non-professional carers. Social workers, who have parallel assessment and 'care management' procedures, should be involved in more complex assessments, and these may be carried out jointly. A full need assessment may require a multi-disciplinary meeting. Risk of self-harm, self-neglect, or harm to others, should be assessed.

Written care plan

For inpatients, or outpatients who need multi-disciplinary input, a care plan should be agreed at a ward round or CPA meeting, with everyone who will be involved in implementing it. The plan should be agreed as far as possible with the patient, and with carers. For other patients, this might simply involve a plan for outpatient treatment being written in the notes after completing a history and examination, though even this should be discussed and agreed with the patient.

Keyworker

The keyworker has responsibility for the coordination of the care programme. If the patient moves to another area, a proper hand-over should be made by the keyworker to another team. The keyworker should be the professional with the closest relationship with the patient; this will often be a CPN or social worker, but could be the psychiatrist in training. Each key worker will usually need to nominate a 'deputy' for periods of sickness or planned leave.

Regular reviews

The care plan should usually be reviewed at least every 6 months, but the keyworker should be able to arrange for a review meeting with others involved in the patient's care if the care plan is not being effectively carried out. A register of names of patients needing reviews should be kept ('CPA register'), and reminders of the need for review issued. There are important implications of this system of reviews for clear, shared documentation of care plan and CPA reviews, and for the supporting information systems.

The CPA in practice

Who should receive the CPA? The CPA applies to all patients under the care of specialist psychiatric services. However, not every patient can or should have multi-disciplinary team reviews. The 1995 NHS Executive document 'Building Bridges' set out a three tiered approach to implementing the CPA (Table 11.3). However, there remain considerable local variations in how far the CPA has been implemented (see 'Mallone Review', NHS Executive 1996).

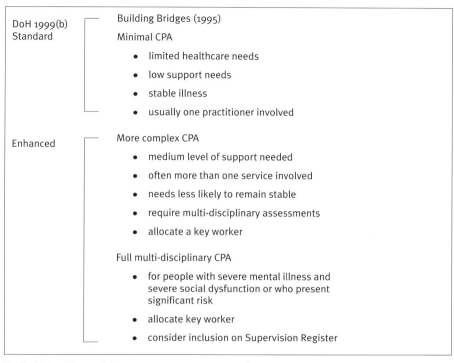

Table 11.3 – Tiers of the care programme approach.

A guidance document which updates the CPA policy was issued together with the National Service Framework (NSF) (Department of Health 1999b). This proposes that all Trusts should simplify the structure of their tiered CPA to a two tier one, with a 'standard' tier equating to the previous 'minimal' tier, and an 'enhanced' tier to include patients previously placed on 'complex' or 'full multi-disciplinary' tiers.

In terms of the timing of the CPA in relation to discharge from hospital, a CPA meeting should take place before discharge to ensure that the necessary community services will be in place. In the case of detained patients, this can also serve as a 'Section 117' meeting, where the aftercare required by Section 117 of the Mental Health Act (1983) is planned. If an adequate care plan cannot be put into practice, the patient should not be discharged.

The Supervision Register

The Supervision Register (SR) is an administrative measure which the government instructed psychiatric services to introduce in 1994. It was felt to be necessary because of concerns, such as those expressed in the report of the Inquiry into the Care of Christopher Clunis, that the CPA was not being provided for patients 'who may be at greatest risk and need most support'. The SR is intended to apply to a small group of patients who already fall into the 'full multi-disciplinary' tier of the CPA, and in practice may be regarded as the most intensive tier of the CPA (Table 11.4)

The Supervision Register is a list of names, 'held locally by each provider trust, of patients with a severe mental illness who are known to be at significant risk or potentially at significant risk of committing serious violence, or suicide or of serious self-neglect as the result of severe and enduring mental illness'. The register should include the names of the patient, the Responsible Medical Officer (RMO), and keyworker as well as the nature of the risk, and basic CPA details of the CPA (date of registration, components of the care plan, and review date). In practice only a small proportion of patients on each team's caseload, that is those who represent the highest risk, will be on the SR if resources are to be especially targeted to them.

The requirement was strongly criticised by professionals and service users (Caldicott 1994, Harrison 1994). Among other criticisms it was suggested that the difficulty of accurately predicting risk would limit its effectiveness, and it could result in stigmatization of patients and affect their civil liberties.

Trusts will be permitted to discontinue SRs from April 2001 providing risk assessment, the importance of which is strongly emphasized in the new guidance, is being effectively carried out for patients on the CPA.

The 1995 Zito Trust Report, 'Learning the Lessons'

The 1995 report produced by the Zito Trust, 'Learning the Lessons' (of which a second edition was published in 1996), summarizes the terms of references and the recommendations of 36 inquiries into homicides involving the mentally ill which occurred between 1985 and 1996. It usefully organizes the recommendations under headings that include health services, social services, monitoring and inspection, GPs and inpatient care. It provides essential and salutary reading for all mental health service managers and clinicians (Shepherd 1996), as well as the best single source detailing the relevance of individual inquires for all services.

- Consider as the most intensive tier of the CPA
- Applies to those 'known to be at significant risk or potentially at significant risk of committing serious violence, or suicide or of serious self-neglect as the result of severe and enduring mental illness'
- Requires allocation of a key worker and a risk assessment

Table 11.4 – Key features of the Supervision Register.

The 1995 Mental Health (Patients in the Community) Act/Supervised Discharge Orders

Supervised Discharge Orders (SDO) were introduced by the Mental Health (Patients in the Community) Act (1995), which amends the Mental Health Act (1983). The Order complements, but is different from, the Supervision Register. It allows the RMO, who is treating a patient under Sections 3, 37, 47 or 48 of the Mental Health Act (MHA) 1983, to apply for powers of formal supervision of the patient after discharge from hospital, which will be exercised by a 'supervisor', typically a CPN acting as a keyworker (Table 11.5).

The application is made by the RMO to the provider unit managers. The patient will have already satisfied the conditions for detention under the MHA Sections given above, and in addition the RMO must believe that there will be a substantial risk of serious harm to the patient or to the safety of other people if the patient does not receive aftercare on discharge from hospital, and that the powers of supervised discharge are likely to help ensure that the patient receives aftercare, according to the CPA.

The application by the RMO must be supported by applications from another doctor approved under Section 12(2), who could be the consultant providing community care ('Community RMO') if different from the RMO, or the GP, **and** from an Approved Social Worker. The application must always include an agreed care plan.

The SDO only takes effect once the patient is both discharged from hospital, and discharged from detention, so it does not apply while the patient is on leave of absence (Section 17). The patient has a right of appeal to a Mental Health Review Tribunal. SDO last for 6 months, and like Section 3 the RMO can apply to renew it for 6 months, then for 1 year at a time. The patient can be required to reside in a particular place, to attend at set times for medical treatment, occupation, education or training, and the supervisor must be allowed access to the place of residence to see the patient. In these respects the legal powers are similar to those of a Guardianship Order.

- Amendment to 1983 Mental Health Act
- Allows legal supervision of patients after discharge
- Requires 'substantial risk' to or by patient
- 'Supervisor' has power to 'take or convey' patient
- Similar to Guardianship Order

Table 11.5 – Key features of supervised discharge orders.

Though the procedure is elaborate, the powers are limited, and may be unusable or ineffective, as they will be if the patient is determined not to cooperate with the care plan. They may restrict civil liberties without making it possible to deliver better care. There may be a small group of patients who are currently very difficult to care for who will respond to the more assertive treatment the supervisor can provide using SDO. Since its recent introduction the SDO has been relatively little used.

The 'Spectrum of Care'

The booklet issued by the Department of Health in 1996 (along with four other guidance documents) supplemented previous guidance given in the Health of the Nation Key Area Handbook (1994) and summarized the components of care that should be offered to people with mental illness on a local level (Table 11.6).

The 1996 NHS Executive report on 24-h nursed care

Launched at the same time as the 'Spectrum of Care' the NHS Executive Report on 24-h nursed care focused on the needs of the 'new long stay' group. Numbering at least 5000 in England and Wales, these people include many who respond only partially to acute treatment and who remain substantially disabled. The NHS Executive report makes clear that when patients require facilities which offer 24-h nursing care, this is an NHS responsibility, as it was in the days when many more long-stay wards in psychiatric institutions were provided (Table 11.7).

The report also gives recommendations on the location, size, design, staffing, and treatment appropriate for such settings. It makes clear that a local needs assessment exercise should be carried out by each health authority, followed by a strategy for the planned expansion of 24-h nursed care. The central message of this document is 'whatever the ambiguities with other client groups, there should be no doubt that providing fully for this client group is a NHS responsibility'.

The National Service Framework

A new policy framework for adult mental health services, the national Service Framework (NSF), was introduced in October 1999 (Department of Health 1999a). The NSF covers a wide range of mental health issues, but the CPA remains central to the care of those with SMI. The NSF establishes broad principles for the organization of services, and also sets specific standards. Those relating to the CPA are that care offered as part of the CPA should focus on optimizing engagement, anticipating or preventing crises, and reducing risks; that service users should receive copies of their care plan, which should include crisis plans and advise to GPs; and that service users should be able to access the necessary services 24 h a day.

	ACUTE/EMERGENCY CARE	REHABILITATION/CONTINUING CARE
Home-based	sector teams	domiciliary services
	sustainable out-of-hours cover	key workers care management and Care
	intensive home support	Programme Approach
Daycare	day hospitals	drop-in centres
		support groups
		employment groups
		daycare
Residential support	crisis accommodation	ordinary housing
	acute units	unstaffed group homes
	local secure units	adult placement schemes
		residential care schemes
		mental nursing homes
		24-h nursed NHS accommodation
		medium secure units
		high-secure units

Table 11.6 – Key components of the 'Spectrum of Care'.

Twenty-four-hour nursed care is for people with severe and enduring mental illness who need:

- Daily mental state monitor
- Frequent monitoring of risk
- Supervision of medication
- Assistance with self-care and daily living
- Support to access with daycare/rehabilitation
- Skilled management of challenging behaviour
- Ongoing evening and weekend active support

Table 11.7 – Defining the client group for 24-h nursed care.

Putting policy into practice

In writing this chapter we are reminded of the volume of recent guidance, the rapid-fire nature of its release and the confusing variety of terminology used. In practice, the central difficulty faced in implementing reasonable care is often the split between the provisions of the Care Programme Approach and care management. In fact, the spirit behind both of these is almost identical. In each case the key worker/care manager has similar goals and responsibilities, as shown in Table 11.8.

The goal of integrated social and health care which effectively and efficiently meets the needs of the severely mentally ill remains far from being widely realised. Recent policies and guidance in the UK have generally made a contribution to this goal. However, local solutions to overcome considerable practical difficulties in implementation and major alterations in traditional practices will only be achieved by professionals inspired with vision and energy working in services given adequate time and resources. Inquiries will continue to highlight the repeated lessons described by Lelliot et al. (1997) (table 11.9) until this implementation is achieved.

- Design care package
- Identify patients (case finding)
- Assess needs
- Coordinate service delivery
- Monitor service delivery
- Evaluate effectiveness of services
- Modify care package
- Repeat cycle unless services no longer needed

Table 11.8 – Core tasks of key worker/care manager.

- Theme 1 – Poor communication between agencies (7); particularly between health and social services (5), between mental health services and housing departments (3) and between specialist mental health services and GPs (3). A related theme to this was that of poor joint working (4), which was at all levels from commissioning and strategy (2) to multi-disciplinary care delivery (3).

- Theme 2 – Problems with discharge from hospital (5). This particularly related to failure to follow Section 117 procedures, assess need, develop an aftercare plan and communicate this adequately to other agencies.

- Theme 3 – Poor assessment of risk of violence (6). This emphasized particularly the need for better and more training in risk assessment (4) and the importance of disclosure of risk factors to those with a need to know.

- Theme 4 – Liaison with police and probation services (5). This related both to the involvement of police in receiving or providing information about people receiving care from mental health services (2) and the better involvement of mental healthcare workers in diversion from custody services (3).

Table 11.9 – Key themes arising in enquiries into mental health services.

- Theme 5 – Confidentiality and professional ethics (4). These were reported as barriers particularly between health and social services (2) and between mental health services and the police (2).

- Theme 6 – Adequacy and allocation of resources (9). The inadequacy of, or the need to protect, numbers of residential care places in London (including hospital beds) was a common theme (8). Specific mention was made of short-stay admission beds (4), medium secure provision (4), and the importance of maintaining a wide range of community-based residential services (4) with DoH guidance on levels of provision. Comment was also made on the inadequacy of numbers of community workers (2) and of provision of daycare services (2). Allocation of resources was commented on both between competing groups e.g. children, elderly, etc. (1), between health and social care (1), between areas of high and low need (2) and for the targeting of the most severely ill (3); as was the need for bridging money or ring-fencing of money as services move from a hospital to a community focus (2).

Note: the numbers in parentheses indicate the number of separate reports in which they figure (maximum = 10).

Source: London in the context of mental health policy, Lelliott et al. (1997), Bernard Audini, Sonia Johnson and Hilary Guite, in Johnson et al. (1997).

Table 11.9 *continued* – Key themes arising in enquiries into mental health services.

References

Audit Commission. Making a Reality of Community Care. London: HMSO, 1986.

Caldicott F (1994) Supervision Registers: the College's response. Psychiatric Bulletin; 18: 385–386.

Challis D. Case Management in Community Care. Aldershot: Gower, 1986.

Department of Health. Building Bridges: A Guide to Inter-agency Working for the Care and Protection of Severely Mentally Ill People. London: Department of Health, 1995.

Department of Health. The Care Programme Approach for People with a Mental Illness Referred to as the Specialist Psychiatric Services. hc (90)23/LASSL(90)11. London: Department of Health, 1990.

Department of Health (1999a) The national service framework for mental health. http://www.doh.gov.uk/nsf/mentalhealth.htm

Department of Health (1999b) Effective care co-ordination in mental health services. Modernizing mental health services. London: Department of Health.

Griffiths R. Community Care: An Agenda for Action. London: HMSO, 1988.

Harrison K (1994) Supervision in the community. New Law Journal; 144: 1017.

Holloway F (ed.) Supervision Registers. Recent government policy and legislation. , Psychiatric Bulletin 1994; 18: 593–596.

House of Commons. The National Health Service and Community Care Act. London: HMSO, 1990.

House of Commons. Second Report from the Social Services Committee, Session 1984–85, Community Care. London: HMSO, 1985.

Johnson S, Brooks L, Thornicroft G et al. London's Mental Health. London: King's Fund, 1997.

Kingdon D. Care Programme Approach. Recent government policy and legislation. Psychiatric Bulletin 1994; 18: 68–70.

Lelliott P, Audini B, Johnson S, Guite H. London in the Context of Mental Health Policy. In Johnson S et al. (eds), London's Mental Health. London: King's Fund, 1997.

NHS Executive. 24 Hour Nursed Care for People with Severe and Enduring Mental Illness. Leeds: NHS Executive, 1996a.

NHS Executive. An Audit Pack for Monitoring the Care Programme Approach. Monitoring Tool. (HSG(96)/LASSL (96)16. Leeds: NHS Executive, 1996b.

NHS Executive. Guidance on Supervised Discharge (Aftercare Under Supervision) and Related Provisions. HSG(96)11. London: NHS Executive, 1996c.

NHS Executive. Guidance on the Discharge of Mentally Disordered People and Their Continuing Care in the Community. Health Service Guidelines HSG(94)27. London: NHS Executive, 1994.

NHS Executive. Review of Purchasing of Mental Health Services by Health Authorities in England. Leeds: NHS Executive, 1996d.

Onyett S. Case Management in Mental Health. London: Chapman & Hall, 1992.

Patmore C, Weaver T. Community Mental Health Teams: Lessons for Planners and Managers. London: Good Practices in Mental Health, 1991.

Peck E, Smith H, Barker I, Henderson G (1997) The obstacles to and the opportunities for the development of mental health services in London. The perceptions of managers. Johnson S, Ramsay R, Thornicroft G, Brooks L, Elliott P, Peck E, Smith H, Chisholm D, Audini B, Knapp M, Goldberg D. London's Mental Health. The Report to the Kings Fund London commission. London Kings Fund 1997.

Shepherd D. Learning the Lessons, 2nd edn. London: Zito Trust, 1996.

Spectrum of Care. Local Services for People with Mental Health Problems. NHS Executive. London: Department of Health, 1996.

12

MODELS OF MENTAL HEALTHCARE FOR THE ELDERLY

Sube Banerjee

INTRODUCTION

The need to identify effective models of care for the elderly mentally ill is driven by the economic, social care and healthcare challenges presented by the ageing worldwide population (WHO 1991). Developing countries are projected to experience a massive increase in the numbers of older people (Prince 1997), both in relative and absolute terms. However, the situation in the UK, which is shared by much of the more developed world, is an increase in the oldest old (those over 75 and those over 85) in whom are concentrated high levels of physical and psychiatric morbidity and, therefore, the greatest need (OECD 1988).

This chapter summarizes the organization and delivery of mental healthcare for older people in the UK and exemplifies the issues relating to more developed countries. What becomes quickly evident is the lack of hard evidence on which to base decisions concerning the purchasing and provision of services – in this old age psychiatry shares much in common with the rest of psychiatry in particular and medicine in general. Nevertheless, services for those over the age of 65 make up an increasingly important, if often less vocal, part of mental health services as a whole. People over this age make up around one-third of all new admissions and re-admissions to mental health beds in England (DHSS 1988), and this proportion appears to be on the increase (figure 1) (Philpot and Banerjee 1997).

THE CONTEXT OF CARE FOR THE ELDERLY

Before considering models of mental healthcare for the elderly it is first necessary to consider the matrix of care into which such services fit. This is of particular importance since the nature of the problems of the elderly mean that individuals are much more likely to have complex co-morbidity and multiple service use (see Chapter 7).

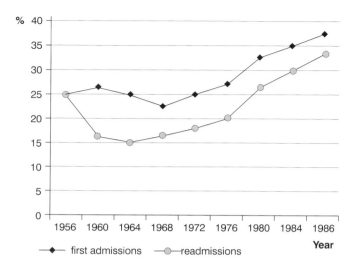

Figure 12.1 – Percentage of first admissions and readmissions to mental health beds aged 65 or more

This is one of the major differences of older as opposed to younger populations with mental health problems and it forms an important part of the rationale for the provision of specialist services for the elderly. Care for older people is provided by a complex web of formal and informal services, which are summarized in Table 12.1.

The nature of older people's disorders and disabilities varies little from place to place once age is taken into account. Older people throughout the world have high levels of acute and chronic medical illnesses – they have depression, dementia and anxiety; and have impairment, disability and handicap. The lack of variability between developed countries in the age-specific prevalence rates of dementia in the elderly is one of the most striking findings in psychiatric epidemiology (Hofman et al. 1991). In broad terms, services are also remarkably similar in developed countries; there are what one would term health services, social services, and the support of families and communities. However, the detail of these services varies greatly in their content, comprehensiveness, accessibility and funding.

It is almost axiomatic that it is the issue of cost that has prompted policy-makers throughout the world to start to take notice of the challenges presented by the elderly. This is as much the case in developing countries as it is in the developed world (Kalache 1991). The comprehensive costs for society of caring for the elderly include health and social care and the opportunity costs to families who take on a caring role. The language that accompanies these debates, such as 'demographic time bomb', 'the economic tidal wave of the aged' and most succinctly 'burden', seem symptomatic of the profound fears raised by this subject.

INFORMAL CARE	FORMAL CARE
• Spouse • Children • Other family • Neighbours • Friends • Volunteers • Church groups • Others (e.g. those who deliver the milk or the post	**Social Services** • Home care • Day centres • Respite care • Residential care • Nursing home care **Health Services** • Primary healthcare • Old age psychiatry • Geriatric medicine • Other secondary care • NHS continuing care **Voluntary sector** • Daycare • Advocacy • Residential care **Private Sector** • Home care • Daycare • Residential care • Nursing home care

Table 12.1 – Informal and formal care provided to elderly people.

Where then does old age psychiatry fit into this matrix? The answer in most countries is 'nowhere at all'. Specific old age psychiatric services are available for only a tiny proportion of the world's population. The UK remains probably the only country in the world to have developed a comprehensive nationwide old age psychiatric service. It is striking that even within the European Community it is only the UK that recognizes the speciality as a discrete entity for the higher training of psychiatrists.

In other countries the same mental health problems exist, so who manages them? The answer, of course, depends on the specific services available in each country. Older people with mental health problems may be managed by generic psychiatrists, primary care physicians, geriatricians or neurologists depending on the disorder and local conditions (EuroCARE – EC study of carers of people with dementia – unpublished data). However, the most likely answer to the question is that they are not actively managed at all. There is strong evidence for low levels of recognition and active management of depression in elderly populations (Waxman and Carner 1984, Macdonald 1986, Rapp and Davis 1989, Banerjee and Macdonald 1996). With respect to dementia it can be argued that arrival at an accurate diagnosis is only a very minor part of helping a family to care for someone with cognitive impairment, yet the outreach elements of hospital-based geriatric medicine and neurology are almost non-existent with a few notable exceptions such as Aged Care Assessment Teams in Australia (Ames and Flynn 1994).

This is perhaps the most compelling argument for the establishment of old age psychiatric services. Without them, older people with treatable disorder causing immense decrease in quality of life for the person and for their carers, increased mortality, and profound economic burden are denied effective management because they are left to rely on services whose primary interest is not the mental health of the elderly.

DEVELOPMENT OF OLD AGE PSYCHIATRY IN THE UK

Specialist services for the elderly mentally ill in the UK developed from asylum psychiatry. Up to the late 1960s, the elderly mentally ill either were left in the community with no active treatment or were cared for as inpatients in the asylums, only rarely receiving outpatient care. Their care was largely undifferentiated from that of other mentally ill patients and general psychiatrists managed these patients alongside their younger ones. Patients suffering from chronic or progressive disorders such as intractable functional disorder or dementia ended up warehoused on the asylums' long-stay or 'back wards', or on the equivalent wards run by geriatric medicine, with little active input. There is clear evidence that this particularly disadvantaged the elderly. A survey of three mental hospitals in London in the late 1940s and 1950s reported a lack of precision in diagnosing dementia and cases of acute confusion and frequent misdiagnosis of affective disorders (Norris 1959).

The main factors that seem to have motivated the pioneers of old age psychiatry to develop specialist services include: the increasing need for psychiatric care in the elderly due to increased life expectancy; growing research-based knowledge about late-onset mental disorders, and the perceived success of geriatric medicine (Wattis 1994). The separation of mental healthcare for the elderly from that for other adults, therefore, seems to have its roots more in a need to overcome institutional age-related prejudice, to improve care, and the presence of dementia as a specific disorder of later life, rather than in any biological disconjunction occurring at the age of 65 (Murphy and Banerjee 1993).

Jolley (1995) commented that the speciality developed without recourse to randomized controlled trials of treatment methods or service structures but from a pragmatic approach based on a passionate advocacy for the client group and a struggle to identify funding and facilities. This candid statement delineates the strengths and weaknesses implicit in the development of old age psychiatric services in the UK and in other countries. The UK blueprint for service provision has been held up by its more vocal proponents as a universal way forward with little critical appraisal. It may be argued that response to questions of development has been somewhat stereotyped, with the UK point of view summarized as 'the same but more of it please'. In short, the service model is a product of evangelism rather than evidence. It is important to note that in this old age psychiatry varies little from any other arm of psychiatry in particular, or medicine and surgery in general.

Probably the first unit specifically for the study and treatment of the elderly mentally ill was Gresham Ward at the Bethlem Royal Hospital, London, which was opened in 1949 with 40 beds for patients with functional disorder over the age of 60. The work of its consultant Felix Post was instrumental in providing clear evidence of the difference between depression and dementia in the elderly and the possibility of successful treatment. The first comprehensive old age psychiatric service to be established was probably that at Goodmayes Hospital in London's eastern suburbs (Arie 1970). The underpinning principles upon which this service was based included: (1) ease of accessibility; (2) flexibility; (3) assessments being made at the patients home; and (4) management of the patient in close co-operation with general practitioners (GPs) and other interested parties. This model of service, with its comprehensiveness and strong community focus remains the basis for old age psychiatric services provided in the UK.

During the late 1970s it became NHS policy to provide at least one psychiatric consultant with a specific role for the care of the elderly in each health district. Consequently the number of old age psychiatrists in the UK grew from about 20 in 1973 to over 370 in 1992 (Banerjee et al. 1993). In addition, these posts have become increasingly filled by people working full-time in the speciality, rather than those devoting a few sessions to the subject.

Even with these comprehensive and ubiquitous services, the majority of elderly people with depression and dementia do not have contact with old age psychiatry services. Instead they are maintained at home or in residential settings by a combination of their families, friends, neighbours, primary healthcare teams, social services, and private and voluntary care providing organizations. For people with dementia, up to now this has been a tenable position if it is accepted that primary heathcare services and secondary care other than old age psychiatry have the ability accurately to make a diagnosis of dementia and to refer on to appropriate services. One of the most useful pieces of information in the planning of services for people with dementia would be the proportion of the demented who require specialist old age psychiatric input. These data are not available and there are arguments about what criteria should be used for referral to, and acceptance for treatment by, old age psychiatric services. Arguments range from the most inclusive 'all people with dementia should be seen by an old age psychiatrist' to the most exclusive 'only people with severe behavioural disorder or complicated psychopathology in dementia should be seen by old age psychiatric services'. There is no good evidence with which to estimate the proportion of those people with dementia in the community who would benefit from contact with old age psychiatry services. Data from the Camberwell Dementia Case Register suggest that only about 10% of those with dementia in the community come to the notice of old age psychiatric services (Holmes et al. 1995).

The caveat 'up to now' in the preceding paragraph is caused by the recent licensing in the UK of the first drugs for the treatment of Alzheimer's disease. These are anti-cholinesterases with modest efficacy in improving cognitive function in those with mild-to-moderate Alzheimer's disease and a benign side-effect profile when compared with other potential compounds such as tacrine (Rogers and Friedhoff 1996) (see Chapter 7). The impact of these compounds and those which are due to follow in the near future may be profound. At present few people with Alzheimer's disease are assessed and managed by secondary care services, but it has been widely suggested that such treatment should be initiated only by specialists such as old age psychiatrists, neurologists and geriatricians. If this is to be the case then there would be a massive increase in the workload of specialist services in completing the detailed assessments needed to decide whether to initiate treatment and to monitor response. It is likely that other unmet need in people with dementia would also be uncovered, requiring further specialist input. Present resources will not be able to meet this demand. The case of anti-Alzheimer's drugs presents a very unusual situation in medicine, that of a medication becoming available for a disease for which hitherto there has been no medical treatment. For old age psychiatric services to take on a role in the provision of such drugs needs careful consideration. In particular, the non-drug costs (increased referrals, assessments, investigations and follow-up appointments) need to be taken into account and provided for as well as the drug costs.

For depression the position is more clear. Around 6% of those elderly people with serious depression identified by community surveys in the UK are receiving old age psychiatric services (Waterreus et al. 1994). This would be perfectly reasonable if those with depression were being effectively managed within primary care, but this does not seem to be the case. Community studies have consistently demonstrated that less than 15% of older people with depression of such a severity that intervention would be warranted are receiving any form of active management of this depression (Blanchard et al. 1994). There is, therefore, a clear discontinuity along the pathway from recognition to action on the part of primary care. It is unclear whether this is due to a lack of recognition (Williamson et al. 1964), or due to recognition not being linked to action (Macdonald 1986), but important contributory factors are likely to be the knowledge, attitudes and behaviours of: primary healthcare; the older people themselves; and those of the society in which we live.

Given the sheer size of the public health burden of depression in primary care it is not a feasible contention to hold that all people with depression should be referred to and managed by specialist old age psychiatrists. A more feasible and sustainable approach might be for old age psychiatrists to transfer skills and competence in this area to primary healthcare teams. This requires an understanding of where the blocks are and a commitment to address them. This is likely to need effective public education, as well as education focussed on primary and secondary healthcare services, if the situation is to be changed so that older people with depression can be offered treatment for depression, and helped to understand the potential benefits of accepting treatment. Psychiatrists need training in how best to transfer skills and competence. Such an approach is only likely to be effective if it is jointly owned by primary and secondary care, if its benefits are clear, and if its costs (in terms of time and effort) are perceived as reasonable.

ELEMENTS OF SERVICE ORGANIZATION

As noted above it is UK policy that all districts should have at least one specialist old age psychiatry consultant post. Data held by the Royal College of Psychiatrists' Faculty of Old Age Psychiatry suggest that is the case. In addition these posts are increasingly filled by single-speciality doctors rather than those whose time is split between old age and general psychiatry. However, this seemingly rosy statement needs to be interpreted with caution as many of the posts are poorly resourced with unsustainably large catchment areas and workloads. The recommendations set out by the Royal College of Psychiatrists suggest that no consultant should be responsible for a catchment area with more than 10 000 people over the age of 65 (RCP 1992), a reduction from the previous recommendation of one consultant per 22 000 over 65s (RCP 1987). Also, the extent to which these posts are vacant or filled by locums is striking. For example, in South London in October 1996, 20% of old age psychiatric consultant posts were either vacant or filled by a locum (Philpot and Banerjee 1997).

Despite the 'top-down' drive to homogeneity, which includes the Royal College of Psychiatrists' recommendations, methods of service delivery vary markedly. This is sustainable because of the lack of any comparative evaluation (in terms of effectiveness and cost) of the different models of care. Services will also differ because of the variation in organization and service provision of local authority social services and the voluntary and private sectors. This matrix of service providers changes area by area and, therefore, adaptability to local circumstances is necessary for old age mental health services. There are nonetheless common elements. Services generally include: an inpatient assessment/treatment unit; long-stay accommodation; daycare and some form of non-hospital assessment provision. It is within these broad groupings that the variation occurs.

An old age psychiatric service is a complex system; it is also a delicate system, so that dysfunction in any one of the constituent parts will result in the other components suffering. The extent of this damage is proportional to the amount of capacity in the system, the tighter the system is stretched the greater the damage. Recent health service cost cutting or 'efficiency-savings' have left little spare capacity to respond to new challenges such as those posed by the introduction of anti-Alzheimer's drugs.

Inpatient assessment/treatment units

A unit for the inpatient assessment and treatment of people with functional and/or organic mental disorder who cannot be managed in the community is a central component of all old age psychiatric services. Inpatient units may be separated into organic (dementia and sometimes delirium) and functional (the rest) wards or may be integrated. There is no evidence that supports one or the other approach. However, there may be difficulties in identifying which form of disorder an individual has on admission and there is also a substantial degree of co-morbidity of organic and functional disorder in the elderly. Additionally, there may be particular concerns if the quality of care varies between the two units, for example as a result of a perceived difference in attractiveness of working with one group or the other.

Access to inpatient care is almost invariably based on geographical catchment area which has the advantage of ensuring that patients, no matter how difficult the problems they present, have an identifiable team to take responsibility for their care. However, the principal disadvantage is the lack of choice for users, carers and primary care of who provides the services.

Acute inpatient units have increasingly been sited in district general hospitals (DGH) rather than in specialist hospitals with the re-provision of mental healthcare away from the asylums (Shulman and Arie 1991). This may have advantages in terms of ease access to medical help, which is of importance to the old age psychiatric population given their high level of physical morbidity. However, problems may arise when old age psychiatry is the only psychiatric speciality in a DGH with the provision of on-site psychiatric cover. Any division of old age psychiatry from the rest of psychiatry can lead to isolation and marginalization, and increased cost due to the maintenance to twin sites and a lack of flexibility in medical and nursing cover.

Units vary in their integration with geriatric medicine, from joint assessment wards in DGH with dual responsibility and care, through DGH or mental hospital units with good mutual liaison links, to wards in isolated mental hospitals with little or no contact with geriatric medicine. In the 1970s the Department of Health and

Social Security (DHSS 1970) advocated the establishment of wards managed jointly by geriatricians and old age psychiatrists in order that patients with delirium and acute onset or deterioration of dementia, or those in whom mental and physical problems were interrelated, could benefit from joint management. The reality has been that, despite a few successful examples, these joint facilities are very uncommon. It is likely that the majority of old age psychiatric and geriatric patients do not need such an approach, but for a minority it may be very useful.

The argument for the development of formal links between geriatric medicine and old age psychiatry in terms of liaison and training are strong. Co-morbidity of physical and mental disorder is so common that effective liaison is needed so that old age psychiatric patients can receive good quality attention to their physical health needs and, just as importantly, so that geriatric patients can have their mental health needs adequately addressed. Local factors such as the geographical situation of the two services, the level of local service provision in each speciality, and the personal relationship of the clinicians involved will again determine the extent of liaison. The increasing separation of mental health services away from general medical services in the UK by their being managed by different NHS Trusts must not be allowed to interfere with effective joint working.

NHS Continuing Care

The provision of 'long-stay' or continuing care psychiatric places has undergone the most marked of changes within old age psychiatry and is subject to the widest variation with the closure of the asylums. Three main groups of older patients needing such care can be identified: (1) people with dementia who have severe intractable behavioural disorders; (2) people with treatment resistant functional disorder first occurring after the age of 65; and (3) 'graduates' from general services with early onset functional disorder who reach the age of 65. Current NHS psychiatric continuing care provision makes up only a tiny and diminishing proportion of all long-term care whereas the asylums provided free care to a wider population than that catered for by re-provided services.

Long-term care may be provided in mental hospitals, in DGH, in NHS community units, in collaborative ventures between health services and housing associations, by social services, and by the voluntary and independent sectors. Government policy and funding in the 1980s and 1990s favoured 'market solutions' with a consequent increase in independent sector nursing and residential homes. The numbers of these have increased markedly over the past 15 years as NHS long-stay beds and to a lesser extent social service provision have decreased (Bebbington and Darton 1995). The consequence of this has been to provide NHS Continuing Care places only to those who can not be placed elsewhere. This results in the small number of remaining NHS Continuing Care beds being filled with the most challenging patients, requiring high levels of skilled staffing.

The closure of the large mental hospitals left an opportunity for innovation in the provision of long-stay accommodation, including joint ventures and private sector solutions with more or less health service input. There has been a distressing stream of 'disaster stories' of mismanaged relocation of long-term care for the elderly with high mortality and questions concerning quality of care on transfer such as the re-provision from Park Prewitt and Napsbury (Review Panel 1997). Where there is the decision to invest in clinical and environmental quality such as in the 'domuses' in Lewisham and North Southwark, there is evidence that this can be effective and rewarding (Lindesay et al. 1991). The 'domus' philosophy centres upon creating homes for individuals with severe dementia and challenging behaviour in the community which maximize autonomy and privacy, while providing the skilled support needed for patients and staff. However, such quality comes at an increased cost (Beecham et al. 1993), and this is a cost that few health purchasers have been prepared to consider.

Whatever the model of provision adopted there is a need for adequate health service-based resources to be purchased in order that therapeutic activity can be pursued and so that quality of care can be assured. Re-provision into small, autonomous and poorly supervised units in the community can lead to negative outcomes such as increased mortality and decreased quality of life. Cost savings could end in the re-creation of units with the same poverty of environment and care that characterized the worst of the asylums.

The availability of, and entry criteria into, NHS Continuing Care beds are issues of particular concern. Finance is a crucial consideration as NHS provision is free but Social Service or private provision is means-tested. This may, therefore, require the liquidation of patients' assets, including the sale of property. With pressures on budgets, or scarcity of beds, or strong views on the part of carers and relatives, disputes over responsibility for providing care will arise. Valid and reliable criteria to identify the need for NHS continuing care would reduce such 'border disputes'. Unfortunately no such clinically applicable criteria exist, and there are clear questions about whether they can be developed at all. This revolves around the lack of clearly definable distinction between health and social care needs which might, therefore, separate means-tested from free placement. The Royal Commission on Long-term Care for the Elderly has considered this and the other complex and important issues raised by the challenge of long-term care which are of great and increasing concern to all developed countries. Any solution is likely to be politically challenging and will have an important impact on old age psychiatric and social services as well as on the general population.

Community assessment and treatment

Traditional service delivery combines first assessment either in an outpatient clinic or at home by means of GP-requested consultant domiciliary visit (DV) with outpatient clinic or Community Psychiatric Nurse (CPN) follow-up. Outpatient assessment may be a particularly flawed approach for the elderly compared with home visits for four main reasons: (1) difficulties in attending clinics due to disability; (2) transporting elderly people with dementia to unfamiliar surroundings may exacerbate disorientation and behavioural disturbance and so compromise the assessment; (3) an inability to assess true level of functioning within patients' own homes; and (4) decreased access to information (e.g. medicine bottles and district nursing notes) and informants such as neighbours. Many services have, therefore, almost entirely done away with hospital-based outpatient assessment and follow up for these reasons. The reasons why some pursue the traditional model of service delivery are unclear and unresearched but may include clinician unwillingness to alter established patterns of behaviour or the assumption that a home-based service is more costly in time and resources.

Daycare is an important element of community care for older people with mental health problems and may be provided by social services, the voluntary sector or by health services. Although many services include high cost old age psychiatric day hospitals, there is no good evidence to inform whether purchasing a day hospital is a reasonable use of scarce resources. The available data when scrutinized seems to largely consist of assertion and anecdote (Fasey 1994, Howard 1994). However, the cost–benefit equation is likely to be least compelling for those day hospitals with relatively high costs and low throughput. It also seems important to ensure that day hospitals are not dupli-cating a service that could be provided at no cost (at least to health services) or a lower cost by social service or voluntary sector day centres (such as meals, company and social support).

Community old age psychiatry includes some of the most advanced models of true multi-disciplinary working in psychiatry such as the 'Guy's model' described below (Collighan et al. 1993). The way in which community teams work has been identified as one of the most contentious issues in old age psychiatric service provision (Denning 1992). The only team members common to both inpatient and community services are usually the medical staff. Community Teams vary from those consisting only of CPN to those with involvement of social workers, occupational therapists, psychologists, physiotherapists, case managers and speech therapists.

Access to these services is subject to considerable variation. A closed system, with referrals only coming to the consultant and only accepted from GPs and other hospital consultants, is particularly problematic for the elderly given their multiple service contacts, especially with social and voluntary services and resi-dential care. Forcing all referrals though the GP is a way of managing demand but it is particularly inimical to the effective multi-agency working demanded by the mental health problems of the elderly. Concerns that open access may 'swamp' services or lead to inappropriate referrals do not seem to be borne out by the small amount of research-based evidence available (Macdonald et al. 1994).

Who should carry out initial community assessments and formulate management plans? Some declare that only doctors are capable of these functions but there does not appear to be any empirical evidence to support this view. Others state that with training and supervision a team member of any professional background can make an accurate initial assessment. This is supported by evidence from systematic research that suggests that non-doctor team members are as accurate in assigning psychiatric diagnoses to those on whom they have completed new assessments, as are medical team members (Collighan et al. 1993). With respect to the formulation of management plans there is no clear evidence of the best way to achieve this. However, the complex needs of the elderly might point to the utility of multidisciplinary input.

Research demonstrating the efficacy and cost-effectiveness of community old age psychiatric services is almost entirely absent as is any scientific comparison of the different forms of service delivery outlined above. The exception is the 'Guys model' of multidisciplinary open access generic team working (Collinghan et al. 1993), which is at least supported by limited evidence of efficacy in the treatment of depression in the frail elderly (Banerjee et al. 1996). This lack of evidence does not mean that other forms of service provision are not effective, but it does make clear the need for studies evaluating the effectiveness and relative cost effectiveness of differing models so that rational decisions can be made about service purchasing and provision.

References

Ames D, Flynn E. Dementia services: an Australian View. In Burns A, Levy R (eds), Dementia. London: Chapman & Hall, 1994.

Arie T. The first year of the Goodmayes psychiatric service for old people. Lancet 1970; ii: 1175–1182.

Banerjee S, Lindesay J, Murphy E. Psychogeriatricians and general practitioners – a national survey. Psychiatric Bulletin 1993; 17: 592–594.

Banerjee S, Macdonald A. Mental disorder in an elderly home care population: associations with health and social service use. British Journal of Psychiatry 1996; 168: 750–756.

Banerjee S, Shamash K, Macdonald A et al. Randomised controlled trial of effect of intervention by psychogeriatric team on depression in frail elderly people at home. British Medical Journal 1996; 313: 1058–1061.

Bebbington AC, Darton RA. The supply of long-stay facilities for elderly people in London. PSSRU Discussion Paper 1139/3. Canterbury: University of Kent, 1995.

Beecham J, Cambridge P, Hallam A et al. The costs of domus care. International Journal of Geriatric Psychiatry 1993; 10: 827–832.

Blanchard M, Waterraus A, Mann A. The nature of depression among older people in inner London, and their contact with primary care. British Journal of Psychiatry 1994; 164: 396–402.

Collighan G, Macdonald A, Herzberg J. An evaluation of the multidisciplinary approach to psychiatric diagnosis in elderly people. British Medical Journal 1993; 306: 821–824.

Denning T. Community psychiatry of old age: a UK perspective. International Journal of Geriatric Psychiatry 1992; 7: 757–766.

Department of Health and Social Security. Mental Health Statistics for England, Booklet 12: Mental Illness Hospitals and Units, Diagnostic Data. London: HMSO, 1988.

Department of Health and Social Security. Psychogeriatric Assessment Units, HM(70)11. London: HMSO, 1970.

Fasey C. The day hospital in old age psychiatry; the case against. International Journal of Geriatric Psychiatry 1994; 9: 519–523.

Hofman PM, Rocca WA, Brayne C et al. The prevalence of dementia in Europe: a collaborative study of 1980–1990. Eurodem Prevalence Research Group. International Journal of Epidemiology 1991; 20: 736–748.

Holmes C, Cooper B, Levy R. Dementia known to mental health services: first findings of a case register for a defined elderly population. International Journal of Geriatric Psychiatry 1995; 10: 875–881.

Howard R. Day hospitals: the case in favour. International Journal of Geriatric Psychiatry 1994; 9: 525–529.

Jolley DJ. The first year of the Goodmayes psychiatric service for old people. Commentary. International Journal of Geriatric Psychiatry 1995; 10: 930–932.

Kalache A. Ageing is one-third World problem too. International Journal of Geriatric Psychiatry 1991; 6: 617–618.

Lindesay J, Briggs K, Lawes M et al. The domus philosophy. A comparative evaluation of a new approach to residential care for the demented elderly. International Journal of Geriatric Psychiatry 1991; 6: 727–736.

Macdonald AJD. Do general practitioners 'miss' depression in elderly patients? British Medical Journal 1986; 292: 1365–1368.

Macdonald A, Goddard C, Poynton A. Impact of 'open access' to specialist services, the case of community psychogeriatrics. International Journal of Geriatric Psychiatry 1994; 9: 709–714.

Murphy E, Banerjee S. The organisation of old-age psychiatry service. Reviews in Clinical Gerontology 1993; 3: 367–378.

Norris V. Mental Illness in London. Maudsley Monographs no. 6. London: Chapman & Hall, 1959.

Organisation for Economic Co-operation and Development. Ageing Population: The Social Policy Implications. Paris: OECD, 1988.

Philpot M, Banerjee S. Mental health services for older people in London. In Johnson S, Ramsey R, Thornicroft G et al. (eds), London's Mental Health. London: King's Fund, 1997.

Prince M. The need for research on dementia in developing countries. Tropical Medicine and International Health 1997; 2: 993–1000.

Rapp SR, Davis KM. Geriatric depression: physicians' knowledge, perceptions and diagnostic practices. Gerontologist 1989; 29: 252–257.

The Review Panel. Report of the Review Panel into the deaths of Eight Patients Following their Transfer from Napsbury Hospital to Elmstead House Nursing Home. London: Barnet Health Authority, 1997.

Rogers SL, Friedhoff LT. The efficacy and safety of donepezil in patients with Alzheimer's disease: results of a US multicentre, randomised, double-blind, placebo-controlled trial. Dementia 1996; 7: 293–303.

The Royal College of Psychiatrists. Guidelines for regional advisors on consultant posts in old age psychiatry. Psychiatric Bulletin 1987; 11: 240–242.

The Royal College of Psychiatrists. Mental Health of the Nation. London: Royal College of Psychiatrists, 1992.

Shulman K, Arie T. UK survey of psychiatric services for the elderly: direction for developing services. Canadian Journal of Psychiatry 1991; 36: 169–175.

Waterreus A, Blanchard M, Mann A. Community psychiatric nurses for the elderly: well tolerated, few side-effects and effective in the treatment of depression. Journal of Clinical Nursing 1994; 3: 299–306.

Wattis JP. The pattern of psychogeriatric services. In Copeland JRM, Blazer DG (eds), Principles and Practice of Geriatric Psychiatry. Chichester: Wiley, 1994.

Waxman HM, Carner EA. Physicians' recognition, diagnosis, and treatment of mental disorders in elderly medical patients. Gerontologist 1984; 24: 593–597.

Williamson J, Stokoe IH, Gray S et al. Old people at home: their unmet needs. Lancet 1964; i: 1117–1120.

World Health Organisation. World Health Statistics Annual 1990. Geneva: WHO, 1991.

13

FORENSIC PSYCHIATRY SERVICES

Huw Stone and Amanda Taylor

INTRODUCTION

Forensic psychiatry services should be one part of a 'spectrum' of psychiatric care, extending from community and primary healthcare to high secure hospitals. Forensic psychiatry has often been viewed as only being part of the secure end of the spectrum. However, we believe that it is as relevant to community psychiatry as it is to maximum secure care in a special hospital, with for example, the issues of risk assessment and risk-management. Forensic psychiatry services in the UK differ from the rest of the world and vary even within the UK, with different legislations produce differing services. For example, in Scotland the definition of Mental Disorder in the 1984 Mental Health Act does not include the category of Psychopathic Disorder, as it does in England and Wales.

The development of forensic psychiatry services seems to depend to a large degree on the legal code of the particular country. An example is the Hospital Order within the Mental Health Acts of England and Wales, Scotland and Northern Ireland. This allows an individual found guilty of a criminal offence to be sent to hospital by the courts for treatment if this is believed to be the most appropriate disposal. In the USA and Canada, where equivalent legislation does not exist, such an individual could only receive treatment in a psychiatric hospital if found Not Guilty by Reason of Insanity. Therefore, in the UK there has been a continuing growth in forensic psychiatry services as part of the psychiatric services within the NHS, but in North America much more treatment is provided within the prison system. For a detailed comparison of forensic psychiatry services in various countries, see Harding (1993). This chapter focuses on forensic psychiatry services in England and Wales to illustrate the role of forensic psychiatry in a system providing comprehensive mental health services.

Historical perspective

In 1957 the report of the Royal Commission on the Law relating to Mental Illness and Mental Deficiency suggested that dangerous patients should be looked after in a few hospitals. Before the passing of the subsequent 1959 Mental Health Act, the Ministry of Health urged hospital boards to provide adequate security precautions for some patients. The hospitals also noted that not all of these patients would have been before the courts. The 1959 Mental Health Act is widely regarded as an innovative and enlightened piece of legislation which changed the practice of psychiatry in the UK and in other countries who have used it as a model for their own mental health legislation (Bluglass 1984). The term 'forensic psychiatry' was first used in the UK in the 1920s by Norwood-East (Bowden 1991); however, psychiatrists did not adopt it until the 1960s. Even consultants in Special Hospitals did not refer to themselves as forensic psychiatrists (Partridge 1953). Throughout the 1960s the Ministry of Health advocated secure hospital units. However, it was not until two reports were published during that decade that the impetus to develop the forensic psychiatry services began. These reports came from different directions: the first was the Report of the Working Party on the Special Hospitals (Emery Report) (Ministry of Health 1961), which was set up after the passing of the 1959 Mental Health Act to advise on the place of the Special Hospitals within that Act. These were the three maximum-security hospitals that were taken under the direct control of the Ministry of Health. The second was the Report of the Working Party of the Organisation of the Prison Health Service (Gwynne Report) (Home Office 1964) on the future of the Prison Medical Service. The Emery Report went beyond the recommendations for Special Hospitals alone and recommended secure units in each region whose security fell short of that provided by Special Hospitals. They were concerned that if no suitable local facilities were provided then the courts would simply not use new legislation under the 1959 Act. This allowed those convicted of crimes to be sent to hospital for treatment under a hospital order. The Gwynne Report suggested the appointment of 'consultant forensic psychiatrists'. These were to be joint appointments between the Home Office and the Ministry of Health. It was suggested that they would work in local prisons and provide outpatient services to psychiatric hospitals. It is generally accepted that these posts resulted in the later development of forensic psychiatry in the UK. The outcome of these appointments has been reviewed by one of the Home Office and Ministry of Health joint appointees (Faulk 1992).

In the 1970s the case of the poisoner Graham Young (Bowden 1995) led to the setting up of the Committee on Mentally Abnormal Offenders (Butler Committee) (Home Office and DHSS 1975) which proposed services for mentally disordered offenders (Table 13.1). In parallel, the Working Party on Security in NHS Psychiatric Hospitals was set up (Glancy Report) (Department of Health and Social Security 1974) (Table 13.2). These two reports in their separate ways provided the impetus to set up regionally based forensic psychiatry services outside Special Hospitals. Often the joint appointed forensic psychiatrist led the development of services. However, there were critics of these developments, particularly Scott (1974) (Table 13.3). It is enlightening to consider how many of these suggested criticisms have come true today. A programme of building medium secure units began in some regions before others.

- Secure hospital units in each region
- Units would operate as part of regional forensic psychiatry services
- Interagency collaboration with social services, probation services and criminal justice system
- Patients in units would not require special hospital but would be unsuitable for open wards
- Forty beds per million population

Interim Report and Report of Committee on Mentally Disordered Offenders (1974, 1975).

Table 13.1 – The Butler Report's recommendations.

- Security
    - Should not be excessive, otherwise it could defeat the aims of treatment
    - Unobtrusive, since a secure boundary was not necessary
    - Unit divided into smaller wards of varying security
- High staffing levels
- Clear operational policies to help staff manage patients
- Occupational, educational and recreational facilities were necessary
- Number of beds in each region of 20 per million population

Report of the Working Party on Security in NHS Psychiatric Hospitals (1974).

Table 13.2 – Glancy Report.

- Would not relieve overcrowding in Special Hospitals
- Would not help long-term prison inmates who were mentally abnormal
- Could prevent therapeutic developments in prisons
- They would be expensive to construct and run
- It would be difficult to find enough skilled nurses
- They could be too selective
- Psychiatric facilities in prisons should be improved instead

Scott (1974).

Table 13.3 – Criticisms of regional secure units.

The proposed level of provision was 20 beds per million population, giving 1000 beds for England and Wales. A quick method of providing medium secure beds was to open a converted ward as an interim medium secure unit (ISU) while plans were drawn up for purpose built regional secure units. Three interim secure units were opened during the late 1970s.

The 1980s was the decade of expansion of regional secure unit services. When the decade opened there were three interim secure units in existence, by its close there were 655 NHS medium secure unit beds in 12 of the 14 regions of England. Lessons learned from the early interim secure units were used to inform those developing regional secure units (Treasaden 1985) (Table 13.4). There have been a number of reviews of practice in regional secure units, including those by Snowden (1985), Bullard and Bond (1988), Smith (1991) and Mendelson (1992 a, b). During the late 1980s private sector companies moved to the fill the gap in services with the opening of some private low/medium secure units. The other major change in secure care during this decade came in July 1989 when control of the four Special Hospitals came under the Special Hospitals Service Authority (SHSA). The aim of this change was to link the Special Hospitals more closely with the NHS. The SHSA was also given the role of developing longer-term policy for the Special Hospitals in the future.

The early 1990s saw forensic psychiatry move up the political agenda. The end of the 1980s had seen the killing of a psychiatric social worker by a psychiatric patient (Department of Health and Social Security 1988). This case led, in part, to the development of the Care Programme Approach (CPA). At the same time the Royal College of Psychiatrists produced a document on the care of potentially dangerous patients (Royal College of Psychiatrists 1991). During the early 1990s there were

---

- 25% of patients came from local psychiatric hospitals that were unable to manage the patients because of aggressive behaviour

- 66% of patients were transferred either from prison or from special hospital

- Two-thirds of patients had a functional psychosis

- The usual reason for admission was violence to others

- The length of stay was usually 6–12 months

- Treatment regimes included conventional psychiatric treatment and rehabilitation

- Most units used a graduated system of increasing time off the unit

- Most patients were either discharged to the community or to an open ward of a local psychiatric hospital

Table 13.4 – Clinical experience from four interim secure units (Treasaden 1985).

reviews of forensic psychiatry services from various sources. In 1992, The National Association for Mental Health (MIND) produced the document 'Treatment, Care and Security' (Bynoe 1992). This suggested that local district services were no longer orientated to meeting the needs of mentally ill offenders. Second, the medical services within prisons were well below the standard found in NHS psychiatric hospitals. Third, the number of places at medium secure unit level was insufficient and, finally, Special Hospitals were unable to eradicate serious flaws in their organization and performance. MIND recommended interventions at various levels in the Criminal Justice System, low security units and moving high secure units from the Special Hospitals. At the same time The Review of the Services for Mentally Disordered Offenders and other Disturbed Psychiatric Patients (Reed Committee) was completed (Department of Health and Home Office 1992). This produced a range of documents including those of hospital, prison and community services. The final summary report contained no fewer than 276 separate recommendations. In 1990 the Home Office and DHSS joint circular 66/90 was produced. This encouraged prison medical officers to transfer mentally disordered inmates from prison to hospital. The response to this has been demonstrated by the Home Office's own statistics which show that from 1990 to 1995 the number of patients transferred from prison to hospital increased from 325 to 725 (Home Office 1996). The majority of these transfers was under Section 48 of the Mental Health Act, to medium secure unit beds. This had the effect of saturating the NHS medium secure provision. As the NHS has been slow to respond to the need for further medium secure beds, there has been an increase in private sector secure units.

To bring the Special Hospitals into the 'purchaser–provider' NHS, in 1996 their management was shifted from the SHSA to each of the three hospitals, which became Special Health Authorities, and these became the providers of high secure care. The purchasing of this care was taken on by the High Security Psychiatric Services Commissioning Board (HSPSCB). It was intended that these changes would help those patients, who it was believed were inappropriately placed in Special Hospitals, to move to lower security within the NHS (NHS Executive 1995). One of the last acts of the SHSA was to produce a summary of work that had been done over the 6 years of its existence, which described the needs of patients in Special Hospital. It also suggested a strategy for long-term medium security (SHSA 1995). In 1997 the government White Paper 'The New NHS' recommended that a number of specialized services should be commissioned (rather than purchased) by Regional Specialised Commissioning Groups (RSCG), instead of Health Authorities. The Department of Health announced in 1998 that from April 2000 both high and medium secure care would be commissioned by the RSCG. In addition, it was suggested that Special Hospitals should become part of established mental health trusts.

Another characteristic of the 1990s has been the public enquiries related to psychiatric care, which have ranged from Special Hospital care (Department of Health

1992, 1999) to community care, e.g. North-East Thames RHA and South-East Thames RHA (1992). Bingley (1996) and Petch and Bradley (1997) have reviewed the subject of the enquiries into homicides by psychiatric patients. Current forensic psychiatry services have been reviewed by Exworthy (1998).

DIAGNOSES OF PATIENTS WITHIN FORENSIC SERVICES

In general, forensic psychiatrists assess and manage patients with the same diagnoses as general psychiatrists, although there is a greater proportion of patients with resistant schizophrenia and personality disorder. Their skills lie in the assessment of risk, the understanding and management of offending behaviour related to mental disorder and an understanding of how psychiatry relates to the law and the criminal justice system.

Referrals to forensic psychiatry services

In the only study of patients referred to a regional forensic service, 40% had a diagnosis of personality disorder amounting to the legal category of psychopathic disorder. Approximately one-fifth of the patients had schizophrenia and substance misuse was present in over one-quarter. One feature of the group was the presence of co-morbidity which often makes forensic patients more difficult to assess and, therefore, to manage. Approximately one-third of the patients referred had not offended but were proving to be too difficult to be managed in general or open psychiatric wards because of disturbed, unpredictable and dangerous behaviour. Only 7.5% of all the patients referred were offered secure care (Mendelson 1992a, b).

Personality disorder

About 10% of patients detained in medium secure units are detained under the legal category of psychopathic disorder compared with 1% in general psychiatric wards and 25% in Special Hospitals (Department of Health and Home Office 1994). This presumably reflects the resources available to manage these patients. The Reed Report into Psychopathic Disorder (Department of Health and Home Office 1994) recommended that specialized placements should be made available for these patients. More importantly, it recommended that more research should be conducted into the management of patients with personality disorders. The Special Hospitals have responded by developing specialist therapeutic units within conditions of maximum security for young people (under 35 years of age). Within the prison service there is one facility, HMP Grendon, that has been developed as a therapeutic community to treat specially selected inmates who suffer from personality disorders (Gender and Players 1994). There have also been small 'special units' developed within specific prisons to manage similar prisoners who are not considered suitable for transfer to hospital. The work of these is well described by Dolan and Coid (1994). The diversion from custody to hospital of this group of prisoners remains controversial. The Reed Report into Psychopathic Disorder recommended greater use of Section 38 of the Mental Health Act 1983 to assess whether patients with personality disorder were suitable for treatment. Patients can now be detained under Section 38 for up to 12 months, instead of 6 months, which it is hoped will further encourage its use. Legislation was introduced by the Crime Sentences Act 1997 which allows this group of patients to receive a prison sentence combined with a period of time in hospital ('The Hybrid Order'). Until it is widely used, its implications on the management of such patients and the resources available to treat them, will not be known. The government has made it clear that separate facilities and legislation will be created to manage those people with severe personality disorder, whether they have offended or not (Hansard 1999).

Schizophrenia

About 50–60% of inpatients within all levels of secure care will be suffering from schizophrenia and a large proportion of these are referred because they have failed to respond to treatment and their illness places them at risk of violence. Studies have indicated that more than 50% of Special Hospital patients are treatment resistant and this has been shown to be one of the factors in determining their length of stay in conditions of maximum security. Clozapine and other new generation antipsychotic medication have been used in this group and The Special Hospitals Treatment Resistant Schizophrenia Research Group (1996) has described its use. The group highlights one of the concerns about the use of these medications in violent schizophrenics, namely, the risk of rebound psychosis following abrupt cessation of clozapine. This has serious implications for these patients when they eventually move into the community where patients' compliance may fluctuate. The group is planning a long-term follow-up of these patients, but more importantly is promoting clinical trials for the seriously mentally ill within a special hospital setting.

RISK ASSESSMENT

The purpose of risk assessment

Psychiatrists are expected by the general population to determine which patients are a risk to themselves or to others. This forms an essential part of the psychiatric assessment for detention under the Mental Health Act. The assessment of this risk has to be part of the decision-making process inherent in the clinical management of patients such as when patients should be admitted to hospital or discharged. The introduction of the Care Programme Approach and the Supervision Register was, at least in part, as a result of poor decision-making in several notable cases. This in turn has led to demands that psychiatrists should be more rigorous in their assessment of risk and decision-making. Traditionally forensic psychiatrists were considered to have expertise in assessing risk because they frequently managed patients who have offended or been violent. However, the expectations are now that all psychiatrists should be able to assess and manage risk.

Risk versus dangerousness

It has been suggested that the concept of dangerousness should now be replaced by that of risk. Reasons for this include the fact that dangerousness is viewed as an inherent characteristic of the patient which remains static. The assessment of dangerousness is subjective whereas that of risk can be more objective. Risk invites further definition depending upon other characteristics of the individual as well as their environment. Risk changes over time often according to circumstances. It also allows for definition of the type of risk including severity and potential victims whereas dangerousness is a more fixed concept.

The psychiatrists role in risk assessment

Psychiatrists have regarded the assessment of risk of suicide as part of their normal clinical practice and have to consider the risk a patient poses to others when detaining a patient under the Mental Health Act. Psychiatrists have been considered to be generally poor in making these predictions and tend to be over cautious. Some studies have shown that psychiatrists' predictions are correct in about 30% of cases (Monahan 1984). However, Lidz (1993) found that psychiatrists assessing patients in an emergency room were correct in their predictions of violence about 60% of the time. Psychiatrists are no better or no worse than any other professional in their assessment. Steadman and Coccozza (1974) reported on the outcomes of the release of 967 patients who had been detained in a hospital for the criminally insane, as they were considered dangerous. Their release was directed by the US Supreme Court following an appeal by one of the patients that his detention was unlawful. Only 3% were re-admitted to similar hospitals in the first year and only 20% were assaultive in the 4 years following release.

Clinical aspects of risk assessment.

The risk factors for violence in the mentally ill can be divided into the dispositional, historical, illness-related and contextual (Monahan 1993). The first two tend to be static; the second two are changeable. As a result, they are particularly important in reducing risk.

Dispositional factors include gender, age, socio-economic and marital status, intellectual functioning and personality traits. The risk of violence in the female mentally ill population appears to have been underestimated in the past because of the low rates of violence in females in the general population. Three studies of inpatient hospital violence reported no differences between the sexes (Klassen and O'Connor 1994). The Macarthur Risk Assessment study showed that self-reported violence in ex-psychiatric patients was equal in males and females (Steadman 1991). Most studies of patients have found differences in age, in either inpatient or community settings, where violence is commoner in younger people. However, this difference does not appear as marked in patient populations as it is in the general population. Violence tends to be generally associated with lower socio-economic groups. The same is true for mental illness because such patients drift down the economic scales. Generally being involved in a stable relationship is not associated with violence however there has been one study, which suggests that marriage is associated with violence in an inpatient setting (McNeil 1988).

Offending is included within the diagnostic criteria for some personality disorders which automatically suggests some link. However, it appears that it is only certain traits that may be associated with violence. There have only been two empirical studies of borderline personality disorder and the disposition to violence (Snyder et al. 1986, Stone 1990). These have suggested that anger and impulsivity may at times result in violence. Antisocial or dissocial personality disorder in the absence of a history of violent or aggressive behaviour does not necessarily indicate a risk of future violence. The relationship of a low IQ to violent behaviour is unknown and it has been suggested that it is more appropriate to consider the effects of limited coping skills, misinterpretation and impulse control rather than to rely on the levels of intellectual functioning.

Historical factors include personal, forensic and psychiatric histories. A history of separation from parents and childhood conduct disorder increases the risk of recidivism in a forensic psychiatric population (Harris et al. 1993). A history of treatment for a previous mental disorder is not predictive of violence (Link et al. 1992, Swanson 1994). The best predictor of violent behaviour is a past history of violence however it is measured, i.e. whether self-reported or by recorded arrests. Observing violence in childhood or being the victim of violence also appears to be associated with violent behaviour in psychiatric patients (Klassen and O'Connor 1988).

Contextual factors include the patients current life situation, their social supports, their current emotional state, perceived stresses, means for violence including their access to weapons, threats and substance abuse. These factors are particularly important because they can be altered to reduce the risk. It has been shown that those who perceive hostility from their social supports, particularly from significant others, are more likely to be violent. It is also clear from investigations that mothers not only bear the responsibility of being the carer of a mentally ill child but are at increased risk of repeated violence from them (Estroff and Zimmer 1994). Sixty percent of the victims of violence of the mentally ill were immediate family members in one study and only 9% strangers (Hafner and Boker 1973). The chronically mentally ill tend to have impoverished social networks and this along with conflict within the relationships that do exist may predispose to violence.

Certain emotional states that predispose to violent behaviour include: fear, jealousy and anger. Access to weapons increases the risk of violence as in the general population.

Illness-related factors include specific psychopathology, the treatability of the disorder and co-morbidity. The association between mental illness and violence had been thought to be insignificant by criminologists. However, there have been well-publicized inquiries into homicides committed by psychiatric patients that have led the public to question the association. Research by psychiatrists now confirms the link between mental illness and violence. Studies of patients presenting for the first time with symptoms of schizophrenia show that up to 30% admit to some violence in the previous month (Johnstone et al. 1986). Studies of remand prisoners charged with homicide in Brixton prison, such as that reported by Wessely showed that 8% suffered from schizophrenia (Taylor 1984, Wessely 1997)

It has also been recognized for some time that characteristic psychopathology is associated with an increased risk of violence by mentally ill patients. One of the first studies to demonstrate this came from the then Federal Republic of Germany in the 1970s (Hafner and Boker 1973). This large study included four control groups and sought to identify whether violent offending was higher in those with mental illness, particularly schizophrenia. As part of that work the authors discovered that the type of delusions that a patient described could predict whether they would act on those delusions. The violent group was more likely to have experienced delusions which were systematized with themes such as morbid jealousy and persecution rather than delusional mood. Since then it has been recognized that patients may be more willing to act on delusions rather than command hallucinations. This appears to have at least face validity since anyone may be supposed to respond to what they believe rather than what they hear. Taylor (1993) describes the relationship of delusions to a patient's behaviour in more detail.

The specific type of psychopathology described by Hafner and Boker has been taken further by Link and Steuve (1994). They have described specific symptoms that predict whether a mentally ill person may be violent. They have called these 'threat/control override' symptoms. These symptoms are said to occur when someone with mental illness experiences threatening delusions and hallucinations and their internal controls are compromised. In this situation they suggest that violence appears more understandable. In a later multi-site community survey four of these symptoms were used to determine whether people had experienced threat/control override symptoms. They were:

1. A belief of being controlled against the person's will.

2. A belief that others were plotting against the person and trying to harm or poison him.

3. Symptoms of thought interference or withdrawal.

4. Belief that the person was being followed.

This study was known as the Epidemiological Catchment Area (ECA) survey (Swanson et al. 1990, 1996). That survey found that when one or more of the above symptoms were present, then the risk that the person had been violent in the previous year was doubled.

The co-morbidity of substance misuse with mental disorder significantly increases the risk of violence (Swanson et al. 1990). This has been illustrated by the ECA survey (Swanson et al. 1996), which discovered that the base rates of violence for individuals without mental illness or substance abuse was 2% in the previous year. The presence of schizophrenia or a major affective disorder increased the risk of violence in the previous year by four times to 8%. However, co-morbidity of substance abuse with schizophrenia or affective disorder produced a 16-fold increase so that about 30% had committed violence in the previous year. This work emphasizes the importance of recognizing and effectively treating substance abuse disorders in patients with severe mental illness.

PRACTICAL RISK ASSESSMENT

The Department of Health guidelines on risk assessment (The Department of Health and Social Security 1991) state that the following are necessary to make an accurate assessment of risk.

1. Ensuring that relevant information is available regarding the patients past behaviour, present mental state and social functioning. It advised liaison with other agencies to achieve this.

2. Conducting a full assessment of risk. The guidelines quote the case of Kim Kirkman (W Midlands RHA 1991) and suggested the following factors should be considered.

- Past history of the patient.

- Self reporting by the patient.

- Observed behaviour of the patient.

- Discrepancies between what is reported and what is observed.

- Psychological and if appropriate, physiological test.
- Statistics from studies of related cases.
- Predictive indicators derived from research.

3. Defining situations and circumstances known to present increased risk.

4. Seeking expert help. It recommended that 'expert forensic help' should be available to local psychiatric teams.

The Royal College of Psychiatrists (1996) has produced a document on the assessment of risk. It suggest that a formulation should be made based on specific information such as that in table 5 and all other items of history and mental state. The formulation should specify factors that would increase risk and those that would decrease it. It is, therefore, suggested that the formulation should define the risks more clearly, including plans that could reduce the risk.

It is important that information sources are clearly identified and that as many sources as possible are used. This will include third-party information, previous records, witness statements and information from other agencies. There have been concerns in the past about the sharing of information and the possible breaching of confidentiality but it is vital if risk assessment is to be effective. Information may be passed onto someone else if either the patient gives consent or on a 'need to know' basis in certain circumstances as described by General Medical Council (1995).

Problems with risk assessments

Inquiries into homicides committed by psychiatric patients have highlighted situations in which care has failed. The conclusions of these have shown that poor communication between agencies, inadequate information available and undervaluing the history of violence have all led to a poor assessment of risk and failure to provide adequate care. It is very important that any incident particularly a violent one is well documented including the circumstances surrounding it and that this

---

- Previous violence including a forensic history
- Previous self-harming or suicidal behaviour
- History that indicates a chaotic lifestyle, including poor employment and relationship records, and changes of address
- History of substance misuse
- History of poor compliance with psychiatric treatment or difficulties engaging with services
- Precipitants of any previous violence including changes in mental state

Table 5 – Information required for risk assessment.

should be passed on to other agencies. Lipsedge (1995) describes the reasons why disasters can occur in mental health services. Other than those reasons already stated they include an undue emphasis on the civil liberties of patients at the expense of increased risk of suicidal and homicidal behaviour, a failure to properly implement the Mental Health Act and a tendency to take a 'cross-sectional' view of cases rather than a longitudinal view.

RISK MANAGEMENT

The concept of risk-management is a relatively new one in the field of medicine and specifically psychiatry. It has been suggested that risk assessment alone will not achieve anything unless it is accompanied by subsequent management of the risk identified (Monahan and Steadman 1994). Snowden (1997) has discussed the concept and use of the words 'risk-management'. He describes the history of risk-management from its use in the 1960s by insurance companies in the USA where it was developed to control expenditure on insurance claims. Clearly, the way in which it is currently used is very different. Walker (1996) describes the need for a balance between the risk of harm to others and the civil liberties of the individual. For example, it is well recognized that an individual convicted of several offences of violence is at greater risk of future violence and if that person were to be detained in prison indefinitely, then this risk would be reduced, but at the expense of his civil liberties. Chiswick (1995) is almost certainly correct when he suggests that risk-management is already part of the clinical work of all psychiatrists.

The work that has been done on describing risk-management could be loosely grouped under three headings: clinical, risk-management systems and criminological.

Clinical

Gunn (1993, 1996) has provided one of the clearest descriptions of the clinical process of risk-management. Gunn emphasizes the context of the risk and poses the question in what circumstances is the individual dangerous? Risk or danger-ousness is not an entity that an individual possesses which can be measured. It varies according to the situation in which the individual finds himself. Gunn divides the clinical management of risk under three headings: security, supervision and support.

Security extends from no care to the maximum security provided by a special hospital. The factors that determine the level of security include:

1. Seriousness of previous aggressive behaviour.

2. Severity of mental disorder.

3. Type of mental disorder and its prognosis.

4. How long the risk of aggressive behaviour will continue to be present.

5. Likelihood of the return of aggressive behaviour.

6. Range of therapeutic and educational services available.

Supervision involves the continuing assessment of the risk to others and is relevant to all levels of security including the community. The number and the skills of the supervising staff determine the type of supervision provided. In higher levels of security, supervision of inpatients will include monitoring their compliance with medication and visual monitoring of patient's movements and availability of potential weapons. While outpatient supervision will concentrate more on providing clear boundaries on limits of behaviour or non-cooperation with treatment.

Gunn's view of support is that he believes there should be trust established between patient and supervisor. He likens this to the psychotherapists use of the term 'transference'.

Gunn has also described risk assessment as a form of 'clinical judgement' (Gunn 1996). He says that it is better to try to forget prediction and concentrate instead on management. If the time-scale is reduced to a more manageable length, for example, 2 weeks, then by using information gained about a patient, in particular the psychopathology and social circumstances in which violence occurs, then the risk can be reduced. In this way Gunn suggests assessment merges into management.

Snowden (1997) takes the clinical description of risk-management a stage further and has attempted to operationalize it. He describes the three parts of the process, risk identification, risk assessment and clinical risk-management. Identifying the risk includes recognizing violence to others or to self and self-neglect. Snowden then suggests that the risk assessment should assess each of these identified risks in terms of the likelihood of it occurring and its severity. He emphasizes the importance of review including written reports. This report should include the history of risk in individual patients, for example, specific phenomenology, early warning signs, treatment changes which decrease risk and relevant advice from the psychiatric literature. Finally, clinical risk-management involves the development of treatment strategies, which would include physical treatments, such as medication, psychological treatments and social interventions. Snowden emphasizes the need for complete packages of treatment including psychosocial interventions, which has echoes of the Care Programme Approach.

In a review of this subject, Mullen (1997) states that good clinical management is essential to reduce the risk of violence. He concludes: 'In the long run maintaining a therapeutic alliance, particularly with the difficult and objectionable patients, which promotes treatment compliance and maintains the necessary social and interpersonal supports, is a greater contribution to reducing violence than the finest skills in risk assessment'.

Risk management systems

Carson has been one of the leading proponents of adopting a more actuarial style of managing risk by carefully considering the clinical decisions that make up risk-management. In his five-part model of risk (Carson 1996) the individual dangerousness of the patient is only one part of the model. Carson includes the situational factors that can increase or decrease the risk that an individual poses. The third part of his model is 'risk as decision-making'. He suggests that not taking a risk decision is as important as taking a decision that has harmful consequences. For example, the decision not to discharge a patient can be as wrong or poorly made as a decision to discharge him without appropriate aftercare. The final parts of the model are decision management and system management. The former includes the need for decision-makers to have proper training, help in making decisions, and feedback and guidance on the results of decisions that are made. The latter suggests the need for individual organizations such as mental health services, social services, housing, etc. to develop clear procedures and policies on the management of risk.

Carson has also suggested that risk-management should be more pro-active involving the establishment of a framework and standards for decision-making rather than only finding a way of reducing the likelihood and seriousness of the consequence of decision (Carson 1995). He emphasizes that the plethora of enquiries that have resulted from homicides by mentally ill patients in the community has led to a rather one-sided view of risk decisions, which are only seen in terms of the failures. He makes the valid point that the benefits from taking risk decisions must be clearly emphasized. The risk decision has to also be viewed and understood in the context of a time-scale. For example, if a risk decision results in a harmful outcome 10 years later is this as blameworthy as if the same outcome had occurred ten weeks after the decision was made? Carson also emphasizes the need to learn from the implementation of risk-management strategies and advises against trying to devise and describe more risk factors that cannot be changed. For example, an individual's past history of violent behaviour, while this risk factor may predict future violence, it is not amenable to change.

Criminological

Walker has described in some detail, over a number of years, the criminological and ethical problems encountered in assessment and management of risk (Walker 1978, 1991, 1996). He has highlighted in particular the difficulties in prediction. This includes the fact that the less frequent an outcome to be predicted occurs, the less accurately will samples predict. Second, it is difficult to study serious violence offences in the population since the more serious the offence the longer the person will spend in prison and hospital and this will affect any attempt to describe the true incidence of repeat offending in this group. One way round this problem is to try and use longer follow-ups.

Several probation services have recently attempted to describe the processes of risk assessment and risk-management (Institute for the Study and Treatment of Delinquency 1995). These concentrate on the risk of serious violence in offenders, who may or may not have a recognizable mental disorder. One such document emphasizes the need for risk assessment to be seen as part of a dynamic process, which depends greatly on the quality of information available (Hampshire Probation Service 1995). Using relevant information about an offender it is possible to draw up an intervention plan to try and influence the circumstances in which the offender may cause harm to others in the future.

Legal provisions in risk-management

The decision to admit a patient to hospital under the Mental Health Act 1983 involves an assessment of the existence of a mental disorder and whether they are a risk to their own health or safety or a risk to the safety of others. The issue of risk to others is more clearly defined in the case of a Restriction Order under Section 41 of the Mental Health Act. The single criterion for adding a Restriction Order to a Hospital Order is to 'protect the public from the risk of serious harm'. The trial judge having heard medical evidence makes the decision whether it is needed.

There are ways in which the Mental Health Act 1983 is used to manage mentally disordered patients once they are discharged in to the community.

1. Patients on Restriction Orders are usually conditionally discharged. The conditions can include: residence, attendance at psychiatric outpatients, attendance at social supervisor and often compliance with medication. If any of these conditions are broken the patient can be immediately recalled to hospital. The effectiveness of supervision of conditionally discharged patients was investigated by the Home Office's Research and Statistics Department (Home Office 1995). A sample of patients who were conditionally discharged between 1985 and 1989 was surveyed to measure the effectiveness and quality of supervision. Some patients and supervisors were also interviewed. The patients valued the following:

   - Help when first discharged after years in hospital.

   - Long-term moral and practical support from their social supervisor.

   - Psychiatric supervision, which guaranteed treatment if needed and a bed in hospital if required.

Psychiatrists believed that statutory supervision had reduced the likelihood of aggressive behaviour in the majority of mentally ill patients but only in the minority of personality disordered patients. In the latter it was more difficult to monitor and predict their behaviour. Psychiatrists believed that in the case of mentally ill patients the statutory supervision ensured closer monitoring of their mental state and treatment and improved their compliance. In only 9% of patients were there problems in ensuring compliance with medication.

Amongst those patients who were recalled to hospital, only one-quarter had committed an offence or showed any suggestion of risk to the public. Only 5% of conditionally discharged patients are re-convicted of very serious offences in the first 5 years after discharge. When these cases were reviewed, it appeared that it was seldom possible to have foreseen the serious offending and taken preventative action.

The research emphasized how important a relationship of trust, support and openness is with patients. This confirms the views of other authors on the subject (Gunn 1993, Grounds 1994).

2. Patients admitted to hospital under a treatment or hospital order can now be discharged on trial leave for up to 12 months. Conditions can be attached to this trial leave in similar way to the discharge of a restricted patient. It remains to be seen if this provision improves the supervision of patients in the community.

3. Patients can be admitted into Guardianship Orders under Section 7 of the Mental Health Act or as an alternative to a hospital order under Section 37 of the Mental Health Act. Although the named guardian can place conditions on the patient, it is well recognized that little can be done to enforce them if the patient refuses to comply.

4. The Supervised Discharge Order was introduced in 1996. It is discussed, along with supervision registers and the Care Programme Approach, in Chapter 11.

LIAISON WITH OTHER AGENCIES

The Butler Committee recommended that mentally disordered offenders should be dealt with other than through the courts (Home Office and Department of Health and Social Security 1975) and Home Office Circular 66/90 reiterated this. A further Home Office Circular 12/95 reported on the progress made and highlighted the importance of interagency working and in particular information sharing. The Review of Health and Social Services for Mentally Disordered Offenders (Reed Committee) (DoH and Home Office 1992) made a number of similar recommendations that mentally disordered offenders should receive care and treatment from health and social services rather than in custody. The report recommended that forensic and general psychiatric services should develop closer links and that all psychiatric services should develop closer working relationships with other agencies, in particular with the probation service, social services and the police. The report recommended the development of court diversion schemes. It also recommended the use of CPA for mentally disordered prisoners to ensure they receive appropriate care on release.

Probation services

Probation officers play a key role in the assessment and management of mentally disordered offenders. Research indicates that about 20% of probation clients have some sort of mental illness (Pritchard et al. 1992). As a result, psychiatric clinics have been set up in some areas in probation offices and hostels. Their function is to assess risk and mental state, to advise on management and prepare reports for court. These clinics have improved compliance with supervision and treatment, probably because they are part of the probation service rather than attached to a hospital (Huckle 1996). Psychiatric services also provide liaison and advice to bail hostels and although the Reed Report recommended the creation of probation hostels specifically for mentally disordered offenders, only one is currently in existence in London. An Inner London study has recognized the need for specific bail place-ments for those with mental disorder who come before the courts to reduce the number of them being remanded in custody for their own safety and for reports (Kennedy et al. 1997).

Court diversion schemes

The Home Office Circular 66/90 (1990) stated 'a mentally disordered offender should never be remanded to prison simply to receive medical treatment or assessment'. Studies of remand prisoners have shown that up to 10% of this popu-lation suffer from schizophrenia which has been thought to be partly due to the practice of remanding the mentally ill into custody for psychiatric reports to be prepared. Court Diversion Schemes were, therefore, originally developed to avoid the practice of remanding mentally disordered offenders to prison and to direct them to the appropriate services. There have been concerns about where the offenders are diverted to and whether services are available for this group in the long-term (Exworthy and Parrott 1997) The research into diversion schemes have shown that between 10 and 26% of cases seen in these schemes are actually diverted to hospital. In the case of two London services this only represented 1.7 and 5% of all admissions to local psychiatric units. The result of diversion schemes has been to significantly reduce the time mentally disordered offenders spend in custody (James and Hamilton 1991, Joseph and Potter 1993b). Court Diversion schemes can operate in a variety of ways. The first English scheme to be reported on ran with a psychiatrist providing two sessions to the local magistrate's courts. Defendants were either seen on the day they first appeared or were remanded in custody until the psychiatrist next visited. The referral criterion were 'those defendants perceived by any court official as requiring a psychiatric assessment who might be, or who already had been, remanded into custody for a medical report' (Joseph and Potter

1993a). Alternative diversion schemes involve community psychiatric nurses as the key person who assesses the offenders either in the courts or prior to their appearance in court at the police station. The community nurse then advises the police, highlights vulnerable or mentally ill defendants and refers onto the appropriate agency.

Prison psychiatry

Despite efforts to divert mentally disordered offenders from the criminal justice system large numbers still remain within prison. A study of 5% of the UK sentenced prisoner population suggests that 38% have a psychiatric diagnosis, between 750 and 1400 prisoners may require hospital inpatient care and up to 30% of these require maximum secure care (Gunn et al. 1991). Further epidemiological research undertaken by the Office for National Statistics (Singleton et al. 1998) has demonstrated even higher levels of psychiatric morbidity within the prison population, although this study did not address the issue of the number who would require treatment in hospital. Forensic and general psychiatrists provide clinics in prisons offering advice on diagnosis, management and the transfer of patients to hospital, if required. An example of such a service is that in Cardiff Prison as described by Huckle and Williams (1994). One of the major problems of working in prisons is the time mentally ill prisoners have to wait for a bed in a psychiatric hospital. An audit of psychiatric services at one English prison revealed that prisoners had to wait an average of 3–6 weeks before they could be transferred, which is much longer than the standard recommended by the Reed Committee of 3 days (Resnick 1995). In general, mentally ill prisoners tend to be held in prisons of a higher security and have fewer opportunities for parole.

One of the targets of the Health of the Nation Report (Department of Health 1993) was to reduce the number of suicides. This is particularly relevant to those working in prisons where suicide is one of the major risks for mentally disordered prisoners. It is eight times more common in the prison population than in the general population and the annual rate of suicide in prisons has almost doubled between 1972 and 1987 (Dooley 1990). Prisoners who successfully commit suicide tend to have a history of drug or alcohol misuse, previous self-harm and psychiatric disorder. However, most are unpredictable and in contrast to the general population, only a minority is mentally ill at the time. Deliberate self-harm is also very common particularly among the younger prison population. Prisons now have policies for dealing with suicidal prisoners or those at risk of self-harm, which often will involve assessment by a visiting psychiatrist. Isolation of the prisoner in a strip cell has been the commonest form of management of suicide risk. This practice has been condemned by HM Chief Inspector of Prisons who has recommended more time out of the cell for prisoners, improved standards of hygiene and better access to voluntary schemes such as the Samaritans (Home Office 1990).

FUTURE FORENSIC PSYCHIATRY SERVICES

Having witnessed the move of general psychiatry from the asylums to the community over the past 30 years, perhaps the time has come for similar changes in forensic psychiatry services. Support for this idea comes from a recent article on the future of forensic psychiatry by Grounds (1996). He recognized that whereas the Butler Committee was responsible for the development of regional forensic psychiatry services, the Reed Committee should have done the same for district forensic psychiatry services, but did not. Grounds listed a number of tasks to be completed before such services could be developed. These include education, integrating principles of risk assessment and management into community teams, developing a model of a district forensic psychiatry service and training. Grounds suggests the need for academic developments in forensic psychiatry, beyond that of service orientated research. To achieve this, better training for academics is needed.

Chiswick (1996) described a broader view of the future. He concentrated on three areas. First, research that he believes should be less service directed. Second, service developments with the need for local forensic psychiatry services. Third, the law, changes in which will not prevent further homicides by the mentally ill in the community. Chiswick ends with three cautionary points.

- We are not as skilled as we would like to be in preventing relapse or influencing other factors which could reduce violence.

- Even if we were more skilled the infrastructure required is absent.

- Even if both these were present the law would impede us.

The Reed Report (1992) highlighted the need for long-stay medium secure unit beds. The Royal College of Psychiatrists considers there is a need for 1500 medium secure unit beds and 750 long-term medium secure unit beds for England and Wales. These would be distributed according to population requirements. The High Security Psychiatric Services Commissioning Board had, as part of its remit, responsibility for the development of long-term medium secure units (NHS Executive 1995). It invited tenders for three particular patient groups which they viewed as a priority for long-term medium security (HSPS Commissioning Board 1996).

- Men with learning disabilities.

- Men with enduring mental illness.

- Women patients.

Since then, the Department of Health has identified a fourth priority group: people with personality disorders. It is clear that future government policy on the Special Hospitals will be directed at integrating maximum secure care into generic mental health services, because these hospitals are viewed as both geographically and professionally isolated (Hansard 1998). A further pressure on NHS resources is likely come about as a result of changes in the provision of healthcare in prisons. This is one of the recommendations made by the Home Office/NHS working group on the future of prison healthcare.

The often-suggested 'seamless service' in forensic psychiatry can only exist when specialist forensic psychiatry services are provided at a district as well as regional level. This fact is recognized in The Royal College of Psychiatrists Consultant manpower recommendations and by the NHS Executive, which in 1995 estimated the need for all secure beds in England and Wales (Table 13.6). District forensic psychiatry services would work with local community mental health teams. The suggested fragmentation of the Special Hospitals, with smaller more local high secure units, could mark the beginning of the de-institutionalization of forensic psychiatry. Unless this happens, we run the risk of forensic psychiatry and community mental health services moving further apart and not closer, to the detriment of a group of patients who require well coordinated and integrated care for their own well-being and the safety of others.

- High security – 850
- Medium security (less than 24 months duration) – 1390
- Longer term medium security – 940
- Long-term low security (more than 24 months) – 2120

Table 13.6 – Number of secure beds needed in England and Wales (NHS Executive 1995).

References

Bingley W. Hospital inquiries: have we learned anything? Criminal Behaviour and Mental Health 1996; (suppl.): 5–10.

Bluglass R. A Guide to the Mental Health Act. London: Churchill Livingstone, 1984.

Bowden P. Graham Young (1947–90): the St Albans' Poisoner: his life and times. Criminal Behaviour and Mental Health 1996; (suppl.): 17–24.

Bowden P. Pioneers in forensic psychiatry: William Norwood East. Journal of Forensic Psychiatry 1991; 2: 59–78.

Bullard H, Bond M. Secure units, why they are needed. Medicine, Science and The Law 1988; 28: 312–318.

Bynoe I. Treatment and Care in Security. London: Mind, 1992.

Carson D. Developing models of risk to aid cooperation between law and psychiatry. Criminal Behaviour and Mental Health 1996; 6: 6–10.

Carson D. From Risk Assessment to Risk Management. Managing Risk: Achieving the Possible. London: ISTD, 1995, pp. 75–78.

Chiswick D. Dangerousness. In Chiswick D, Cope R (eds), Seminars in Practical Forensic Psychiatry. London: Gaskell, 1995, pp. 210–242.

Chiswick D. Forensic psychiatry 2000 and beyond: peering into the abyss. Criminal Behaviour and Mental Health 1996; (suppl.): 33–42.

Department of Health. Health Service Guidelines, (94) 5, 1994.

Department of Health. Report of the Committee of Inquiry into Complaints about Ashworth Hospital Cm 2028 I and II. London: HMSO, 1992.

Department of Health. Report of the Committee of Inquiry into the Personality Disorder Unit, Ashworth Special Hospital. Cmnd. 4194. London: HMSO, 1999.

Department of Health. The Health of the Nation. London: HMSO, 1993.

Department and Health and Social Security. Health Circular (90) 23, 1991.

Department of Health and Home Office. Report of the Working Group on Psychopathic Disorder. London: HMSO, 1994.

Department of Health and Home Office. Review of Health and Social Services for Mentally Disordered Offenders and Others Requiring Similar Services (The Reed Report). Final Summary Report. Cmnd. 2088. London: HMSO, 1992.

Department of Health and Social Security. Report of the Committee of Inquiry into the Care and After-care of Miss Sharon Campbell, Cmnd. 440. London: HMSO, 1988.

Department of Health and Social Security. Revised Report of the Working Party on Security in NHS Psychiatric Hospitals (Glancy Report). London: DHSS, 1974.

Dolan B, Coid J. Psychopathic and Antisocial Personality Disorders: Treatment and Research Issues. London: Gaskell, 1994.

Dooley E. Prison suicides in England and Wales 1972–1987. British Journal of Psychiatry 1990; 156: 40–45.

Estroff SE, Zimmer C. Social Networks, social support and violence. In Monahan J, Steadman H (eds), Violence and Mental Disorder. Chicago: University of Chicago Press, 1994, pp. 259–295.

Exworthy T. Institutions and services in forensic psychiatry. Journal of Forensic Psychiatry 1988; 9: 395–412.

Exworthy T, Parrott J. Comparative evaluation of a diversion from custody scheme. Journal of Forensic Psychiatry 1997; 8: 406–416.

Faulk M. 1971: an audit of dreams. Journal of Forensic Psychiatry 1992; 3: 1–3.

General Medical Council. Confidentiality. London: GMC, 1995.

Grounds AT. Forensic psychiatry for the millennium. Journal of Forensic Psychiatry 1996; 7: 221–227.

Grounds AT. Risk assessment and management in a clinical context. In Crichton JM (ed.), Psychiatric Patient Violence: Risk and Response. London: Duckworth, 1994, pp. 43–59.

Gunn J. Dangerousness. In Gunn J, Taylor P (eds), Forensic Psychiatry: Clinical, Legal and Ethical Issues. London: Butterworth-Heinemann, 1993, pp. 624–664.

Gunn J. The management and discharge of violent patients. In Walker N (ed.), Dangerous People. London: Blackstone, 1996.

Gunn J, Maden A, Swinton M. Treatment needs of prisoners with psychiatric disorders. British Medical Journal 1991; 303: 338–341.

Hafner and Boker. Crimes of Violence by Mentally Abnormal Offenders [1973], trans. H Marshall. Cambridge: Cambridge University Press, 1984.

Hampshire Probation Service. Recognising and Reducing Risk. Hampshire Probation Service, 1995.

Hansard. 15 February 1999, Col. 605.

Hansard. Special Hospitals, 9 April 1998, pp. 902–912.

Harding T. A comparative survey of medico-legal systems. In Gunn J, Taylor P (eds), Forensic Psychiatry: Clinical, Legal and Ethical Issues. London: Butterworth-Heinemann, 1993, pp. 118–166.

Harris et al. Violent recidivism of mentally disordered offenders: the development of a statistical prediction instrument: Criminal Justice and Behaviour 1993; 20: 315–335.

Home Office. Report of a Review by HM Inspector of Prisons for England and Wales of suicide and Self Harm in Prison Service Establishments in England and Wales. London: HMSO, 1990.

Home Office. Report of the Working Party on the Organisations of the Prison Medical Service (Gwynn Report). London: HMSO, 1964.

Home Office. Statistics of Mentally Disordered Offenders, England and Wales 1995. Statistical Bulletin, 20/96, 1996.

Home Office. The Supervision of Restricted Patients in the Community. Home Office Research and Statistics Department Research Findings no. 19. London: Home Office, 1995.

Home Office and Department of Health and Social Security. Circular 66/90, 1990.

Home Office and Department of Health and Social Security. Circular 12/95, 1995.

Home Office and Department of Health and Social Security. Report of the Committee on Mentally Abnormal Offenders (Butler Report). Cmnd. 6244. London: HMSO, 1975.

Huckle P, Tavier, Scarf. Psychiatric clinic in probation offices in South Wales. Psychiatric Bulletin 1996; 20: 205–206.

Huckle P, Williams T. Providing a forensic psychiatric service to Cardiff Prison. Psychiatric Bulletin 1994; 18: 670–672.

Institute for the Treatment and Study of Delinquency. Managing Risk: Achieving the Possible. London: ISTD, 1995, pp. 75–78.

James D, Hamilton L. Setting up psychiatric liaison schemes to magistrates courts: problems and practicalities. Medicine Science and the Law 1992; 32: 167–176.

Johnstone E, Crowe T, Johnson A et al. Northwick Park study of first episodes of schizophrenia. 1: Presentation of the illness and problems relating to admission. British Journal of Psychiatry 1986; 148: 115–120.

Joseph PL, Potter M. Diversion from custody I: Psychiatric assessment at the magistrates court. British Journal of Psychiatry 1993a: 162: 325–330.

Joseph PL, Potter M. Diversion from custody II: Effect on hospital and prison resources. British Journal of Psychiatry 1993b: 162: 330–334.

Kennedy M, Truman C, Keyes S and Cameron A. Supported bail for mentally vulnerable defendants. Howard Journal 1997; 36: 158–169.

Klassen D, O'Connor WA. Demographic and case history variables. In Monahan J, Steadman H (eds), Violence and Mental Disorder. Chicago: University of Chicago Press, 1994, pp. 229–258.

Klassen D, O'Connor WA. Predicting violence in schizophrenic and non schizophrenic patients. Journal of Community Psychology 1988; 16: 217–227.

Lidz CW, Mulvey E, Gardner W. The accuracy of predictions of violence to others. Journal of the American Medical Association 1993; 269: 1007–1011.

Link BG, Stueve A. Psychotic symptoms and the violent/illegal behaviour of mental patients compared to community controls. In Monahan J, Steadman H (eds), Violence and Mental Disorder. Chicago: University of Chicago Press, 1994, pp. 137–159.

Link BG et al. The violent and illegal behaviour of mental patients reconsidered. American Sociological Review 1992; 57: 275–292.

Lipsedge M. Psychiatry: reducing risk in clinical practice. In Vincent C (ed.), Clinical Risk Management. London: BMJ Publ., 1995.

McNeil J, Freenfield. Predictors of violence in civilly committed acute psychiatric patients. American Journal of Psychiatry 1988; 145: 965–970.

Mendelson EF. A survey of practice at a regional forensic service: what do forensic psychiatrists do? 1: Characteristics of cases and distribution of work. British Journal of Psychiatry 1992a; 160: 769–772.

Mendelson EF. A survey of practice at a regional forensic service: what do forensic psychiatrists do? 2: Treatment, court reports and outcome. British Journal of Psychiatry 1992b; 160: 773–776.

Mental Health Act Commission. Report of the Royal Commission on Law Relating to Mental Illness and Mental Deficiency (1954–57). Cmnd. 169. London: HMSO, 1957.

Ministry of Health. Special Hospitals: Report of a Working Party [Emery Report]. London: Ministry of Health, 1961.

Monahan J. Mental disorder and violence: another look. In Hodgins S (ed.), Mental Disorder and Crime. London: Sage, 1993, pp. 287–302.

Monahan J. The prediction of violent behaviour: toward a second generation of theory and policy. American Journal of Psychiatry 1984; 141: 10–15.

Monahan J, Steadman HJ. Violence and Mental Disorder. London: University of Chicago Press, 1994.

Mullen PE. Assessing risk of interpersonal violence in the mentally ill. Advances in Psychiatric Treatment 1997; 3, 166–173.

NHS Executive. Health Service Guidelines (94) 27, 1994.

NHS Executive. High Security Psychiatric Services: Changes in Funding and Organisation. London: Department of Health, 1995.

North-East Thames RHA and South-East Thames RHA. The Report of the Inquiry into the Care and Treatment of Christopher Clunis. London: HMSO, 1994.

Partridge R. Broadmoor. London: Chatto & Windus, 1953.

Petch E, Bradley C. Learning the lessons from homicide enquiries: adding insult to injury? Journal of Forensic Psychiatry 1997; 8: 161–184.

Pritchard et al. Mental illness, drug and alcohol abuse and HIV risk behaviour in 214 young adult probation clients. Social Work and Social Services Review 1992; 3: 227–242.

Resnick J. Waiting for treatment, an audit of psychiatric services at Bullingdon Prison. Journal of Forensic Psychiatry 1995; 1: 305–316.

Royal College of Psychiatrists. Assessment and clinical management of risk of harm to other people. Council Report no. 53, 1996.

Royal College of Psychiatrists. Community Treatment Orders – A Discussion Document. London: Royal College of Psychiatrists, 1987.

Royal College of Psychiatrists. Good medical practice in the aftercare of potentially violent or vulnerable patients discharged from inpatient psychiatric treatment. Council Report no. 12, 1991.

Royal College of Psychiatrists. Supervision Registers: The College's Response. Psychiatric Bulletin 1994; 18: 385–388.

Scott PD. Solutions to the problem of the dangerous offender. British Medical Journal 1974; 4: 640–641.

Singleton N, Meltzer H, Gatward R. Psychiatric Morbidity among Prisoners. London: HMSO for Office of National Statistics, 1998.

Smith J, Parker J, Donovan M. Female admissions to a regional secure unit. Journal of Forensic Psychiatry 1991; 2: 95–102.

Snowden PR. A survey of the regional secure unit programme. British Journal of Psychiatry 1985; 147: 499–507.

Snowden PR. Practical aspects of clinical risk assessment and management. British Journal of Psychiatry 1997; 170 (suppl. 32): 32–34.

Snyder et al. Selective behavioural features of patients with borderline personality traits. Suicide and Life Threatening Behaviour 1986; 16: 28–39.

The Special Hospitals Service Authority. Service Strategies for Secure Care. London: SHSA, 1995.

The Special Hospitals Treatment Resistant Schizophrenia Research Group. Schizophrenia, violence, clozapine and risperidone. British Journal of Psychiatry 1996; 169 (suppl. 31): 21–30.

Steadman H, Coccozza J. Careers of the Criminally Insane. Lexington: Lexington Books, 1984.

Stone M. Abuse and abusiveness in borderline personality disorder. In Links PS (ed.), Family Environment and Borderline Personality Disorder. Washington, DC: American Psychiatric Press, 1990, pp. 131–148.

Swanson JW, Borum R, Swartz MS, Monahan J. Psychotic symptoms and disorders and the risk of violent behaviour in the community. Criminal Behaviour and Mental Health 1996; 6: 309–329.

Swanson JW, Holzer CE, Ganju VK, Jono RT. Violence and psychiatric disorder in the community: evidence from epidemiological catchment area surveys. Hospital and Community Psychiatry 1990; 41: 761–770.

Swanson JW. Mental disorder and substance abuse and community violence: an epidemiological approach. In Monahan J, Steadman H (eds), Violence and Mental Disorder. Chicago: University of Chicago Press, 1994, pp. 101–136.

Taylor PJ et al. Delusions and violence. In Monahan J, Steadman H (eds), Violence and Mental Disorder. Chicago: University of Chicago Press, 1994, pp. 161–182.

Taylor PJ, Gunn J. Violence and Psychosis 1: Risks of violence among psychotic men. British Medical Journal 1984; 288: 1945–1949.

Taylor PJ. Psychosis, violence and crime. In Gunn J, Taylor PJ (eds), Forensic Psychiatry: Clinical, Legal and Ethical Issues. London: Butterworth-Heinemann, 1993, pp. 329–372.

Treasaden I. Current practice in regional interim secure units. In Gostin L (ed.), Secure Provision: A Review of Special Services for the Mentally Ill and Mentally Handicapped in England and Wales. London: Tavistock, 1985, pp. 176–207.

Walker N. Dangerous mistakes. British Journal of Psychiatry 1991; 158: 752–757.

Walker N. Dangerous people. International Journal of Law and Psychiatry 1978; 1: 37–50.

Walker N (ed.). Dangerous People. London: Blackstone, 1996.

Wessley S. The epidemiology of crime violence and schizophrenia. British Journal of Psychiatry 1997; 170 (suppl. 32): 8–11.

West Midlands Regional Health Authority. Report of the Panel of Inquiry Appointed by the West Midlands Regional Health Authority, South Birmingham Health Authority and the Special Hospitals Service Authority to Investigate the Case of Kim Kirkman. Birmingham: West Midlands Regional Health Authority, 1991.

14

SERVICES FOR SEVERE
SOMATOFORM DISORDERS

Eleanor J. Feldman

INTRODUCTION

This chapter discusses the provision of specialist liaison psychiatry services for patients with the most severe forms of somatoform disorders and conversion disorders. Chapter 6 has already described the kinds of problems that present, the degrees of major disability that such patients experience, and their clinical needs. In this chapter, I will now focus on the principles of patient management, the various models of service that exist, and consider the issues involved in planning a service, including how to assess need.

PRINCIPLES OF PATIENT MANAGEMENT

The exclusion of organic pathology is an appropriate first step following presentation of somatic symptoms, but should not in itself form the basis of a diagnosis of somatoform disorder. Psychiatric assessment is valuable to look for the presence of treatable depression and/or anxiety states which can present with somatic symptoms, and to assess for personality difficulties and other psychiatric co-morbidity that will have a crucial bearing on prognosis. If a patient refuses psychiatric referral, the general practitioner (GP) or physician should at minimum attempt to look for uncomplicated depression and/or anxiety disorder as the majority of patients with unexplained medical symptoms fall into this treatable group (see Chapters 3 and 4). For those with major personality difficulties, the goal of treatment is the prevention of iatrogenic harm by containing the involvement of other specialists for the investigation of, or intervention for, medically benign symptoms. This is no mean feat, but some GPs and senior physicians have developed skills in this area. Junior physicians are not usually able to contain these patients as they are too prone to the anxiety that something organic has been missed, and under too much time pressure in their clinics, to continue to see these patients and yet, from their perspective, to 'do nothing' (in the form of further investigations or prescribing); furthermore, juniors cannot provide the continuity needed for firm consistent management. Often, these patients will continue to have repeated unfruitful medical consultations, inappropriate investigations, inappropriate drug treatment, repeated hospital admissions, and sometimes harmful operative procedures.

Where a specialist liaison psychiatry service exists, the main contribution of the psychiatrist beyond assessment and treatment of any tractable condition is to attempt to support the GP or physician involved in minimizing further specialist involvement and, thereby, prevent iatrogenic harm.

HOW SERVICES ARE CONSTRUCTED

Across the UK there are only a handful of liaison psychiatry specialist units, and many of these are too small to provide more than a rudimentary service for the full range of severe problems encountered. There is, therefore, only a small fund of UK clinical experience to draw upon, and little systematic research in the form of controlled treatment trials, apart from the management of chronic pain and chronic fatigue syndrome (see below). Provision of liaison psychiatry services is better in some other European countries (Huyse 1991), but probably the most widely available service provision is in North America.

MODELS OF CARE

Care by GPs and physicians

In many cases, patients with chronic somatoform disorders do not engage in psychiatric care, although they can sometimes be persuaded to have an assessment. This is partly because the patients have strong defences against a psychological explanation for their problems, and partly because general psychiatric services do not have the skills or structures to offer much to these patients. Chronic somatization disorder (formerly known as Briquet's syndrome) has an estimated prevalence of at least 4 per 1000 population (Deighton and Nicol 1985, Swartz et al. 1986, Escobar et al. 1987). Thus, all GPs will have a few of these patients on their list and all hospital specialists will have encountered such patients.

Specialist psychiatric care

Patients with chronic somatization should ideally receive psychiatric attention in the general hospital setting where they have presented for other specialist care. For this to be realistically achieved, there needs to be a specialist liaison psychiatry service and a consultant liaison psychiatrist who has the confidence of the local physicians and surgeons. Such confidence is not automatically given, and will take time and shared experience to accrue. Education of referrers in the recognition of suitable patients and referral techniques is a major task for any liaison service. In the early stages of the development of a service there is a need to focus on the immediate priorities of providing good core services for deliberate self harm patients (see Chapter 16), acute behavioural emergencies, and establishing a reputation for helpful and effective treatment of the majority of patients referred. It would seem inadvisable to attempt to build a new service around a small number of the most-difficult-to-treat patients. It is, therefore, only in the more long-established liaison psychiatry services that the problems of the most disabled somatizing patients can begin to be systematically addressed.

In the main, general adult mental health sector services have little to offer this patient group, particularly as the care demands of patients with other severe mental illnesses have increased. The skills and experience needed to manage severe somatizing patients will not have been acquired without higher training or senior experience in liaison work which is not widely available. Patients referred to a general adult mental health service will often be sent back with the opinion that there is no psychiatric disorder, plus inappropriate suggestions for further physical investigations. The multidisciplinary teams of general psychiatry services do not have the right skill and experience mix: physiotherapists will not be members of such teams, occupational therapists will not have experience of working more with severe physical disability and pain, and clinical psychologists experienced in cognitive behavioural work with somatizing patients are in very short supply. Finally, close cooperation is needed with the general hospitals to facilitate patient acceptance of referral and then to coordinate all the non-psychiatric specialist care, making liaison specialist teams best placed for this role.

Liaison or consultation

Two models by which mental health services can work with general hospital patients are generally described: liaison involves a mental health professional who functions as part of a general medical/surgical firm, goes to regular meetings and ward rounds, and so relatively quickly becomes well-known and trusted by the team; consultation involves the mental health professional coming to see patients and advise on an ad hoc basis, without explicitly making any other relationship with the medical/surgical team. As the liaison model is so time-consuming, most services follow the consultation model, but most liaison psychiatrists will have one specific area of liaison work and most would agree that this is the most rewarding way of providing psychiatric care. Over the years of providing a helpful service, the benefits of the liaison-type relationship with a wider group of general hospital specialists will develop, simply through familiarity and growing respect on both sides.

A service targeting the very disabled chronic somatizers would benefit from following the liaison model and identifying a partnership with an interested general hospital specialist who is seeing a lot of these patients. Patients with chronic somatoform disorders and chronic conversion disorders accumulate in any service that attempts to help people with intractable, but not life-threatening, symptoms such as pain clinics and neurological rehabilitation services; in many teaching hospitals there will be senior physicians who will see these patients because they give the ultimate medical opinions. The capacity to develop a successful liaison is largely determined by the interest and willingness of the partner physician or surgeon.

Out- and inpatient care

The majority of patients will be seen as outpatients, but some will warrant in patient care because of the degree of their disability or other complicating problems. Very few liaison psychiatry services in the UK have their own inpatient beds. House (1994) describes an example of an inpatient liaison service in Leeds, and Lipowski (1988) has described an inpatient unit and treatment program for somatizing patients in Toronto. House comments that patients with chronic and usually severe somatization need admission to treat immobility, loss of other functions, drug overuse or associated mood disorder. These patients require special nursing skills and a therapeutic milieu that cannot be provided on general psychiatric wards (Egan-Morris et al. 1994). Shorter et al. (1992) observe, from the experience of a case series of 92 somatizing patients treated as inpatients on Lipowski's specialist unit, that patients without co-morbid depression have a worse prognosis and tend to have an earlier age of onset, whereas those with depression do better in general as this is a more readily treatable element. Those with a childhood history do particularly poorly.

Secondary and tertiary services

Liaison psychiatry services are by nature tertiary services as their priority is to provide psychiatric care to the patients of the general hospitals. However, the specialist skills offered by such a service can appropriately be made available to referrals from general practice. There is no doubt that GPs can be educated to make very appropriate referrals and they very much appreciate such services. Problems will arise if these services are unfunded and not separately recognized in contracts, but count as ordinary mental health activity. Consultations with this patient group whose problems are complex involve senior staff and take longer than the average general psychiatry consultation. Treatments on the whole will be psychotherapeutic. Extra demands may be small to start with but soon snowball and place staff under extreme pressure that is not sustainable. Savings made in general practice and general hospital budgets as a result of effective treatments for these resource-consuming disorders is generally not reinvested in the mental health services. Rectifying strategic errors of this type is painful for all.

PLANNING A SERVICE FOR SEVERE SOMATOFORM DISORDERS

As indicated above, a liaison service should be relatively well established and provide satisfactory core services before embarking upon providing any new specific service for a severely disabled and difficult to help minority. As part of routine work in a liaison mental health services, the clinician will see many somatizing patients, and the majority will be readily treatable with a combination of antidepressants and/or cognitive behavioural therapy. A starting point for a service for the more severe and intractable cases might be to select a liaison model, linking perhaps with a pain clinic and provide outpatient care as a tertiary service. Later additions could include an inpatient service and broadening of acceptance of referrals from GPs. Each phase should happen in a planned way, with identification of resources required and agreement for funding. The key elements in a planning process are described below.

Responding to the local need

The starting point for any planning is likely to be a clinicians understanding of local need and how this could be met. The process which follows must include a precise definition of the client group and an estimate, using all available sources, of the levels of need and demand for services. A number of practical questions must be addressed at this stage: how will demand be managed? will there be a waiting list, and/or restricted referral acceptance?; what will be the treatment aims?; what treatments will be provided?; which staff will be providing them and where?; what will be the arrangements for supervision, training and research? Some of these points are elaborated below.

Balancing need, demand and provision

It is important that activity matches resources; experience in this area is that there is a very substantial unmet need. Benjamin and Bridges (1994) have estimated that a health district with a population of 250 000 will contain at least 250 residents with the most severe and chronic disorders. As many as 25 000 are likely to have recurrent or persistent problems of somatization. Hospital-based data indicate that chronic somatizing patients are extremely common in a broad range of medical and surgical settings, with the highest prevalence estimates involving pain clinics (Benjamin and Bridges 1994). Local clinic prevalence data is advisable in the planning phase as figures from other centres will not take into account the idiosyncrasies of local practice that affect referral patterns. It should also be noted that demand is a dynamic phenomenon that tends to increase with supply; hence, it needs to be recognized that it may be necessary to have a phased expansion of the service as it develops.

Once need has been estimated, this has to be related to what resources are required to meet it. It is difficult to estimate this accurately without experience of the service once started. In my own service based around the provision of cognitive behavioural therapy for chronic fatigue syndrome, my first year service figures indicated that for every one session of consultant psychiatrist time spent in face-to-face contact assessing this patient group, there needed to be a corresponding 3.3 sessions of cognitive therapist time in face-to-face patient contact to keep up with the demand for therapy. Thus, the best way to estimate annual activity is through piloting a service and monitoring it closely.

How will demand be managed?

Given a situation of considerable unmet need, a skills shortage and limited finance, demand must be managed. There are two main ways this is done in a health service that is free at the point of delivery: by waiting list or by restricted referral acceptance. Most services utilize both to a greater or lesser degree. The latter is desirable where it minimizes abortive assessments, that is cases where patients fail to attend or are unsuitable for the approach provided. The potential for such wasted appointments of a senior clinician's time is great with this patient group and the way in which referrals are made can reduce this wastage considerably. Hence, clear guidance on referral and close working relationships with referrers are desirable.

What will be the treatment aims?

Treatments should not only be evidence based in areas where such evidence exists, but also should allow for work at the boundaries of knowledge and experience to progress with appropriate scientific evaluation. Service providers need to evaluate the literature for the patient group for whom they intend to provide a service and decide what the end points of treatment and the specialist service involvement are. A patient may have chronic problems, but that does not mean that a highly specialized expensive service is always going to be the most appropriate care provider for that patient. For the most severe chronic somatizing patients, the end point of treatment may have little to do with changing the patient and everything to do with modifying the attitudes and behaviours of those around the patient, particularly the other involved health professionals.

Which staff will be providing treatment?

Ideally multidisciplinary teams for outpatients will need to include sessions from a consultant liaison psychiatrist, an experienced cognitive behaviour therapist (usually a clinical psychologist or senior clinical nurse specialist) and sessions from occupational therapy and physiotherapy. This team may be an amalgam of mental health staff and general hospital staff, depending on the skills and interests of existing staff. Similarly, inpatient services will need the range of skills above, plus nursing staff who will be confident in managing patients with combined physical and mental health problems.

What will be the arrangements for supervision, training and research?

There is a need for postgraduate training in this area and specialist liaison services invariably have trainees from all disciplines wanting supervised experience. Senior clinicians need to ensure that trainees are properly supervised and not left with cases beyond their competence. Patients entering these services will only have one chance of expert help and have often had a poor experience of care in other services. There is a need to disseminate skills at all levels and liaison service providers find themselves teaching and training across disciplines and specialties. As a young subspecialty working at the interface with general hospitals, there is much that is unexplored and many opportunities for research. New services should recognize the need to properly evaluate changes at the boundaries of knowledge and experience as they are introduced, and this means that research as well as audit are integral to service development. Hence, a service will benefit from senior clinicians with academic skills who have time and support for teaching, audit and research.

Where will patients be seen?

There are a number of options, depending on local circumstances, but as a rule it is best to see outpatients in the same clinical setting as the referring specialty. This helps break down barriers to referral and facilitates an integrated holistic approach to the patient. If this is not practical, then at least it is advisable to use clinic rooms on the general hospital site. Preferably these rooms should have windows and not be too small as patients undergoing therapy need to feel as relaxed and comfortable as possible. Further developments may include day-patient and inpatient services, again preferably in the same clinical setting as the referring specialty.

Justifying the use of resources

It is important to be clear about the evidence for health gain. Often, treatments at the developing edge of clinical practice are without stringent scientific evidence to prove their worth and the best that can be achieved are case reports and descriptions of good examples of existing services and their follow up results. While there is good evidence for psychological intervention in irritable bowel syndrome and for the milder forms of hypochondriasis, effective treatments for the more severe and chronic disorders are less well researched with the exception of chronic pain (e.g. Malone and Strube 1988, Benjamin 1989) and chronic fatigue syndrome (Sharpe et al. 1996, Deale et al. 1997), where randomized controlled trials show significant health gains.

The cost of any service is of crucial importance in a publicly funded system; the strongest financial argument in favour of a service for chronic somatization is likely to be the cost offsets that can be achieved by reducing wasteful specialist consultations and interventions. All studies that examine inpatient investigation and treatment, particularly surgery, show that this is the most costly unnecessary care that might be obviated. It should be noted that financial savings accrue to the budgets of the general hospitals and GPs, not to those of the mental health services.

Some studies of treatments for chronic pain have looked at the cost efficiency of interventions. For example, Jacobs (1987), working in California in the 1980s, reports on the use by adult male patients of hospital and clinic resources before and after their involvement in psychologist-directed programmes of stress management, pain control, vocational rehabilitation and coping skill training. Patients in all programmes showed reductions in health care utilization, particularly inpatient hospital stays: after 1 year, hospital days were down by 72% compared with pretreatment levels; and at 3 years hospital days remained at 47% of pretreatment levels.

With respect to clinical populations other than chronic pain patients, the available literature also indicates cost savings of liaison services. Smith et al. (1986) in the USA undertook a controlled study of 38 patients with chronic somatization randomly assigned to treatment or control, and followed up for 18 months. The treatment group received education about their disorder and recommendations to the physician, who was encouraged to serve as the primary physician of the patient with the disorder. All physicians were advised to make regular scheduled appointments with each patient at roughly monthly intervals, and not to see the patient on demand. Other recommendations included the patient having a physical examination at each visit, and physicians were advised against hospital admission, diagnostic procedures, surgery and laboratory tests purely for reassurance purposes. Following this intervention, the quarterly healthcare charges in the treatment group declined by 53%, but there was no change in the controls. This was a crossover study: at 9 months the control group was entered for treatment, where after their quarterly charges declined by 49%. Average quarterly costs of all healthcare fell from $2681 to $1606. In both groups, the majority of the cost reductions were attributable to decreased hospital admission.

There has not been a equivalent controlled study in the UK, but Williams and House (1994) describe a case seen in Leeds where a similar intervention reduced costs for one patient from a total of over £10 000 a year to a little over £2000 a year; this particular patient had had 77 hospital admissions over 25 years, with 856 days spent in hospital, costing over £250 000. No physical diagnoses had ever satisfactorily explained her symptoms and over the years until this intervention, she was getting more symptoms, seeing more hospital specialists and being prescribed more drugs, including opiates.

Shaw and Creed (1991) report an economic analysis of a liaison service in Manchester, pointing out the costs of general hospital investigations prior to referral to a liaison psychiatrist in depressed patients who present with somatic symptoms; they find that median cost was £286 (range £25–2300). These patients are not such a severe and chronic group, and can be helped considerably by psychiatric treatment. Patients such as this, and those with somatized anxiety and panic disorder, will form the bulk of patients with unexplained physical symptoms referred to a liaison service. For every one severe chronic somatization case there will be about 15 patients with more tractable conditions (RCPRCP 1995)

A local project will often carry greater weight than research from other centres, partly because all the clinicians concerned in the research will have had first hand experience of an effective service, and partly because it has been demonstrated that the local clinical conditions favour the service. For example, Bass et al. in Oxford have just completed a study of biofeedback in chronic constipation showing considerable savings by helping patients who then do not need major abdominal surgery (personal communication). The research makes a strong case on clinical and financial grounds for the funding of a nurse who will undertake the biofeedback. The savings from surgery will more than pay for the costs of the nurse.

Implications for other services

The provision of a new service will have implications for other healthcare providers who should be considered in consultation with representatives of colleagues in primary care, in the general hospitals and in the general mental health services. There is likely to be most support for the development of these services from GPs and the hospital specialists who are most involved with chronic somatizers. They would wish to see benefits to patients, efficiency gains and no increase in overall costs to their budgets.

Generally, liaison services need to operate in partnership with a clinician from the general hospital who will play a key role in facilitating negotiations with the management of the general hospital and who will be a long-term collaborator in the service. It is important that this is made explicit at the outset.

SUMMARY

Mental health liaison services to general hospitals provide a valuable resource for the cost-effective management of disorders which can otherwise result in considerable disability to the individual and inappropriate as well as costly care to health services. Across the UK and internationally, with the possible exception of North America, such services are poorly developed. However, models of care and treatment packages exist to guide planners and inform the development of effective services.

References

Bass C and Benjamin S. The management of chronic somatization. British Journal of Psychiatry 1993; 162: 472–80.

Benjamin S and Bridges K. The need for specialised services for chronic somatisers. In Benjamin S, House A, Jenkins P (eds), Liaison Psychiatry. Defining Needs and Planning Services. London: Gaskell, 1994.

Benjamin S. Psychological treatment of chronic pain: a selective review. Journal of Psychosomatic Research 1989; 33: 121–131.

Deale A, Chalder T, Marks I, Wessely S. Cognitive behaviour therapy for the chronic fatigue syndrome: a randomised controlled trial. American Journal of Psychiatry 1997; 154: 408–414.

Deighton CM, Nicol AR. Abnormal illness behaviour in young women in a primary care setting: is Briquet's syndrome a useful category? Psychological Medicine 1985; 15: 515–520.

Egan-Morris E, Morris R, House A. The role of the nurse in consultation–liaison psychiatry. In Benjamin S, House A, Jenkins P (eds), Liaison Psychiatry. Defining Needs and Planning Services. London: Gaskell, 1994.

Escobar JI, Golding JM, Hough RL, Karno M, Burnam MA, Wells KB. Somatisation in the community: relationship to disability and use of services. American Journal of Public Health 1987; 77: 837–840.

House A. Liaison psychiatry in a large teaching hospital: the service at Leeds General Infirmary. In Benjamin S, House A, Jenkins P (eds), Liaison Psychiatry. Defining Needs and Planning Services. London: Gaskell, 1994.

Huyse FJ. European consultation–liaison psychiatry workgroup. Consultation–liaison psychiatry: does it help to get organised? General Hospital Psychiatry 1991; 13: 133–187.

Jacobs DF. Cost-effectiveness of specialised psychological programs for reducing hospital stays and outpatient visits. Journal of Clinical Psychology 1987; 43: 729–735.

Lipowski ZJ. An inpatient program for persistent somatisers. Canadian Journal of Psychiatry 1988; 33: 275–278.

Malone MD, Strube M. Meta-analysis of non-medical treatments for chronic pain. Pain 1988; 34: 231–244.

Royal College of Physicians and the Royal College of Psychiatrists. The Psychological Care of Medical Patients. Recognition of Need and Service Provision. Report CR35. London: Royal College of Physicians and the Royal College of Psychiatrists, 1995.

Sharpe M, Hawton K, Simkin S, Surawy C, Hackmann A, Klimes I, Peto T, Warrell D, Seagroatt V. Cognitive Behaviour Therapy for the chronic fatigue syndrome: a randomised controlled trial. British Medical Journal 1996; 312: 22–26.

Shaw J, Creed F. The cost of somatisation. Journal of Psychosomatic Research 1991; 35: 307–312.

Shorter E, Abbey SE, Gillies LA, Singh M, Lipowski ZJ. Inpatient treatment of persistent somatisation. Psychosomatics 1992; 33: 295–301.

Smith GR, Monson RA, Ray DC. Psychiatric consultation in somatisation disorder. A randomised controlled study. New England Journal of Medicine 1986; 314: 1407–1413.

Swartz M, Blazer D, George L, Landerman R. Somatisation disorder in a community population. American Journal of Psychiatry 1986; 143: 1403–1408.

Williams C, House A. Reducing the costs of chronic somatisation. Irish Journal of Psychological Medicine 1994; 11: 79–82.

15

PSYCHOLOGICAL APPROACHES TO PSYCHOTIC ILLNESS

Zaffer Iqbal and Max Birchwood

INTRODUCTION

The development in recent years of evidence-based psychological interventions for the treatment of severe mental illnesses allow the mental health clinician greater opportunity to provide effective services which complement traditionally employed pharmacotherapy regimes.

The development of such interventions for psychotic disorders has been particularly pronounced in recent years. The marriage of interventions within a case management framework using resources of an appropriate service infrastructure is, we believe, the next step and challenge for the new millennium. Continuity of care is a critical component of case management, alongside engagement and maintenance of treatment for patients and their carers. This requires a clear psychological formulation of the determinants of engagement and treatment cooperation. We will outline the main difficulties associated with these factors.

Specific approaches can be implemented for the family management of psychosis, prediction and prevention of relapse, and the cognitive management of delusions and auditory hallucinations. These interventions are highly skilled, requiring expertise and professional training backgrounds. In this chapter we will provide an overview of these three areas of clinical research, highlighting the theoretical basis for each approach, and providing a discussion of the clinical framework involved in service delivery and its efficacy.

FAMILY INTERVENTION

Overview

The nature of the interaction between family members and the person with schizophrenia has received broad documentation as being a significant factor in the course of a schizophrenic illness (Faloon, 1988; Leff, 1989; Tarrier, 1989). The major impetus for the interest in family intervention has been the development of the concept of expressed emotion (EE) (Brown et al. 1972). EE is a composite of several aspects of the relative's attitudes and behaviours to the patient. These are: number of critical comments, marked emotional over-involvement, hostility, warmth and positive affect. Living with a high EE relative proves to be a powerful predictor of early relapse in schizophrenia, and this finding has been replicated across various international studies (Koenigsberg & Handley, 1988; Kuipers & Bebbington, 1988). It is argued that living with a high EE relative produces ambient stress and over-stimulation which cumulatively result in relapse.

The critical features of EE continue to elude researchers in spite of prodigious effort. Criticism by relatives is acknowledged to be associated with long-standing social impairment (Vaughn, 1986) and maladaptive behaviours (Brown et al. 1972), especially unpredictable behaviour (Greenley, 1986), all of which create burdens for the family. The stability of EE is questionable. Following an acute admission, the EE of relatives has been reported in some cases as becoming both less (Hogarty et al. 1991) and more critical (Tarrier et al. 1988) than at the earlier more acute stage. It is suggested (Kuipers & Bebbington, 1988) that EE stability is dependent upon the interaction between the relatives' ability to cope and their current circumstances. Furthermore it is proposed (Birchwood & Smith, 1987) that EE contains a 'state' element which is sensitive to the developing interactions between the patient and individual family members, during the period that the family are coming to terms with the emergence of schizophrenia. The coping styles and strategies employed by relatives (figure 1), in response to the behavioural changes in the family member with first-episode schizophrenia, and whether these changes have any bearing upon family burden as well as on the patient's social impairment, behavioural disturbance and progress of illness, were investigated by Birchwood and Cochrane (1990). The results provided significant indications that styles of coping were associated with perceived control or burden: relatives making greater use of coercive, avoidant and disorganised coping styles experienced less perceived control, more stress and greater burden.

The supposed temporal stability of EE has been questioned by a series of studies in which up to 25% of high EE families changed to low EE independent of intervention (Hogarty et al. 1991; Tarrier et al. 1988). Although low EE relatives tend to stay low a minority 'spontaneously' revert to high EE. The coping style of a family member can aid clarification as to whether high or low EE is observed (Birchwood & Cochrane, 1990; Smith et al. 1993). This led Kuipers and Bebbington to argue that several groups of relatives may exist (Kuipers & Bebbington, 1988): a low EE (good coping) group who remain low irrespective of changing circumstances; a high EE (poor coping) group with multiple problems who cope poorly, and a vacillating group of low EE (poor coping) relatives who may change to high EE dependent upon circumstances.

Coping Strategy: COERCION

Symptoms:	'I would laugh at him to show him how stupid they are… I'd try to bring him to his senses and I'd say… "just watch the TV there's nothing going to happen!".'
Withdrawal:	'I'd tell him "buck yourself up" but he just ignored me so I'd say "for crying out loud help yourself and buck yourself up, people are being kind…".'
Slowness:	'I'd say "for crying out loud, I'll do it myself… you're so slow you drive me up the wall".'

Coping Strategy: AVOIDANCE

Symptoms:	'I just leave him, whatever you say you won't convince him… if I try he only gets aggressive and I don't want that again.'
Withdrawal:	'I knew he was bad and did not want to force him to do things because I knew it would make him worse or even violent… I used to force him out but he would end up coming back because of some incident… I don't push him now because I don't want people to see him while he is ill.'
Loss of independence:	'I usually do everything for him to keep the peace… my husband tries but he (son) goes on at him until he ends up doing it.'

Coping Strategy: IGNORE/ACCEPT

Symptoms:	'I was worried but thought it was a phase he was going through… I would ask him if he was all right then leave it at that… I didn't want to make a fuss about it.'
Withdrawal:	'With such a lot in the family we hardly noticed he wasn't doing very much and was quieter than usual… we ignored it really, left him to his own devices.'
Loss of independence:	'We saw it as part of his illness… we do as many things for him as he wants… we leave him time on his own.'

Coping Strategy: COLLUSION

Symptoms:	'I sometimes pretended to hear the voices as well, to reassure him that he was not the only one.'
Withdrawal:	'I tell her who is coming to the door so if its someone she doesn't want to see it gives her time to get upstairs.'
Loss of independence:	'I do most things she asks… I tell her that I don't mind… and I won't make her do things she doesn't want to… I don't want her to have this terrible illness again.'

Coping Strategy: CONSTRUCTIVE

Symptoms:	'I'd say, "just don't listen to them try to forget them"… I'd try and distract her whenever I can.'
Withdrawal:	I try to draw him into conversations all the time… I rattle on at him in the hope he will find something of interest… I suggest little jobs for him to do to get him going rather than sitting here moping.'
Loss of independence:	'I comment on it, tell her that she's doing wrong… its a matter of 'restraining' her; by pointing out where she's going wrong in the hope that she will gradually improve.'

Coping Strategy: RESIGNATION

Symptoms:	'I'd say good God there's nothing (poison) in the tea, I poured it myself… it made no difference so I just ignore him now.'
Withdrawal:	'I just ignored it and left him to it in the end… I used to call him again and again, he said he'd get up soon, he never did, so in the end I just left him to it.'
Loss of independence:	'I used to get annoyed and have a go at him… its hopeless, there's nothing you can do about it… I'm resigned to it now, I just take each day as it comes.'

Coping Strategy: REASSURANCE

Symptoms:	'I tried to reassure him that there was too much love around him, nobody could get him… I always react in this way though I put it in different ways each time.'

Figure 15.1 – Examples of coping strategies (Birchwood and Cochrane 1990)

Hence, any service utilising the EE framework would require regular EE assessments if an intervention based on EE is to be provided.

A potential problem for service provision, due to the dynamic nature of EE, is that the difficulties of families with low EE profiles may be overlooked as clinicians concentrate their efforts on relatives with high EE. Regardless of the level of EE observed, relatives will be faced by similar problems of stigma, isolation and the burden of caring for someone with a severe mental illness (Kuipers & Bebbington, 1988; Hatfield, 1978; Barraclough & Tarrier, 1990). Comparisons of the needs of high and low EE families demonstrate that although some two-thirds of high EE relatives reported marked levels of stress, burden and coping difficulty (Leff & Vaughn, 1985) in contrast to about one third of low EE families, a core group of low EE families existed whose needs did not fit the low EE model (Smith et al. 1993). This subgroup reported high stress or burden or impaired coping and patients were in many cases operating in an 'impaired' social range. The lack of significant differences between this subgroup and the remainder of the low EE group suggest that other factors are also involved. Prudence dictates that, although the major measure of family intervention is relapse, multiple outcome indices should be used (e.g. social functioning, the relatives burden of caring for a mentally ill person and patient and relatives' satisfaction with the intervention strategies)(Birchwood & Smith, 1987; Smith & Birchwood, 1990; Goldstein & Kopeikin, 1981) thus providing a broader focus than that derived solely from the EE literature.

Clinical implications of EE research

Clearly high EE families will be a major focus of a family intervention service as high EE is strongly associated with relapse and comprises certain types of behaviour, e.g. critical, overinvolved and rejecting. Adopting the high EE index as an entry qualification will limit a family intervention to only engaging patients and families at the point of admission, at which high EE can be most reliably detected (Tarrier et al. 1988). Besides the limits which attempting to recruit individuals and their families at admission will evidently bring, patients who are not regularly admitted will be overlooked although high EE families are liable to exist in this population to an unknown degree. Furthermore, it has also been suggested that patients and families who have little contact with services may have an equal (if not greater) need for EE focused intervention that those who receive regular input (Smith & Birchwood, 1990).

The measure of success in many of the family intervention studies outlined has been reduction in the risk of relapse. However, there is a frequent failure to examine whether high EE predicts poor social outcome or if low EE suggests that families possess the skills required for social reintegration and maintenance of well-being. Certain studies have observed that some low EE families have attempted to cope with a challenging family member by using disengagement and distancing strategies (Vaughn, 1986; Smith & Birchwood, 1990). By concentrating on reducing the risk of relapse the professional may neglect the needs of the family coping with the significant burden and stress of caring for a relative with a severe mental illness. Evidence suggests that good patient outcome, in terms of social adjustment as well as relapse, is related to successful family coping strategies and a lack of family burden. Hence expansion of the family intervention service' remit to enable relatives to cope by assessing the needs and well-being of the family may significantly increase the success of such an intervention.

Family intervention: core ingredients

Several guidelines have been suggested (Leff & Vaughn, 1985) for effective family interventions to reduce the risk of relapse. Firstly, intervention should focus upon relatives and patients although individual patient work is useful. Secondly, education, e.g. eliciting and discussing information regarding the onset, course and outcome of the illness, is probably useful in an extensive long-term programme. Finally, it is suggested that interventions should be integrated with other psychiatric resources and attempt to increase drug conformity if needs be. Regimes such as problem solving and goal setting as well as social skills training are recommended.

Initial assessments of the patient and individual relatives, can be performed using the Camberwell Family Interview (Leff & Vaughn, 1985). This covers areas such as distress, coping strategies, knowledge of the illness, relationship with the patient/relative, and 'areas of strength', e.g. social supports, positive relationships, etc. Further assessments can be carried out to produce a summary of the individual's problems, needs and strengths. Additional assessments of the patient include information about present symptomatology and social functioning. This can be done by using inventories such as the Symptom-Related Behaviour Disturbance Scale (SBDS), the Symptom Rating Test (SRT), and the Social Functioning Scale (SFS) (Smith & Birchwood, 1993).

Before addressing practical issues it would be prudent to examine the efficacy of introducing a family intervention service alongside conventional therapies. A comparison of the relapse rates of several family intervention studies alongside other treatments is detailed below (table 1).

Outcome studies

Overall, it can be confidently stated that the rates of relapse over 1–2 years produced by family intervention are lower than those for standard treatment. The studies outlined show little difference between relapse and length of family intervention although it has been argued that an intervention period of 12–24 months would provide the most beneficial outcome in preventing relapse (Penn & Mueser, 1996) (Table 15.1).

STUDY		FOLLOW-UP	
	N	9 OR 12 MONTHS	24 MONTHS
Goldstein & Kopeikin (1981)			
family intervention	25	0*	—
routine treatment	28	16*	—
Leff et al (1982, 1989)			
family intervention	12	8	20
routine treatment	12	50	78
family therapy	12	8	—
relatives group	6	17	—
Kottgen et al (1984)			
family intervention	15	33	—
control (high EE)	14	43	—
control (low EE)	20	20	—
Falloon et al (1985)			
family intervention	18	6	17
individual intervention	18	44	83
Hogarty et al (1991)			
family intervention	21	19	—
social skills training	20	20	—
combined interventions	20	0	—
control	17	41	—
Tarrier et al (1988)			
family intervention	25	12	33
education only	14	43	57
routine treatment	15	53	60
Vaughn et al (1992)			
family intervention/education	18	41	—
routine treatment	18	65	—
Zhang et al (1994)			
family intervention	28	—	10
routine treatment	22	—	36
McFarlane et al (1995)			
multiple relative family intervention	83	—	16
single relative family intervention	89	—	27

*Study with 6 month follow-up period. (All subjects medicated unless stated).

Table 15.1 – Relapse rates from family intervention studies.

Service implications

Although new drug treatments are relatively easily incorporated into existing treatment regimes, the development of a family intervention service is complex, time consuming, and requires careful planning. The major areas which need to be considered in planning such a service include whether it is clinically and cost effective, how to identify the target clientele; whether they can be effectively engaged; the procedure for patients referred to the service, and the availability of expertise to provide such interventions.

Efficiency and cost effectiveness

As stated earlier the evidence for the efficacy of family interventions in comparison to conventional treatment suggests that the former provide a marked improved in rates of relapse (table 1). The 'optimum' length of intervention is still an issue for contention as longer-term studies have provided impressive results whereas, in general, relapse rates appear to remain unaffected by shorter-term (2 months or less) studies (Penn & Mueser, 1996). However, the successful development of family intervention services, evidence of clinical efficiency must be matched by data on cost effectiveness. It appears that the cost of providing family intervention and follow-up treatment is easily compensated by the decline in the duration of hospital admissions and the lowering of crises intervention required by patients (Tarrier, 1989), and benefits are maintained on follow up (Falloon et al. 1985).

Engaging families

Although the psychosocial difficulties of families in which a member has a severe mental illness are well documented (Kuipers & Bebbington, 1988), the uptake of family intervention services is usually only partial and non-cooperation ranges from 14 to 35% (Smith & Birchwood, 1990). Three main problems are highlighted by recent research (Smith & Birchwood, 1990). Firstly, families may feel threatened by the offer of such a specialised service and may construe this action by the provider as implying that the 'problem' lies within the home. Hence relatives may feel that they are somehow being held responsible for the onset of the patient's illness. Secondly, a number of patients who have recently developed a severe mental illness may hold the view, as may family members, that this episode is only a temporary setback and that long-term support or assistance from services is unwarranted. The distress and anger shown by relatives towards professionals can be associated with denial, by the patient and the family, that the patient may have a psychiatric problem. Finally, it is important that families understand the reasoning behind family intervention and the role they play in this process. Often family members believe that professionals should be able to 'cure' their relative and do not see their role in this process. Similarly, families may perceive their needs as few or having been met by other parts of the service and hence withdraw from such a programme.

Operating a service

The aforementioned issues are addressed in the family service model developed at

All Saints Hospital in Birmingham by Birchwood (1992). The service does not use high EE or admission only entry points but engages potential service users and their families at several entry points including acute admissions, outpatients and medication clinics, day centres and through local voluntary organisations. The service is offered routinely to families as one component of an assertive outreach service. Following acceptance, multiple assessments (Birchwood, 1986; Birchwood & Smith, 1987; Smith & Birchwood, 1987; Birchwood et al. 1989) allow for evaluation of the needs and strengths of each referred family.

The service is promoted within a framework of partnership where the difficulties faced by families are acknowledged and the family are seen as facing problems rather than being a 'problem family'. Emphasis is placed upon enabling families, through the development of expertise from the information and skills provided, to determine the most appropriate way to tackle the problems they face. This will hopefully remove the families reliance upon the professional to provide solutions to emerging problems which then follow. A crucial stage in the service provision is the negotiation of the goals of the intervention with the patient and his/her family which, besides defining these, allows the breakdown of any 'adversarial' problems which may occur between the professional and the family. A further requirement for an effective service is the necessity for integration with other services and key professionals involved with the client and family. This allows continuity of care and integration of the goals of the family intervention with the overall treatment and rehabilitation plans for the individual.

Availability of expertise

The development of an effective family intervention resource will be most successful if it complements multi-disciplinary community mental health services. The depth of professional expertise and experience available can be focused on specific areas of the family work, providing there is a clear agenda to educate all professionals in the necessary skills. A training scheme providing these specialist skills must address the following three areas: the assessment of the needs of individuals and their families; the ability to respond to the information and emotional needs of individuals and their families following the onset of a severe mental illness, and an ability to help families reduce the emotional and practical hardship of such disorders. The development of back-up information materials and a training manual (Smith & Birchwood, 1987) alongside trained 'tutors' on whom professionals can rely for support and supervision is also a necessary requirement. Efforts must be made to ensure that the quality of the service is continued through the provision of ongoing 'in-house' supervision and training.

EARLY DETECTION AND INTERVENTION FOR RELAPSE PREVENTION

Overview

Even an ideal combination of psychosocial interventions and drug therapy does not eliminate the potential for relapse (Hogarty et al. 1991), which can result in the possibility of the individual developing residual symptoms and a greater probability of future regression (McGlashan, 1988), which in turn generally leads to greater social disablement (Birchwood, 1992).

Although the prediction of relapse may still be only modestly effective, research focusing on the detection of early indicators of loss of well-being does allow for early intervention. An investigation of the perceived well-being of patients, with a diagnosis of schizophrenia, attending for maintenance therapy (McCandless-Glincher et al. 1986) suggests that such indicators are useful in the formation of an early intervention strategy. Of the 62 subjects in this study 61 said they could recognise early signs of relapse, and as a result the majority (50 out of 61) initiated some change in behaviour to combat this, e.g. engaging in diversionary activity, seeking professional help, and resuming/increasing their medication. As these subjects had initiated symptom monitoring and a range of resulting responses, it is possible that patterns of prodromal episodes, as precursors to relapse, may be identifiable.

This possibility was investigated in a large scale study in which 145 subjects with a diagnosis of schizophrenia were recruited alongside 80 family members (Herz & Melville, 1980). The main questioned asked was: 'Could you tell that there were changes in your thoughts, feelings or behaviours that might have led you to believe that you were becoming sick and might have to go to hospital?', and was answered in the affirmative by 70% of patients and 93% of relatives. The results of this and a similar British study are detailed in Table 15.2.

Both studies concur in finding dysphoric symptoms the most prevalent. There was agreement between patients in the Herz and Melville study that non-psychotic symptoms such as anxiety, tension and insomnia were part of the 'prodrome', and 50% of subjects felt that characteristic symptoms of the prodrome were repeated at each relapse. Finally, subjects reported the presence of many of the non-psychotic symptoms during the non-acute periods of the illness.

Hirsch and Jolley (1989) investigated the putative prodromes, i.e. neurotic or dysphoric episodes, in a group of 54 schizophrenic patients. In order to increase their ability to recognise dysphoric syndromes, patients and their key workers received a one hour teaching session about schizophrenia which outlined the importance of dysphoric syndromes as a precursor to relapse. All subjects were symptom free at the commencement of the study, and received assessments using the SCL-90 (Derogalis et al. 1973), a self-report psychiatric measure developed for

CATEGORY	Birchwood et al. (1989) (N=42)		Herz & Melville (1980) (N=80)	
	%	RANK*	%	RANK*
Anxiety/Agitation				
Irritable/quick tempered	62	2 (equal)	—	—
Sleep problems	67	1	69	7
tense, afraid, anxious	62	2 (equal)	83	1
Depression/Withdrawal				
Quiet, withdrawn	60	4	50	18
Depressed, low	57	5	76	3
Poor appetite	48	9	53	17
Disinhibition				
Aggression	50	7 (equal)	79	2
Restless	55	6	40	20
Stubborn	36	10 (equal)	—	—
Incipient Psychosis				
Behaves as if hallucinating	50	7 (equal)	60	10
Being laughed at or talked about	36	10 (equal)	14	53.8
"Odd behaviour"	36	10 (equal)	—	—

*There were many other symptoms assessed. percentage reporting only shown for parallel data.

Table 15.2 – Percentage of relatives reporting early signs.

the assessment of psychiatric pathology, and Herz's Early Sign Questionnaire (ESQ) (Herz et al. 1982). All subjects received monthly assessments unless a dysphoric episode was evident. In such cases these questionnaires were administered at each such dysphoric episode and fortnightly thereafter. The requirement for relapse was defined as the emergence of florid symptoms including hallucinations and delusions. Results showed that 73% of relapses were preceded by a prodromal period of dysphoric and neurotic symptoms within a month of relapse. These prodromes included symptoms such as depression, anxiety, interpersonal sensitivity and paranoid symptoms, and were confirmed by the SCL-90.

Although one half of the subjects in this study received maintenance medication and the other half received a placebo, all subjects were given additional medication upon the emergence of dysphoric symptoms. Dysphoric episodes were far more common in the placebo group (76%) as opposed to the medicated group (27%). However, the prompt administration of medication prevents clarification as to whether these dysphoric episodes were part of a reactivation of psychosis (true prodromes), and also whether such cases included 'false positives' possibly related to the use of a placebo. The use of the ESQ which is reproduced in table 2 does underline the importance of symptoms of dysphoria/depression and the general blunting of drives and interest. Recorded experiences such as 'loss of control', 'fear of being alone' and 'puzzlement about objective experience' suggest the operation of psychological factors, which will be discussed below.

The results of the four major prospective studies of prodromal changes outlined by Birchwood (1992) suggest that psychotic relapse is preceded by non-psychotic dysphoric symptoms and low-level psychotic thinking including ideas of reference and paranoid thoughts. However, the clarity of these results is clouded by the use of a targeted medication strategy (Hirsch & Jolley, 1989; Marder et al. 1984) in two of these studies which allows for potential confusion when attempting to decipher between putative prodromes and false positives. It is also suggested that the use of an early intervention strategy may have exaggerated the magnitude of the recorded prodromes. Subjects who do not relapse may develop fluctuations in levels of dysphoric symptoms, fluctuations which are not part of a relapse (i.e. false positives), but which nevertheless may respond to medication if detected (highly likely) during the course of the study. Hence such interventions may reduce the contrast between relapsed and non-relapsed groups.

A further potential complication is the finding that the pattern of prodromal symptoms suggests between-subject variability (Birchwood et al. 1989). Some patients may 'peak' on anxiety symptoms, other on disinhibition, and so on. Similarly, a small proportion may show no prodromal symptoms (Subotnik & Nuechterlian, 1988). The existence of prodromes of psychotic relapse is confirmed by the studies outlined above, although the limitation of group studies is evident from their inability to address the qualitative and quantitative between-subjects variability in early signs and symptoms. This is supported by the finding that greater prediction was possible when patients were compared against their own baseline rather than that of others (Subotnik & Nuechterlian, 1988). Hence, it may be more useful to look at each patient's prodrome as a 'relapse signature' which contains core or common symptoms along with features unique to the patient. Identification of an individual's prodrome can, it is reasonable to assume, increase the overall predictive power of prodromal symptoms.

A psychological model of prodromes

The research outlined above suggests two stages in the relapse process: dysphoria, including anxiety, restlessness and the blunting of drives, followed by low-level psychotic pathology such as suspiciousness, ideas of reference and so on. It has been argued that strong features of the prodrome include 'loss of control', 'fear of going crazy' and 'puzzlement about objective experience' (Hirsch & Jolley, 1989). However, other studies suggest that a set of early symptoms are being overlooked. Some patients report a feeling of over-stimulation where external and internal events invade consciousness (Chapman, 1966). Visual and time distortions are commonplace and the resultant effect leads to feelings of derealisation and depersonalisation (Donlon & Blacker, 1975). Patients often consult physicians with vague and diffuse somatic symptoms which suggest an overactivation of biological systems (Offenkrantz, 1962).

We argue that the patient faced with the myriad of symptoms intrinsic to psychosis attempts to rationalise and search for intent in these experiences in order to provide him/her with meaning and control. Those with little experience of relapse may be puzzled by these perpetual changes and may respond to them with fear and confusion. Patients with greater experience will be aware of the 'danger' represented by the emergence of such symptoms and respond with a sense of foreboding, as they realise that something is about to happen over which they have little or no control, i.e. relapse. Dysphoria may therefore be regarded as a response to the emergence of a threatening or ominous event (the relapse), or a response to the failure to control what may be regarded as a highly dangerous and alarming event. The stress and ominous feelings this may create could accelerate the relapse process (Figure 15.2).

Critical periods

Although little prospective research exists investigating the long-term effects of schizophrenia from first episode onwards, the available findings suggest that positive and negative symptoms stabilise within 24 months and that no further deterioration occurs in about 25% (Thara et al. 1994). This possibility that deterioration reaches a plateau within the first two years of illness was suggested during the earliest days of mental health research (Bleuler, 1978), and has been reinforced by later studies (Carpenter & Strauss, 1991)

It would appear that for many individuals afflicted with severe mental illness, the initial period following the first episode may provide the best possibility for successful secondary prevention. Psychosocial adjustment at this time may play a key role in successful relapse prevention (Birchwood et al. 1997)

Implementation in the clinical setting

As with the development of a family intervention provision, the necessity for close co-operation between patient, carer and professionals is of paramount concern in the early detection and treatment of relapse. In order to reduce detrimental treatment delay we recommend three strategies:

1. A community education programme emphasising the treatment of psychosis and focussing on the professional and voluntary agencies likely to encounter psychosis.

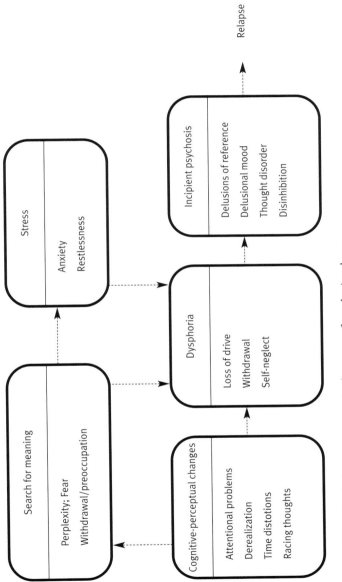

Figure 15.2 – Psychological processes in the stages of psychotic relapse

2. Training general practitioners in the recognition of psychosis and encouraging secondary referral where a psychosis is suspected, although cases which are unclear may require monitoring and support without treatment, through the assignment of a key worker, until the psychosis is confirmed.

3. The provision of services in the home or in a low-stigma setting in order to increase the likelihood of patients and their families accepting early treatment.

Education and engagement of all the parties should be undertaken as part of an 'informed partnership'. Information provided about early intervention and prodromes needs to be incorporated alongside general information about schizophrenia. The responsibility that is being placed upon the individual and relative to recognise components which may constitute a potential relapse and the need for treatment requires succinct explanation. The stability of the relationship provided by the professional will be reflected in the successful engagement and cooperation of the patient with early intervention.

Individuals with a history of repeated relapse or who are at high risk due to factors such as high EE or recovery from a recent relapse or low-dose maintenance medication, may be suitable for early intervention regimes. Patients who receive high doses of maintenance medication may not be suitable for a regime which relies upon increasing drug dosage to combat potential relapse, but may benefit from early intervention procedures based upon psychosocial designs (Penn & Mueser, 1996). In the case of clients receiving very high doses of medication or with severe drug-related symptoms, the likelihood of discriminating a prodrome against such a background would appear to be very difficult. Similarly, the absence of insight may hinder the potential usefulness of an early intervention strategy.

Four potential problem areas have to be addressed if an effective early intervention service is to develop. Firstly, the identification of 'early signs' would require intensive regular monitoring of mental state at least fortnightly, which is rarely possible in clinical practice. Secondly, some patients may choose to conceal their symptoms as relapse approaches and insight declines (Heinrichs et al. 1985). Thirdly, many patients experience residual or persisting symptoms, cognitive deficits or drug side-effects which may obscure the validity of the prodromes. Finally, the characteristics of prodromes may vary from individual to individual and this information may be lost in the use of generalised scales for pathology and group design in research studies. This particular problem may be overcome by the use of precise interviewing techniques when obtaining information from the client, his/her family and close associates. Areas of agreement between the accounts from such individuals may lead to greater accuracy in discriminating a future prodrome.

The use of the Early Signs interview and Early Signs Scale (Birchwood, 1992) provides an ongoing system of monitoring with observations taken on a fortnightly basis, although the frequency of observations can be increased if there is any cause for concern. A sense of ownership over the collected data is to be encouraged and patients can be provided with regularly updated information at each interview in the form of printouts and graphs.

Upon the emergence of a prodrome both the patient and their family will require intensive support and counselling in order to combat the strain that may be associated with the possibility of relapse. The use of stress management techniques, diversionary activities and general support will help alleviate these concerns (Brier & Strauss, 1983), although quick access to such services would be a crucial component of any such intervention. Weekly, daily or even in-patient care, a powerful tool in the repertoire of early intervention work, can be offered not only to alleviate anxiety but also to emphasise the 'shared burden' which needs to be projected for the success of any such service.

Cognitive behaviour therapy

There has been a burgeoning interest in the application of cognitive therapy for people with psychosis. This has focused directly on psychotic symptoms and has challenged the widely held view that it is impossible to 'reason with delusions'. Below we outline this approach drawing upon the techniques outlined by Chadwick et al. (1996).

The cognitive ABC model

The framework for the intervention is based upon Ellis (1962); ABC model (Table 15.3). The model does not purport a causal inference between beliefs and feelings, but rather argues that **A**ntecedents, **B**eliefs and **C**onsequences usually occur as a single experience (Chadwick et al. 1996). Hence this model quite usefully separates out the components of experience implicit in the activation of delusional beliefs and voices.

The 'Beliefs' component of the ABC model includes four cognitions: images, inferences, evaluations and dysfunctional assumptions. 'Image' Bs should always be explored within cognitive therapy practice as they are especially useful with clients who struggle to verbalise beliefs, e.g. an individual who is very anxious about public speaking and is contemplating a forthcoming event might have a sudden image of him or herself fainting on stage. Inference Bs refer to what Beck (1964) described as

A	**B**	**C**
Activating event	**B**eliefs (images, thoughts, beliefs)	Emotional and behavioural **C**onsequences

Table 15.3 – The cognitive ABC model.

automatic thoughts and are predictions or hypotheses of what is happening, will happen or has happened, e.g. I'll fail, people are spying on me, and so on. Inferences occur in abbreviated, often crude language and all go past the factual evidence, e.g. he hates me, the bastards are at it again. Evaluation Bs may be defined as good-bad judgement or a preference as opposed to an inference, e.g. I prefer John to David, other people are bad, etc. Particular importance is given to 'person evaluations' (Chadwick & Birchwood, 1996) which are stable, global and total condemnations of an entire person. They may be made in three ways: self to self where I am making evaluations about myself; self to other where I am evaluating the other, and other to self where the other is making evaluations of me, e.g. I am worthless, other people are bad, and people feel I am bad, respectively.

An ABC perspective on delusions

Delusions within the ABC framework are Bs, that is delusional beliefs based upon the event (A) and may or may not cause distressing Cs. Examples of the major types of delusions within the ABC framework are presented in Table 15.4.

The model will therefore help to clarify whether the delusion is problematic to the client. Additionally, the use of thought chaining to identify the event whose interpretation led to the belief, may uncover further possible dysfunctional beliefs, based upon this primary interpretation. An example of this is outlined below (Chadwick et al. 1996).

> the client infers that the doctor is passing a message to him through his walk – that he, the doctor, sees him as totally inferior, a nothing – that is, he was evaluating the client's entire person. This inferred other-self evaluation will not fully account for the client's experience of shame, because the client might think to himself that the doctor is an ass who's opinion is worth nothing. Further thought chaining revealed that the client accepted the doctor's evaluation of him … he made a negative self evaluation that he as a person was inferior and a nothing. This accounts for the emotional upset and clarifies the two main goals for cognitive therapy – to weaken the delusion and to weaken associated negative evaluative thinking.

The ABC model therefore clarifies the client's reasoning leading to their delusional beliefs. Evidence from the clinical application of this framework suggests that cognitive bias is central to the presence of the individual's delusions, especially when the individual is distressed, angry, anxious, etc. (Ellis, 1962). Hence, standard cognitive distortions (selective attention, overgeneralization, arbitrary inference, personalization) would be observed only when the delusion was present. Inferences which feed delusional interpretation of activating events are influenced by enduring beliefs (evaluations and dysfunctional assumptions). As such, these interpretations do not result solely from 'top-down' influences, i.e. based directly upon what stimulus is

Delusion	Antecedent	Belief	Consequence
Mind Reading	Client cannot find a word, therapist supplies it	She read my mind; I've find her out, I knew it	Elated Pressure to tell people
Paranoid	Car horn sounds outside	They have come for me, to kill me	Fear Runs for flat
Thought broadcast	Client shopping hears man say what he was thinking	My thoughts are being transmitted to others	Panic Escape
Thought insertion	Client has sudden intrusive and shocking thought	It's not mine someone put it in my head with a special machine	Fearful, exposed Urge to hide
Inference	Doctor walks past window, head held high	He thinks he's better than me, he's letting me know	Shame Moves away from window
Grandiose	The Queen says on TV she loves all her children	She means me, she loves me, I am her daughter	Elation
Infestation	Scalp itching	They are biting me, I can't stand it	Anxiety Helplessness
Somatic	Wakes feeling tired, aching Father supports client's admission to hospital Fails to respond to once enjoyed activity	I've got AIDS, I'm going to die He's not my dad, dad wouldn't do it, he's an alien I feel nothing, I am dead	Terror Immobilised Frightened Withdraws clenches fists Emptiness Suicidal
Control	Moves to push daughter out of open window	I didn't do that, they made me do it, they did it, it's not my fault	Reassured Passive

Table 15.4 – A cognitive ABC analysis of delusions.

being responded to by the individual, or 'bottom-up' influences, i.e. based upon the individual's expectations and experience (Chadwick et al. 1996).

An ABC perspective on voices

The major premise (Chadwick & Birchwood, 1996) behind viewing voices from a cognitive ABC perspective is that voices are activating events (As) to which the individual gives meaning (B) and experiences emotional and behavioural reactions (Cs). This novel approach suggests that distress caused by voices are a result of the beliefs held about auditory hallucinations and not just the presence of them (Table 15.5).

Activating event (voice)	Beliefs (images, thoughts, beliefs)	Emotional and behavioural Consequences
Richard hears a voice which says 'hit him'	It is God testing my strength and faith	Does not comply Feel pleased
Jenny hears a voice say 'be careful'	It is the devil, he is watching, waiting to get me	Terror Avoids going to the shops

Table 15.5 – ABC analysis of voices.

The beliefs held about a voice can be reasonably argued to be a type of delusional thinking, and the above approach to voices is actually a cognitive slant to a specific class of delusions, those which are secondary to particular activating events (As), i.e. voices. The major premise of the ABC model of voices is that emotion and coping behaviour are indeed connected to such hallucinations. A secondary assumption is that beliefs *are not* direct interpretations of voice content. Both these hypothesis are supported by robust empirical evidence (Chadwick & Birchwood, 1994, 1995, 1996).

Three categories of consequences (Cs) to voices are suggested (Chadwick et al. 1996): engagement, comprising positive affect and co-operative behaviour such as willing compliance with and seeking to call up the voices; resistance, comprising negative affect and resistant and combative behaviour such as shouting back at and non-compliance with voices, and indifference where the voice is not engaged by the individual which is rare in clinical groups.

Whether the voices are engaged or resisted can be discerned by the individual's beliefs about voices, specifically whether the voices were benevolent or malevolent respectively. However, research suggests that voice content is not always an accurate indicator of the beliefs held about voices. Examples have been cited where what would be assumed to be benevolent voice content is seen by the individual as being highly malevolent, and vice versa (Chadwick et al. 1996). For example, voice content such as 'take care' and 'watch your step' was believed by the patient to have been spoken by evil witches intent on driving him mad. Conversely, voice content suggesting the individual commits suicide was believed to be benevolent. Therefore, the meaning individuals attach to their voice content is fundamental in shaping the responding behavioural and emotional consequences.

Cognitive therapy of delusions and voices: the engagement problem

The major problem in the provision of a psychotherapy for voices and delusions is that of client engagement. Individuals affected with serious mental illness can be difficult to engage at the best of times. Many never attend or do so only during the early sessions before dropping out. Seven major threats to engagement during therapeutic work are outlined below (Chadwick et al. 1996):

1. A failure of therapist empathy

2. Therapist's beliefs about clients

3. Client's blocking beliefs

4. Relationship too threatening

5. Client sees no potential benefit

6. Viewing delusions as facts not beliefs

7. Failing to agree a rationale for questioning the delusion

The ability of the therapist to relate to symptoms such as anxiety, depression and anger which he/she frequently encounters, allow for the development of empathy with the client. However, with psychotic illness the often bizarre and delusional ideas held by the client may threaten the usual empathic process as comprehension in such cases can be difficult. This would be especially so for unusual perceptual experiences, e.g. it would be easier to understand a belief that one is being persecuted (an exaggeration of a common experience) than an experience of passivity. The issue here is that a need for shared experience is not an essential requirement for empathy, but only that the therapist recognises and understands the thinking, feelings and behaviour in such cases. The therapist's understanding should be enhanced by his/her extrapolation of the ways in which clients have made sense of antecedents (As) through the development of specific beliefs and personal meanings (Bs), and the feelings and behaviours (Cs) associated with these.

A related problem with the failure to develop empathy may occur due to the therapist's beliefs about psychosis and the usefulness of psychological therapy in such cases. For example, the belief that psychotic behaviour is discontinuous is likely to influence the therapist's feelings, behaviour and expectations in therapy sessions. There are many other beliefs which therapists may hold that could jeopardise therapy (Chadwick et al. 1996), and such potential problems highlight the necessity for focused supervision which can combat these potential beliefs.

The client's expectations of health care are likely to mould their beliefs about the usefulness of therapy, and sadly their negative experiences of mental health services will in some cases cause clients to not engage in such interventions. Clients often feel that a candid discussion of their delusions and voices may lead to a repetition of previous experience, e.g. a hospital admission, an increase in medication. Clients may feel that the therapist will disregard their beliefs, outlook and experience and regard them as simply 'mad'. Such potential problems can be tackled through the use of a collaborative therapeutic style and enabling the client to comprehend the therapeutic process through education about cognitive therapy. Engaging the client in the therapeutic relationship can be problematic where clients have poor inter-personal skills and find such settings stressful. A related problem could result if individuals combat this anxiety by becoming hyper-vigilant and perceiving threat-ening or rejecting cues from the therapist. Solving these types of problem require forfeiture of some of the more traditional principles of psychotherapy. Initial engagement can be on a more casual basis to put clients at ease; sessions may be more productive if they are shorter and frequent, and the structuring of sessions will counter the problem of lengthy silences.

The viewing of delusions as beliefs (Bs) and not activating events (As) needs to focus on two points: why it is being done and how it is done. Empowering the client to view delusions as beliefs and not facts will allow him/her a way of easing the distress they feel. The therapist does not attempt to persuade the client that he/she is wrong and you, the therapist, is right. Rather the therapist helps the client to draw upon their own doubt and experience in order to look at the belief constructively. Many clients have 'double awareness' of delusions; at times they believe them firmly, yet on other occasions they behave in a way which is contradictory to the delusion, and it is at these times they believe that working with the therapist might ease the problem. Finally, the therapist must accept that it is okay if the client does not alter their belief; the process is one of collaborative empiricism, not indoctrination.

The problem that many therapists face is convincing clients that delusions are beliefs and not actual events. This means that such clients will have no clear objec-tives or motivation to engage in cognitive therapy. The key here is to ensure that both the therapist and client have a common rationale for questioning the delusion. A client will want to address a delusion if they feel it will free them from the distress experienced and allow them to behave differently. The therapist employing the ABC framework clarifies to the client that he/she is experiencing emotional and behavioural problems, and that these are tied to his/her beliefs (delusional and evalu-ative). The next stage is to explore how the client's life would be different if the delusion was false, and hence encourage the client to view the belief as something which causes distress and behaviour which he/she rather not engage in. Once again, the process is critical as although clients experiencing distress will proceed relatively quickly through the ABC assessment, it is not crucial to be able to do this with patients who are deluded. The therapist should oversee a process of gradually moving the client through the conceptual steps in cognitive therapy thereby creating safety as well as insight and motivation. This should appear seamless from the client's perspective although it may be preferable to the therapist to have a graduated process.

Procedures for weakening delusions

The therapists role in disputing the client's delusional system is a four stage process (Chadwick et al. 1996). Firstly, the evidence for the belief is challenged in hierarchical order commencing with the least important evidence inducing the delusion. Secondly, the internal consistency and credibility of the delusional system is questioned. Thirdly, the delusion is reinterpreted into an understandable and personally meaningful alternative response to a specific stimulus experienced by the client (Maher, 1988). Finally, the delusion and alternative explanation are examined in light of the available information.

When challenging the evidence for the beliefs underlying a delusion system, the therapist would begin by eliciting the evidence for the belief. Each piece of evidence would be questioned and an alternative, more reasonable and probable explanation would be offered. The concept of psychological reactance (Maher, 1988), suggests that a too direct approach in attempting to modify delusions will only serve to reinforce the belief, and hence commencing with the weakest belief and working only with evidence for the belief, rather than the belief itself, would aid in overcoming this potential problem (Watts et al. 1973).

The practice of challenging beliefs, besides undermining the confidence in the delusion, will convey aspects of the ABC model to the client and allow for the development of insight into the connection between beliefs, behaviour and affect. This is particularly useful as it will indicate that we all misinterpret events and process selectively in order to allow our experiences to equate with our beliefs. It is important to convey this within the therapeutic situation using everyday examples such as how rival politicians will interpret certain reports in a totally different way, fitting in with their political affiliations. Hence, the therapist offers fresh insight into the client's delusional interpretations, and having considered the alternatives, the client is asked to rate his convictions for each delusional interpretation in the hierarchy of beliefs.

In order to challenge the delusion the therapist relies on the fact that few complex belief systems are watertight. Hence inconsistency and irrationality will be present to some extent in the majority of belief systems. It is important to remember that common reactions to delusions such as thinking that one is going mad and becoming fearful, or that someone is playing a trick and becoming wary and suspicious, allow the therapist a platform from which to work therapeutically with these fears during this stage.

Once the process of reformulating the beliefs has begun and the argument that certain experiences, e.g. trauma, acute pathology, have resulted in a delusion which is psychologically motivated, i.e. it eases puzzlement, the client and therapist may pursue other psychological consequences of the delusion. The evaluative beliefs underlying the delusional system hold the key to the psychological function of the delusion. The therapist will now attempt to connect the evaluative and delusional beliefs and then convey the nature of this connection, e.g. delusion defends against negative self-evaluation. Finally, the evaluative beliefs will be disputed and tested. This further process extends the reinterpretation of the delusion and increases clarity for the client as it provides further psychological motivation for the delusion system. In concluding the client and therapist would assess the delusion and alternative in light of their discussions and the available evidence. For example (Chadwick et al. 1996):

> Terry believed that his appearance was sinister and suspicious, and that he was suspected of various criminal offences for which some form of retaliation was going to be taken. All his evidence for the delusion related to occasions where he had thought some people were suspicious of him and he had experienced strong anxiety and guilt. He took these emotions as proof of his badness, reasoning that if he had done nothing to hide he would not be feeling this way. Although he was never accused of anything by anyone, he always said to himself 'today I was lucky, I got away without being challenged', rather than challenging the delusion.
>
> The event Terry put forward as most integral to the belief took place when he was on a training course. Over the subsequent weeks he saw several police cars. He believed that the police had questioned him and subsequently placed him under surveillance because of his sinister and suspicious appearance. This view was challenged as follows. First, Terry stated that he felt so nervous walking through town that he had 'jumped' on seeing the police car: this may have accounted for the policeman stopping to 'have a word'. Second, the policeman did not ask Terry where he lived or worked and having spoken to him drove off. Terry was certain that he was not followed home. Terry's conclusion (that he was placed under surveillance) therefore did not fit with his own perception of the episode, but made sense only when his delusional belief and affect were 'on line'.

Procedures for working with voices

The need to empower the client and weaken the perceived omnipotence and 'dysfunctional' beliefs about their voices, is an important precursor to using cognitive-behavioural therapy. The associated distress can be overwhelming for the individual and as such he/she will require encouragement and reassurance from the therapist, in re-examining their beliefs about the voices, if the therapy is to be successful. This technique is defined as Coping Strategy Enhancement (CSE) (Chadwick & Birchwood, 1994; Tarrier, 1992). CSE can be used in four ways:

1. To underline the strength and endurance of the individual in attempting to cope with their voices.

2. As a means of underpinning the therapeutic alliance.

3. To develop an understanding of factors that 'cue' the voices.

4. To develop an understanding of the abilities that the person may have to deal with their voices.

CSE would be over-rehearsed by the client in order to develop an automatic response to the voices, but only used selectively as overuse may develop into a form of avoidance and hence fear of the voices. However, if used carefully CSE can be a valuable tool in allowing clients to exercise control over voices once thought to be all powerful.

Assessment of the delusional content of voices, i.e. the personal meaning the voices have for the client, have resulted in the finding that voice identity, purpose, power, knowledge and consequences of compliance and resistance are the significant delusional beliefs held. A semi-structured interview has been constructed specifically for this task (Chadwick & Birchwood, 1994, 1995). Once identified, it is suggested that beliefs concerning voice power, especially those involving compliance and control are challenged initially as this causes less anxiety than beliefs about identity and meaning. If successfully challenged the client will come to view the voices as less powerful and controlling (and hence less distressing), as well as generating implications for other as yet untackled beliefs about identity and meaning, e.g. 'If I can control the voice, can it really be the devil?'

The therapist's major argument is that the beliefs held by the client are reactions to, and attempts to make sense of, the voices. As such a review of the evidence and inconsistency and the use of tests will allow for one of two conclusions: the beliefs are true or that they are reasonable and understandable but mistaken. It is vital that the therapist works collaboratively with the client, drawing out the client's doubts, puzzlement, etc. rather than forcing them to accept a reinterpretation.

In order to increase the clients control over their voices a procedure can be employed in which the client and therapist review situations which start and increase the probability of voices, and then those which stop or reduce them (Chadwick & Birchwood, 1994). An initial assessment provides information as to the cues which induce voices for the client and this information is combined in the following stages:

1. Identify cues that increase and decrease voices.

2. Practice the use of increasing and decreasing cues within a session.

3. Propose the notion that control over the voices requires the ability to be able to increase/decrease the voice at will.

4. In further sessions encourage the client to increase and reduce voice activity for short periods of time.

SUMMARY

In this chapter we have briefly reviewed the rationale, intervention and service implications of three new approaches to the psychological treatment of psychosis.

The evidence for employing interventions to reduce EE within a clinical service comes from the results of family intervention treatments which demonstrate that targeting this particular factor will reduce the risk of potential relapse. However the clinician must be aware of the burden and stress which families experience in such situations, and should aim for good patient outcome and successful family coping and decreased family burden. In developing a family intervention service it is crucial to engage clients and their families effectively if the risk of non-cooperation is to be lowered.

The usefulness of early intervention for relapse prevention lies in the accurate detection of indicators of the loss of well-being and as such requires a system of symptom monitoring and prodrome detection. The overall predictive power of early symptoms is further enhanced by the identification of the individual client's prodrome and specific 'relapse signature'. The development of an early inter-vention service requires intensive and regular symptom monitoring, but also precise interviewing techniques in order to avoid client specific information being lost. Upon the identification of a prodrome the client and family require intensive support and counselling and rapid access to services.

For both family and early intervention service provisions, it is important that the service integrates effectively with existing treatment resources and is reinforced by a training system available to all staff which provides the specialist skills required.

The cognitive behavioural treatment strategies for voices and delusions outlined in this chapter are underpinned by the ABC model, and the crux of these interventions is the 'beliefs' component which is clarified and explored using cognitive therapy. Activating events (As) result in beliefs (Bs) which have emotional and behavioural consequences (Cs). Although this is clearly applicable to delusional beliefs, the approach to auditory hallucinations is no different as beliefs about voices (and not just their presence) cause distress. In order to use this approach the therapist requires a complete understanding of the possible pitfalls and threats to engaging the client.

In attempting to weaken delusions the therapist challenges each belief underlying the delusion in inverse order of their importance, questions the internal consis-tency and credibility of the belief, reinterprets the delusion into an understandable and meaningful alternative response, and jointly with the client, examines the delusion and proposed alternative in light of all the information available. A similar strategy is employed for working with auditory hallucinations, in order to weaken the perceived omnipotence of the voices and also to empower the client, Coping Strategy Enhancement (CSE). This allows the client access to an almost automatic coping mechanism to exercise control over their voices. The therapist's major argument is that beliefs about voices are reactions to, and attempts to make sense of, the auditory hallucinations. Collaborative work between the client and therapist whilst reviewing the evidence and inconsistency underlying the beliefs about voices, will allow for the generation of doubt and the eventual reinterpretation of the beliefs originally held to be true.

In conclusion we have suggested that recent research on the psychosocial approaches to severe mental illness provide robust evidence that, of the underlying abnormal processes and functioning experienced by clients and families, many are 'normal' and can be addressed therapeutically through the use of cognitive–behavioural strategies. Each requires a collaborative partnership between client, carer and service provider which must be implemented in the context of a structure of care in which the client's needs are managed on a long-term basis in conjunction with other treatment modalities.

References

Barraclough C, Tarrier N. Social functioning in schizophrenic patients I. The effects of expressed emotion and family intervention. Soc Psychiatry Psychiatr Epidemiol 1990; 25: 125–129.

Beck AT. Thinking and depression 2: theory and therapy. Arch Gen Psychiatry 1964; 10: 561–571.

Birchwood MJ, Smith J. Expressed emotion and first episodes of schizophrenia. Br J Psychiatry 1987; 152: 859–960.

Birchwood MJ, Cochrane R. Families coping with schizophrenia: coping styles, their origins and correlates. Psychol Med 1990; 20: 857–865.

Birchwood MJ. The control of auditory hallucinations through the use of monoaural auditory input. Br J Psychiatry 1986; 149: 104–107.

Birchwood MJ, Smith J. Schizophrenia and the family. In Orford J (ed). Coping with Disorder in the Family. Beckenham: Croom Helm, 1987.

Birchwood MJ, Smith J, MacMillan JF et al. Predicting relapse in schizophrenia: the development of an 'early signs' monitoring system using patients and families as observers. Psychol Med 1989; 19: 649–656.

Birchwood MJ. Early intervention in schizophrenia: theoretical background and clinical strategies. Br J Clin Psychol 1992; 31: 257–278.

Birchwood MJ, McGorry P, Jackson H. Early intervention in schizophrenia. Br J Psychiatry 1997; 170: 2–5.

Bleuler M. The Schizophrenic Disorders: Long-term Patient and Family Studies (trans. C. Clements). New Haven: Yale University Press, 1978.

Brehm JW. A Theory of Psychological Reactants. New York: Academic Press, 1962.

Brier A, Strauss JS. Self control in psychiatric disorder. Arch Gen Psychiatry 1983; 40: 1141–1145.

Brown GW, Birley JLT, Wing JK. Influence of family life on the course of schizophrenic disorders: a replication. Br J Psychiatry 1972; 121: 241–258.

Carpenter W, Strauss J. The prediction of outcome in schizophrenia V: eleven year follow-up of the IPSS cohort. J Nervous Mental Disease 1991; 179: 517–525.

Chadwick PDJ, Birchwood MJ, Trower P. Cognitive Therapy for Delusions Voices and Paranoia. Chichester: John Wiley, 1996.

Chadwick PDJ, Birchwood MJ. Cognitive therapy for voices. In Haddock G, Slade P (eds), Cognitive Behavioural Interventions for Psychosis. London: Routledge, 1996.

Chadwick PDJ, Birchwood MJ. The omnipotence of voices: a cognitive approach to auditory hallucinations. Br J Psychiatry 1994; 165: 190–201.

Chadwick PDJ, Birchwood MJ. The omnipotence of voices II: the beliefs about voices questionnaire. Br J Psychiatry 1995; 166: 11–19.

Chapman J. The early symptoms of schizophrenia. Br J Psychiatry 1966; 112: 25–251.

Derogatis L, Lipman R, Covi L. SCL-90: an outpatient psychiatric rating scale – preliminary report. Psychopharm Bull 1973; 9: 13–17.

Donlon PT, Blacker KH. Clinical recognition of early schizophrenic decompensation. Disorders Nervous System 1975; 36: 323–330.

Ellis A. Reason and Emotion in Psychotherapy. New York: Lyle Stuart, 1962.

Falloon IRH. Expressed emotion: current status. Psychol Med 1988; 18: 269–274.

Falloon IRH, Boyd JL, McGill CE, Williamson M, Razani J, Moss HB, Gilderman AM, Simpson GM. Family management in the prevention of morbidity of schizophrenia: clinical outcome of a two year longitudinal study. Arch Gen Psychiatry 1985; 42: 887–896.

Goldstein MJ, Kopeikin HS. Short and long term effects of combining drug and family therapy. In Goldstein MJ (ed). New Developments in Interventions with Families of Schizophrenics. San Francisco: Jossey-Bass, 1981.

Greenley JR. Social control and expressed emotion. J Nervous Mental Disease 1986; 174: 24–36.

Hatfield AB. Psychological costs of schizophrenia to the family. Social Work 1978; 25: 355–359.

Heinrichs D, Cohen BP, Carpenter WT. Early insight and the management of schizophrenic decompensation. J Nervous Mental Disease 1985; 173: 133.

Herz MI, Melville C. Relapse in schizophrenia. Am J Psychiatry 1980; 137: 801–812.

Herz MI, Szymonski HV, Simon J. Intermittent medication for stable schizophrenic outpatients. Am J Psychiatry 1982; 139: 918–922.

Hirsch SR, Jolley AG. The dysphoric syndrome in schizophrenia and its implications for relapse. Br J Psychiatry 1989; suppl. 5: 46–50.

Hogarty GE, Anderson C, Reiss D, Kornblith S, Greenwald D, Ulrich R, Carter M. Family psychoeducation, social skills training, and maintenance chemotherapy in the aftercare treatment of schizophrenia, II: two year effects of a controlled study on relapse and adjustment. Arch Gen Psychiatry 1991; 48: 340–347.

Koenigsberg HN, Handley R. Expressed emotion: from predictive index to clinical construct. Am J Psychiatry 1986; 143: 1361–1373.

Kottgen C, Sonnichsen I, Mollenhauer K, Jurth R. Group therapy with the families of schizophrenic patients: results of the Hamburg Camberwell-Family-Interview Study III. Int J Family Psychiatry 1984; 5: 83–94.

Kuipers L, Bebbington P. Expressed emotion research in schizophrenia: theoretical and clinical implications. Psychol Med 1988; 18: 893–909.

Leff J. Controversial issues and growing points in research in relatives' expressed emotion. Int J Soc Psychiatry 1989; 35: 133–145.

Leff J, Kuipers L, Berkowitz R, Eberlien-Vries R, Sturgeon D. A controlled trial of social intervention in the families of schizophrenic patients. Br J Psychiatry 1982; 141: 121–134.

Leff J, Berkowitz R, Shavit N, Strachan A, Glass I, Vaughn C. A trial of family therapy v a relatives group for schizophrenia. Br J Psychiatry 1989; 154: 58–66.

Leff JP, Vaughn CE. Expressed Emotion in Families. New York: Guildford, 1985.

Maher BA. Anomalous experience and delusional thinking: the logic of explanation. In Oltmanns TF, Maher BA (eds). Delusional Beliefs. New York: Wiley, 1988.

Marder SR, Van Putten T, Mintz J, McKenzie J, Labell M, Faltico G, May RP. Costs and benefits of two doses of fluphenazine. Arch Gen Psychiatry 1984; 41: 1025–1029.

McCandless-Glincher L, McKnight S, Hamera E, Smith BL, Peterson K, Plumlee AA. Use of symptoms by schizophrenics to monitor and regulate illness. Hosp Community Psychiatry 1986; 37: 929–933.

McFarlane WR, Lukens E, Link B, Dushay R, Deakins SA, Newmark M, Dunne EJ, Horen B, Toran J. Multiple-family groups and psychoeducation in the treatment of schizophrenia. Arch Gen Psychiatry 1995; 52: 679–687.

McGlashan TH. A selective review of recent North American follow-up studies of schizophrenia. Schizophr Bull 1988; 14: 515–542.

Offenkrantz WC. Multiple somatic complaints as a precursor of schizophrenia. Am J Psychiatry 1962; 119: 258–259.

Penn LP, Mueser KT. Research update on the psychosocial treatment of schizophrenia. Am J Psychiatry 1996; 153: 607–617.

Smith J, Birchwood MJ, Cochrane C, George S. The needs of high and low expressed emotion families: a normative approach. Soc Psychiatry Psychiatr Epidemiol 1993; 28: 11–16.

Smith J, Birchwood MJ. Relatives and patients as partners in the management of schizophrenia. Br J Psychiatry 1990; 156: 654–660.

Smith J, Birchwood MJ. Specific and non-specific effects of an educational intervention with families living with a schizophrenic relative. Br J Psychiatry 1987; 150: 645–652.

Smith J, Birchwood MJ. Understanding Schizophrenia, vols I–IV. Birmingham: Birmingham West Birmingham Health Authority: Health Promotion Unit, 1985.

Subotnik KL, Nuechterlian KH. Prodromal signs and symptoms of schizophrenia relapse. J Abnorm Psychol 1988; 97: 405–412.

Tarrier N. The effect of treating the family to reduce relapse in schizophrenia. J Royal Society Med 1989; 82: 423–424.

Tarrier N. Management and modification of residual positive psychotic symptoms. In Birchwood M, Tarrier N (eds). Innovations in the Psychological Management of Schizophrenia. Chichester: Wiley, 1992.

Tarrier N, Barraclough CD, Vaughn C et al. The community management of schizophrenia: a controlled trial of a behavioural intervention with families to reduce relapse. Br J Psychiatry 1988; 153: 532–542.

Thara R, Henrietta M, Joseph A. Ten year course of schizophrenia – the Madras longitudinal study. Acta Psychiatr Scand 1994; 90: 329–336.

Vaughn C. Patterns of emotional response in families of schizophrenic patients. In Goldstein MJ, Hand I, Halwage K (eds). Treatment of Schizophrenia: Family Assessment and Intervention. Berling: Springer, 1986.

Vaughn K, Doyle M, McConaghy N et al. The Sydney Intervention Trail: a controlled trail of relatives' counselling to reduce schizophrenic relapse. Soc Psychiatry Psychiatry Epidemiol 1992; 27: 16–21.

Watts FN, Powell EG, Austin SV. The modification of abnormal beliefs. Br J Med Psychol 1973; 46: 359–363.

Westermeyer JF, Harrow M, Marengo JT. Risk for suicide in schizophrenia and other psychotic and non-psychotic disorders. J Nervous Mental Disease 1991; 179: 259–266.

Zhang M, Wang M, Li J, Phillips MR. Randomised-control trial of family intervention for 78 first-episode male schizophrenic patients: an 18 month study in Suzhou, Jiangsu. Br J Psychiatry 1994; Suppl. 24: 96–102.

16

SUICIDE PREVENTION

Louis Appleby and Tim Amos

INTRODUCTION

The prevention of suicide is an international health priority. The World Health Organization has the reduction of suicide rates as one of its major targets (WHO 1992). Suicide prevention is a key element of public health policies in many countries (Diekstra 1989). In the UK the prevention of suicide has been a key objective for health services since the publication of *The Health of the Nation* (DoH 1992), the Department of Health's statement of its priorities for the 1990s. In *The Health of the Nation*, mental illness was identified as one of five key areas for health service activity, and three principal targets were specified, two of which concerned suicide. These were:

- a reduction of 15% in the general population suicide rate (from 11.1 per 100 000 population in 1990 to no more than 9.4); and

- a reduction of 33% in the lifetime risk of suicide in people with severe mental illness, from a presumed figure of 15% to 10%

Both targets were to be achieved by 2000, 8 years after their publication and 10 years from the 1990 figures which were used as baseline.

In 1999 *Saving Lives: Our Healthier Nation* was published outlining the Department of Health's priorities into the next century and suggesting a single new target, in the area of mental health, of a reduction in the death rate from suicide (and undetermined injury) by at least a further fifth (20%) by 2010 (DoH 1999).

The setting of these targets can be criticized on several grounds. The figures were largely arbitrary. There was no agreed definition of severe mental illness and no satisfactory way of estimating lifetime risk. They were interpreted by some as ignoring the fact that the main influences on suicide rates this century had been social, large rises occurring at times of high unemployment. They implied that suicide was a satisfactory outcome measure for health service activity, though there is no evidence for this.

Nevertheless, the targets have produced a number of considerable benefits. They have underlined the importance in the UK Health Service of mental illness in general, and of those who suffer from it. They have encouraged services to focus on the mortality associated with mental illness, to consider the needs of those who are at highest risk of this (Morgan 1994), and to view suicide prevention in a more positive way than was previously the case (Morgan 1993). In many parts of the UK, suicide is subject to regular clinical audit. Research funding has also followed.

Nor were the original targets set at a level that could easily be achieved. There have been only two occasions in the past 70 years when the suicide rate has fallen by as much as 15% over 10 years, and on both occasions the baseline rate was substantially higher than in 1992 (ONS 1992). A reduction of 33% in the case of people with severe mental illness is self-evidently a large proportionate change.

Suicide prevention in *The Health of the Nation* is an aim and an outcome, but not a process: there is nothing about how the prevention targets might be achieved. This, however, is not simple omission; it is an accurate reflection of the evidence at the time of publication (Gunnel and Frankel 1994). In *Saving Lives: Our Healthier Nation* there are some suggestions on possible steps but the measures are mostly general and apply to the whole population.

This chapter considers ways in which suicide might be prevented under four broad headings:

- A reduction in the frequency of key risk factors in the general population.

- A reduction in the availability or lethality of common methods of suicide.

- The enhancement of protective factors.

- Specific measures targeted at high-risk groups.

Their relevance to severe mental illness is discussed, and a strategy for suicide prevention by health services is outlined.

REDUCING GENERAL POPULATION RISK FACTORS

The population approach to prevention aims to reduce an outcome, in this case suicide, by reducing the rate of a key risk factor (or factors) in the general population. For this approach to be maximally successful, five conditions need to be satisfied. First, a key population risk factor must be known. Second, it should have a sufficiently strong impact on the suicide rate. Third, its effect should be reasonably direct. Fourth, it should be sufficiently common to be readily targeted.

Fifth, there should be a practicable and effective intervention. Several risk factors for suicide are known, and population approaches based on these might include interventions designed to address social factors such as unemployment, behavioural factors such as alcohol consumption, and medical factors such as depressive illness.

The close link between unemployment and suicide is well known (Sainsbury 1995). Periods of high unemployment this century, such as the 1930s and 1980s, have been associated with high rates of suicide; geographical areas of high unemployment have high suicide rates; recent evidence suggests that the disproportionate increases in younger male suicide seen in the past 20 years did not occur in those countries with the lowest unemployment rates (Pritchard 1996); risk factors for suicide such as deliberate self-harm and depression are more common in unemployed people (Hawton 1996); unemployed people are similarly over-represented in samples of completed suicides (Heikkinen et al. 1995). There is, therefore, evidence for a strong association between unemployment and suicide, but whether the effect is direct is not clear (Platt 1988). For example, unemployment may be interpreted as a broad index of the social environment or, since the unemployed are a high-risk group (Sainsbury et al. 1980), as increasing the numbers of individuals 'at risk' (Low et al. 1981). Furthermore, a reduction in unemployment would rely on political and economic initiatives and even then there is no easily practicable and reliably effective intervention.

Similarly, the link between suicide and alcohol is strong and in part direct. Countries that consume large amounts of alcohol *per capita*, such as those in Eastern Europe and Scandinavia, have high suicide rates, while those that consume small amounts, particularly Muslim countries, have low suicide rates. Within any population suicide is more common in those who misuse alcohol (Adelstein and White 1976); the long-term risk of suicide in alcohol dependence is high (Berglund 1984). Moreover, alcohol can play a direct part in the act of suicide (Ohberg et al. 1996). It may be possible to reduce population consumption by education though research evidence is lacking (Moskowitz 1989). The only measure known to be effective is an increase in price (Kendell et al. 1983a, b), again an intervention that would require considerable political will.

The best known prevention strategy for depression in the community in the UK is the Defeat Depression Campaign, an initiative jointly run by the Royal Colleges of Psychiatrists and of General Practitioners in alliance with other interested groups such as the Samaritans. The campaign was largely one of secondary prevention. It aimed to help the public identify depression in themselves and others and to seek help promptly; it targeted general practitioners, emphasizing the need for them to offer early and adequate treatment. There is some evidence that the campaign had a modest effect on public attitudes (Paykel et al. 1998) and on the reported practice of primary health care staff (Rix et al. 1999). However, changes were limited and for general practitioners further, particularly local, education was recommended.

In summary, there is no doubt that many of the most important influences on the suicide rate are social but the practical problems in using these as the basis of a prevention strategy are huge. It is also possible that the circumstances, behaviour and mood of people with mental illness might be least affected by an approach that sought to influence the population as a whole.

Reducing access to lethal means

In recent years the commonest methods of suicide in the UK have been self-poisoning with drugs and with car exhaust fumes, and hanging. In 1997 there were 1492 suicides due to self-poisoning with drugs, 684 suicides due to CO poisoning, the vast majority due to car exhaust fumes, and 1510 suicides by hanging. All these figures refer to the total of deaths recorded as suicides and those recorded as undetermined. Together these three methods accounted for 3686 deaths in 1997, nearly three-quarters (74%) of the total of 4980 suicides and undetermined deaths in England and Wales (ONS 1998). Reducing access to lethal means is a potentially important route to suicide prevention and represents a particular form of general population strategy. The same approach can also be applied to high-risk groups that tend to employ one method more than others.

The best-known example of the successful withdrawal of a common means of suicide occurred in the UK in the late 1960s and early 1970s, following a change in the domestic gas supply from the toxic coal gas to the relatively non-toxic natural gas. Previously, self-poisoning with domestic gas had been one of the main methods of suicide, being associated with about one-half of all suicides in 1958, the peak year of use. By the mid–1970s the figure was 1 or 2% of suicides per year. There are three points to note about the so-called coal gas story (Kreitman 1976). First, a reduction was seen not only in suicides by domestic gas but in the overall suicide rate; it has been estimated that about 6700 suicides were prevented over the 7 years between 1963 and 1970 (Wells 1981). Second, the effect was transient lasting only until the 1970s. Third, it was incidental to an economic change and not part of any prevention strategy.

Currently, discussion of reducing the population's access to the means of suicide is focussed on two methods of self-poisoning: car exhaust fumes and paracetamol. Asphyxiation by car exhaust fumes has recently been one of the commonest methods of suicide in the UK, while paracetamol accounts for about 150 deaths annually (Spooner and Harvey 1993), and a large and increasing proportion of non-fatal deliberate self-harm (Hawton and Fagg 1992). In the case of car exhaust fumes, three measures are possible. The first is to reduce the toxicity of exhaust gases. In the USA the rate of car exhaust suicides declined following the introduction of emission controls in the mid–1960s (Clarke and Lester 1987). Since legislation in 1993 (ECD 1992), new cars in the UK must be fitted with catalytic converters to detoxify emissions and it remains to be seen whether this will lead to a similar fall in suicide. Initial evidence (Kendell 1998) and case reports (Wagg and Aylwin 1993) are encouraging. The second measure is the alteration of the shape of exhausts themselves to make it more difficult to attach a hosepipe or other conduit. The third measure is the use of devices that shut off the engine when CO levels rise to dangerous levels in the interior of the car.

In the case of paracetamol, four measures have been suggested to reduce access or lethality. The first is to restrict the quantity of paracetamol preparations that can be obtained without medical prescription (Hawton et al. 1996). The problem of over-the-counter access to drugs that can be dangerous in overdose is not new (Kessel 1965), but the rise in paracetamol use in self-harm has emphasized the urgent need for preventive measures, and it appears that fatal overdose from paracetamol is uncommon in countries where the content of each pack is limited (Garnier and Bismuth 1993). The government has recently responded to this suggestion and from 1998, paracetamol has only been available in packs of 16 in shops or 32 tablets in pharmacist supervized chemists. The second measure is to introduce 'blister packs' for all paracetamol preparations – there is evidence that this would reduce the number of tablets taken in an overdose, thus reducing lethality (Hawton et al. 1996). The third measure is the inclusion in paracetamol preparations of a substance such as methionine, which would prevent liver toxicity, the main cause of mortality in overdose. The fourth measure is to develop non-hepatotoxic derivatives of paracetamol (Bray 1993).

Some such measures are likely to reduce suicides by one population group more than another. Reducing car exhaust toxicity, for example, is likely to prevent more suicides among men, particularly young men, because of their greater use of the method, although conversely it may be several years before the type of young men who are now at high risk – unskilled and unemployed – will be driving cars new enough to require catalytic converters. Similarly, there are specific methods that could be the basis of prevention in particular high-risk groups, e.g. firearms and farmers (Farmer and Rohde 1980, Lester 1990).

How could this approach be used to prevent suicide in people with severe mental illness? The most obvious way is in the prescription of psychotropic medication, a common means of suicide and self-poisoning in people in contact with health services (Forster and Frost 1985). There appears to be a link between the number of prescriptions for a certain class of drug and the number of suicides using that method. Data from the UK and Australia support this suggestion. In England between 1964 and 1974, the number of suicides attributed to barbiturates dropped by over one-third mirroring the decrease in the number of prescriptions for barbiturates by 50% (Wells 1981). In Australia the number of suicides by self-poisoning with drugs rose markedly during the 1960s at the same time as a marked increase of sedative drugs were made available to the community. The prescribing of such drugs was restricted by the government from 1967 after which there was a decrease in the number of suicides from drug self-poisoning (Oliver and Hetzel 1973). Although there are no studies to demonstrate effective prevention, it makes good sense for clinicians to prescribe short-term supplies of medication that might be taken in overdose. There has even been a suggestion that prescribing doctors should require the return of unused medication before adding to the patient's stock of potentially lethal agents by writing further prescriptions (Farmer and Pinder 1989). It would also appear to make good sense to prescribe relatively non-toxic compounds whenever there is a risk, and indeed one recent study suggests that some psychiatrists and general practitioners (GPs) do take account of a patient's risk of suicide and use the less toxic antidepressants for the patients prone to suicide (Isacsson et al. 1994). This is, therefore, an argument, for example, for the use of the SSRI rather than tricyclic antidepressants, a subject with economic, legal and perhaps ethical implications (Fradd 1992, Milne et al. 1993, Freemantle et al. 1994). It should be stressed, however, that the main problem concerning antidepressant use and suicide is that their under-use places depressed patients at risk (Isacsson et al 1994) (see Chapter 3).

People with severe mental illness are more likely than the general population to use 'active' or violent methods of suicide such as jumping from buildings or in front of trains, and hanging (Appleby 1992). These methods are more difficult to manipulate but district health services should be aware of suicide 'black spots' in their locality – these are often bridges (Cantor et al. 1989), cliffs (Surtees 1982) or particular stretches of railway lines, including some stations (O'Donnell and Farmer 1992) – and take appropriate steps such as to erect barriers, to use specific designs or even to consider placing an obvious telephone with a free helpline (Glatt 1987). This is also true of psychiatric inpatient wards whose design and location should reflect the high risk of this patient group (Sims and O'Brien 1979, Langley and Bayatti 1984, Salmons 1984, Goh et al. 1989, Lloyd 1995).

ENHANCEMENT OF PROTECTIVE FACTORS

The concept of protective factors in suicide research is one that has parallels in other mental health fields (Rutter 1993). Protective factors are distinct from risk factors and lower risk not by abolishing risk factors but by mitigating their effects. This is important in suicide prevention because most major risk factors, such as age, sex, marital status, employment status, history of mental illness and past self-harm are not open to change. Theoretically, at least, it may be more fruitful to attempt to prevent suicides through protective factors than through risk factors, though most previous research has concentrated on the latter.

To take a crude hypothetical example, losing one's job might be a risk factor for suicide and remaining employed might be a risk factor-based route to prevention.

The protective factor approach would suggest that prevention could be achieved through counterbalancing the effects of job loss; corresponding protective factors might include having a supportive family, winning the national lottery or having access to re-training. None of these is directly concerned with the loss of a job, and each accepts that job loss has occurred. These putative protective factors exert their effect through addressing the consequence of job loss or the mechanism by which it could lead to suicide. The protective factor approach is, therefore, a form of tertiary prevention. To be effective protective factors require risk factors to be present. For example, counselling on alcohol could be a protective factor only if alcohol misuse puts people at higher risk and if counselling is given to those who drink heavily, i.e. rather than to people who drink within normal limits. It is, therefore, implicit in the protective factor approach that suicide prevention strategy should be targeted at those at risk.

One apparently powerful protective factor was illustrated recently for suicide in childbearing women (Appleby 1991, 1996). The rate of mental illness in women following childbirth is high. Of newly delivered mothers, 0.2% experiences an episode of psychotic illness (Pugh et al. 1963, Paffenbarger 1964, Kendell et al. 1987), and most of these are major affective disorders (Meltzer and Kumar 1985, Kendell et al. 1987). A further 10–15% suffer a non-psychotic depressive illness (Pitt 1968, Kumar and Robson 1984, Cox et al. 1993). In the first 3 months following childbirth, women are four times more likely to be admitted to psychiatric hospital than in any preceding period (Kendell et al. 1987). A correspondingly high suicide rate would be predicted.

The rate of suicide in women in the first postnatal year was calculated for a 12 year period from national data on birth, population size and cause-specific mortality. Despite the high rate of mental illness at this time, the standardized mortality ratio (SMR) for suicide was 17, i.e. the rate was one-sixth of that in women in the general population (Appleby 1991). The equivalent SMR in pregnant women, who have a substantial rate of non-psychotic affective disorder (Kumar and Robson 1984, Watson et al. 1984) though not of psychosis (Kendell et al. 1987), was 5, i.e. a 20-fold lowering of the rate was found. These findings were confirmed in a more recent Finnish study (Gissler et al. 1996), and were consistent with previous reports (Barno 1967, Kleiner and Greston 1984, Weir 1984, Platz and Kendell 1988, Syverson et al. 1991). A further study of deliberate self-harm found a low odds ratio associated with childbirth in the previous year (Appleby and Turnbull 1995).

The implication of these findings was that postnatal and pregnant women were protected from mortality by suicide; possible explanations included the close supervision of maternity services, and a protective effect of parenthood. The latter explanation was supported by two studies of 'reasons for living' in the general population and in admitted psychiatric patients, which reported 'child concerns' as an important restraining influence on suicidal behaviour (Linehan et al. 1983). In fact this suggestion was not new: Emile Durkheim, the French social scientist who pioneered the sociological study of suicide attributed the low rate of suicide in married people largely to parenthood rather than marriage *per se* (Durkheim 1952).

If there is a protective effect of parenthood on suicide risk, its significance is likely to go beyond postnatal populations. The protective effect of parenthood may, for example, help to explain the relationship between the increasing divorce rate and the large recent rise in suicide among young men but not young women (Charlton et al. 1992, 1993), the latter being more likely to retain direct responsibility for any children. It may also indicate a mechanism by which people can be protected – in this case, self-worth arising from an awareness of being needed – on which a cognitive clinical intervention might be based, of the kind reported in one study to reduce self-harm in borderline personality disorder (Linehan et al. 1991).

In clinical practice the most important protective factors are likely to be aspects of clinical services as these can be changed in response to perceived risk. However, there is almost no research evidence of suicide prevention in clinical practice on which to base protective services. This is not to say that clinical services do not prevent suicide. It is more a reflection of the relatively low numbers of suicides in one location during the lifetime of a study, the ethical difficulties of randomizing individuals at risk to one treatment group or another, and the problems faced by retrospective studies in ascertaining details of care, particularly from case notes. Nevertheless, it remains a remarkable fact that we know so little about the ability of medical services in general and mental health services in particular to prevent what is arguably the most important complication of psychiatric disorder.

The evidence that does exist is by no means conclusive. There is, for instance, the fall in the suicide rate in the elderly in the UK during the past four decades, particularly in the mid-1950s and 1960s, a period when the number of consultant physicians specializing in geriatric medicine rose sharply. The relationship could be incidental but it raises the possibility that increasing emphasis of services on a particular population subgroup led to better identification of people at risk. Similarly, a fall in suicide in the elderly in Chichester two decades ago was attributed to the development of community mental health services (Walk 1967).

On the other hand, no difference in suicide rates was reported in a US study in which people with severe mental illness received one or other form of community service (Cohen et al. 1990), and another US study found no association between suicide in schizophrenia and the presence or absence of social case work in follow-up (Roy 1982). One UK study identified many hazards of community care but the numbers were too small to ascertain whether the adoption of a new-style psychiatric service had had any influence on the number of suicides in this population (Morgan 1992). An ecological study in the UK failed to find an association between district suicide rates and quantitative estimates of district mental health service provision including number of consultant psychiatrists, community psychiatric

nurses and mental illness beds per 100 000 population, once indices of social deprivation were taken into account (Lewis et al. 1994). One conclusion of this study
was that no simple relationship between mental health service activity and suicide
could be assumed; it could not be expected that suicide would be prevented by
simply increasing overall service provision. Specific interventions were needed,
targeted appropriately.

One example of such an intervention was reported from the Swedish island of
Gotland (Rutz et al. 1992). In 1983 and 1984, GPs on the island received brief
training in the diagnosis and treatment of depression. The following year, a fall in
the suicide rate was found on Gotland but not in the rest of Sweden. The Gotland
study has been widely quoted as demonstrating the crucial importance to suicide
prevention of identifying depression in primary care and the need for appropriate
training, but it can be criticized on a number of grounds. First, suicide prevention
was not a specified aim of the study – indeed suicide rates were examined, apparently as an afterthought, because of a fear that a *rise* could have resulted from the
treatment by GPs of cases of depression which should have been referred to
specialist services. Second, the fall in the suicide rate on Gotland occurred as a
result of only a small fall in the number of suicides. Such changes commonly occur
in areas of small population – the population of Gotland was 56 000 – while it has
been calculated that a population of 13 million people would be required if such a
study were planned with adequate statistical power (assuming a 15% fall in the
suicide rate following intervention). Third, it was possible on Gotland to train 16 of
18 GPs – delivery of training in a larger, urban setting would be more difficult and
the generalizability of the findings is doubtful. Fourth, the suicide rate on Gotland
had risen again within 3 years, which suggested either random fluctuation or a
disappointingly transient effect. Fifth, an intervention delivered through primary
care would be unlikely to have any impact on groups such as young men whose rate
of attendance in primary care before suicide is lower than that of other age/sex
subgroups; and, as young men are a group whose suicide rate has almost doubled in
two decades, they are a particularly important group to reach. Despite such reserva-
tions, however, the Gotland study is virtually the only one to find an association
between a specific health service activity and suicide prevention (Rutz et al. 1997).

TARGETING HIGH-RISK GROUPS

Recent studies of service contacts by people at high risk of suicide have suggested that
an educational intervention aiming to prevent suicide could be more focused on the
recognition, assessment and management of suicide risk itself rather than the broader
question of how to manage depression, and made available to a wider range of
'frontline' health service staff. One of these concerned general practice consultations
by people under 35 years of age who committed suicide in Greater Manchester
during a 2-year period (Appleby et al. 1996). One hundred and sixty-seven suicides
were identified in this age group, and general practice notes were available on 124 of

these. Sixty-one had attended a GP in the 3 months before death. The rate of attendance in the month before death was 27%, consistent with the low figure reported in a previous study (Vassilas and Morgan 1993), but the pattern of attendance in both sexes over 3 months was one of increasing consultation. Twenty-two (15%) attended in the week before death – a 15% reduction is *The Health of the Nation* target for the general population. At the final contact, most had attended for what were broadly defined as psychological reasons, but in no case was significant risk of suicide detected. A study of people attending accident and emergency departments in five hospitals in the North-West Region because of deliberate self-harm similarly found that risk assessment, as recorded in case records, fell below standards set by the Royal College of Psychiatrists in most cases (Amos et al. submitted).

People with mental illness constitute an important high-risk group who should be a key target for service-based suicide prevention strategies, not only because of the high risk associated with most diagnoses, particularly depression, schizophrenia and alcohol dependence (Pokorny 1966, Guze and Robins 1970, Adelstein and White 1976, Roy 1982, Drake et al. 1985, Martin et al. 1985, Allbeck and Wistedt 1986, Sainsbury 1986, Berglund and Nilsson 1987, Monk 1987, Harris and Barraclough 1997, Lonnqvist et al. 1995), but because many suicides occur in close proximity to medical, and particularly mental health service care (Temoche et al. 1964, Flood and Seager 1968, Barraclough et al. 1974, Kraft and Babigian 1976, King and Barraclough 1990, Goldacre et al. 1993). Data from research in the UK show that about 4% of all suicides are current psychiatric inpatients (Appleby et al. 1999), and a further 8% occur in the 3 months following discharge from psychiatric inpatient care; 33% of all suicides in previously admitted patients occur in the 3 months following discharge – a reduction of 33% is *The Health of the Nation* target for people with severe mental illness. About 23% of all suicides have been in contact with psychiatric services in the year before death (Appleby et al. 1999), while 73% have a lifetime history of contact with any services, including accident and emergency departments and general practice, because of psychiatric disorder.

Three established features of suicide in people with mental illness may be used to aid recognition of people at risk. First, patients appear to be at the greatest risk of suicide during the development of an acute illness, at the beginning and at the end of a period of treatment (Copas et al. 1971). There is some evidence that suicide risk is more easily determined in the acute phase of illness than in those who are chronically suicidal (Proul et al. 1997). Second, inpatients are most at risk when they are away from the hospital ward, either because they are on leave or have absconded (Farberow et al. 1971, Crammer 1984). Third, the relationship between hospital staff and patients may make suicide more likely. One study has shown that the most striking feature differentiating a suicide group from two control groups was the high incidence of disturbed relationships with hospital staff resulting in premature discharge, often against medical advice (Flood and Seager 1968). This process is sometimes referred to as malignant alienation and is characterized by a progressive deterioration in the patients' relationship with others, including loss of sympathy and support from members of staff, who tend to construe these patients' behaviour as provocative, unreasonable or over dependent (Morgan 1979, Morgan and Priest 1984, Watts and Morgan 1994). Critics of the concept of malignant alienation suggest that it may lead to the unreasonable blaming of mental health professionals (Davies 1994).

Data from a UK case control study of suicide in previously admitted patients suggests that the training of mental health service staff in the assessment and management of suicide risk could be an important suicide prevention strategy (Dennehy et al. 1996). Suicides were more likely than mentally ill controls to have expressed suicidal ideas in aftercare, according to case-records – this was the only clinical variable significantly associated with suicide. However, suicidal ideas were not recorded in almost half of the suicide group, and in half of those cases in which suicidal ideas were recorded, no change in clinical management occurred. Less than one-third of the suicides were subject to multidisciplinary review under the Care Programme Approach, the centrepiece of mental health service provision in the UK intended to aid identification and monitoring of individuals at risk. These results suggested that services were insufficiently able to recognize, assess and respond to risk, and would benefit from training in these areas.

Why should specialist services find it difficult in clinical practice to identify patients who are likely to kill themselves, particularly as many risk factors for suicide are known? There are at least three answers. First, the risk factors used by clinicians to indicate those patients at highest risk may not be applicable to people with severe mental illness. In the case control study described above, which matched for age, sex and diagnosis, conventional risk factors derived mainly from studies of the general population or all-inclusive patient groups did not distinguish those who had committed suicide. Factors such as being single, unemployment, living alone and substance misuse were common in both groups and seemed to be features of people with severe mental illness in general rather than of those who would kill themselves.

The second reason concerns the over-simplicity of models of risk that are based entirely on risk factors, rather than on a balance of risk factors and protective factors. For example, a person with few risk factors may be at high risk if no protective actions are taken while someone with many risk factors may be at low risk if each is addressed by a comprehensive care plan. Similarly, the clustering of suicides in the immediate post-discharge period is not easily explained by risk factors alone – this should be a period of clinical recovery when risk factors associated with acute illness are reduced. However, it is also a period when services are withdrawn, perhaps abruptly on discharge, and their protective potential, therefore, diminished. If protective services are withdrawn more quickly than risk factors are reduced, the balance of risk and protection is towards greater risk despite clinical recovery. Possible protective factors in mental health service provision include early and intensive follow-up following discharge from inpatient care, direct attempts to encourage compliance with treatment in those who are non-compliant, assertive outreach following non-attendance, referral to specialist services of patients who are misusing alcohol or drugs, and increased supervision through hospital admission, greater frequency of contact or increased medication following accurate assessment of patients at high risk.

Third, suicide is usually viewed as an event when it may be better understood as the end-point of a sequence of events, each indicating increasing risk and, often, offering opportunities for prevention. A typical sequence would be hospital discharge, non-compliance with medication, recurrence of low mood, increasing alcohol consumption, expression of suicidal ideas, and a final event such as the break-up of a relationship. Protective interventions such as those listed above might then be appropriate strategies for prevention.

Such models of cumulative risk composed of illness-related risk factors and service-based protective factors offer the possibility of a detailed understanding of suicide by people with mental illness and of routes to prevention through the targeted activities of mental health and related services. However, it should be stressed that they are at present hypothetical and that data on a large numbers of suicides must be studied before there is a satisfactory evidence base. One source of such data in the UK will be the National Confidential Inquiry into Suicide and Homicide by People with Mental Illness (Appleby et al. 1999).

The Confidential Inquiry into Homicides and Suicides by Mentally Ill People was first established in 1992 by the Department of Health following consultation with the Royal College of Psychiatrists. Its main objective was to enquire into, and record the details of, homicides and suicides committed by people under the care of, or recently discharged by, mental health services in order to recommend measures by which services might reduce the number of such incidents. Its first full report in 1995 made a number of recommendations including: that the risk assessment skills of clinical staff should be strengthened; that there should be an increase in face-to-face contact with patients; that communication between professionals and families should be improved; and that professionals should receive training in the use of legal powers under mental health legislation (Steering Committee 1996).

In 1996, the Inquiry was relocated to the University of Manchester with the same overall aim to reduce avoidable deaths resulting from mental illness. However, specific objectives were identified as: to provide a comprehensive national audit/database of suicides by people with a history of contact with mental health services; to focus on suicides by groups on whom service recommendations are most required because of high risk or problems gaining access to current services, namely current inpatients, patients discharged from inpatient care less than 3 months earlier, patients subject to multidisciplinary review under the care programme approach, patients who have recently failed to attend or been non-compliant with drug treatment, and patients from ethnic minorities; to examine details of the final contact with services before suicide and homicide, particularly the process of risk assessment; to study the antecedents of suicide and homicide; and to develop 'models' of cumulative risk, which would highlight opportunities for prevention.

The Inquiry makes use of the official process of death notification and reporting and receives data on all suicides and probable suicides (open verdicts, deaths from undetermined cause). By checking information on each case against records held by local mental health services and some specialist supra-district services, the Inquiry identifies those with a history of service contact in the year before death (this remains the main inclusion criterion) and the consultant psychiatrist whose team was involved. The latter is asked to hold a multidisciplinary review of the case and to complete a standard questionnaire.

The Inquiry collects information on: priority groups (listed above); demographic information; psychiatric history; details of suicide; inpatient suicides; suicides by outpatients; details of last contact; antecedents of suicide; and the respondent's view on prevention. The questionnaire has been constructed to identify important groups of patients, which appear in only small numbers in most studies, so that they can be studied separately and/or compared with the total sample. Examples include prisoners, diagnostic subgroups, people with a secondary diagnosis of substance misuse or personality disorder, people aged over 65, and people referred to services urgently under Section 136 of the Mental Health Act. The size of the suicide inquiry sample is about 1000 cases per year.

NATIONAL SUICIDE PREVENTION STRATEGIES

In the UK, government policy documents such as *The Health of the Nation* and *Our Healthier Nation* have emphasized the importance of suicide prevention as a public health priority and the National Confidential Inquiry into Suicide and Homicide by People with Mental Illness is one of the strategies aimed at preventing suicide. Other countries have also taken steps to address concerns about suicide. Several countries, e.g. Australia, Finland, Holland, Sweden and USA (Taylor et al. 1997) have established task forces to devise comprehensive national programs for the prevention of suicide. The recommendations of these task forces in general are similar to those made by the World Health Organization (1982) and can be divided into four main categories (Diekstra 1989):

- Implementation of national research programs.

- Improvement of services.

- Provision of information and training on suicide prevention to relevant professional groups, organizations and the general public.

- Formulation of strategies and techniques to deal with special risk groups.

Specific recommendations on research are the development of national and local data collection projects as well as studies to examine risk factors for suicide, particularly the interaction between different risk factors. Improvements to services include training for all health professionals and establishing policies on relevant aspects of both primary and secondary care, for example interagency communication. Training on suicide prevention is also considered essential for other groups, for example teachers and police officers. There are recommendations about the dissemination of information to the general public, particularly on the symptoms of depression and other warnings of suicide, and also on the role of the media. High-risk groups, such as young men, substance misusers, prisoners as well as people with mental illness, are recognized as requiring particular strategies such as provision of special services and active outreach programs.

These recommendations refer to many agencies, with which individuals with mental illness may come into contact, but it is particularly health services that have a major role in preventing suicide in those with severe mental illness.

SUICIDE PREVENTION BY HEALTH SERVICES

Given the scarcity of satisfactory research data at present, what actions can be taken that would be likely to prevent suicide? It is essential to ensure that there is adequate dissemination of what current research evidence is available to all those who might be in a position to prevent suicide, whether they are involved in health service policy and planning or as individual health professionals. The publication of two documents, in the UK in the mid-1990s, aimed to provide such background information and expert guidance. In The Department of Health's *The Prevention of Suicide* (DoH 1994), the management of suicidal patients is discussed from various perspectives, including primary and secondary care, local authorities as well as voluntary bodies such as the Samaritans. Implications of policy for health services are considered, for example, the need for all relevant health professionals to have training and the importance of creating alliances with other agencies such as social services and educational organizations. *Suicide Prevention: The Challenge Confronted* was the first Thematic Review published by the NHS Health Advisory Service (NHSHAS 1994), indicating the importance attached to suicide prevention at a national level by the NHS. The review describes the salient aspects of what is known about suicide risk and its assessment and management, with an emphasis on practical clinical advice. Tables, or check-lists, of key information cover a range of topics from direct advice to health professionals on interview techniques and other key points of risk assessment to important issues for local services, including measures to evaluate and monitor the quality of services.

An example of how regional services can play a role in suicide prevention is the strategy report published by the UK North-West Regional Health Authority in 1996. The report consists of a series of recommendations that could be implemented by health services including health authorities, accident and emergency departments, mental health services and general practitioners. The recommendations were drawn up by a multidisciplinary working party and based on published research evidence and a consensus within the working party on what constituted good clinical practice. They covered five areas: monitoring of suicide, clinical prevention in high-risk groups, training, research and the aftermath of suicide. Each recommendation was designed so that implementation could be easily evaluated. The recommendations are summarized in Table 16.1.

---

1. Suicide monitoring
- Continuous local audit of suicides to identify local patterns
- Regular reviews of 'critical incidents'
- Submission of suitable cases and data to the National Confidential Inquiry into Suicide and Homicide by People with Mental Illness

2. Clinical practice
- Prescribing practice – short-term prescriptions of antidepressant drugs for patients at risk of suicide

- People who carry out deliberate self-harm
    - A trust-wide deliberate self-harm (DSH) planning group to supervisor, monitor and improve quality of care
    - Assessment forms for A&E junior staff and mental health professionals
    - Referral to a specialist alcohol and/or drug service in appropriate cases
    - General practitioners should be notified within one working day of discharge from A&E

- Adolescents and young people
    - Full assessment and treatment service available for young people at risk
    - Adequate facilities to admit suicidal adolescents with severe psychiatric disorders
    - Leaflet on services available to young people in crisis
    - Health education in secondary schools to include identification of depression

- People with mental illness
    - Local operation of the Care Programme Approach to include annual audit
    - Care plans to emphasize first 3 months following discharge
    - Policies on responding to non-attendance and supervision of people at risk

- Elderly people
    - Depressed elderly people who are at risk should be assessed and treated by a locally based old age psychiatry team
    - Elderly patients in primary care with depression and suicidal ideas to be managed in consultation with an old age psychiatry team.

3. Training
- Training in recognition and treatment of depression should be available to all 'front-line' health staff
- Assessment of suicide risk should be specifically included in this training

4. Research – suicide should be a priority for NHS research funding

5. Aftermath of suicide
- Relatives bereaved by suicide to be offered emotional support
- Staff whose patients/clients commit suicide should receive emotional support

---

Table 16.1 – Recommendations to health services on suicide prevention.

CONCLUSION

In summary, social factors are key determinants of suicide rates but have not led to successful initiatives designed to reduce suicide or specifically applicable to people with mental illness who are at risk. On the other hand, clinical practice has not so far been shown to reduce suicide. We have argued for a different understanding of suicide risk in people with mental illness, based on a balance of risk factors and protective factors. Key protective factors will include adequate risk recognition, assessment and management, and widespread training in these skills is likely to be needed.

References

Adelstein A, White G. Alcoholism and mortality. Population Trends 1976; 6: 7–13.

Allebeck P, Wistedt, B. Mortality in schizophrenia. A ten-year follow-up based on the Stockholm County in-patient register. Archives of General Psychiatry 1986; 43: 650–653.

Amos T, Guthrie E, Appleby L, Morton R, Creed F, Ellis R, Tomenson B. Assessment and management of patients following deliberate self-harm: a comparison of five North-West hospitals (submitted).

Appleby L. Suicidal behaviour in childbearing women. International Review of Psychiatry 1996; 8: 107–115.

Appleby L. Suicide during pregnancy and in the first postnatal year. British Medical Journal 1991; 302: 137–140.

Appleby L. Suicide in psychiatric patients: risk and prevention. British Journal of Psychiatry 1992; 161: 749–758.

Appleby L, Amos T, Doyle U, Tomenson B, Woodman M. General practitioners and young suicides. A preventive role for primary care. British Journal of Psychiatry; 1996: 168: 330–333.

Appleby L, Shaw J, Amos T. et al. Safer Services: Report of the National Confidential Inquiry into Suicide and Homicide by People with Mental Illness. London: Department of Health, 1999.

Appleby L, Turnbull G. Parasuicide in the first postnatal year. Psychological Medicine 1995; 25: 1087–1090.

Barno A. Criminal abortion deaths, illegitimate pregnancy deaths, and suicides in pregnancy. Minnesota, 1950–1965. American Journal of Obstetrics and Gynaecology 1967; 98: 356–367.

Barraclough B, Bunch J, Nelson B, Sainsbury P. A hundred cases of suicide: clinical aspects. British Journal of Psychiatry 1974; 125: 355–373.

Berglund M. Suicide in alcoholism. A prospective study of 88 suicides. Archives of General Psychiatry 1984: 41: 888–891.

Berglund M, Nilsson K. Mortality in severe depression. A prospective study including 103 suicides. Acta Psychiatrica Scandinavica 1987; 76: 372–380.

Bray GP. Liver failure induced by paracetamol. Avoidable deaths still occur. British Medical Journal 1993; 306: 157–158.

Cantor CH, Hill MA, McLachlan EK. Suicide and related behaviour from river bridges: a clinical perspective. British Journal of Psychiatry 1989; 155: 829–835.

Charlton J, Kelly S, Dunnell K, Evans B, Jenkins R, Wallis R. Trends in suicide deaths in England and Wales. Population Trends 1992; 69: 10–16.

Charlton J, Kelly S, Dunnell K, Evans B, Jenkins R. Suicide deaths in England and Wales: trends in factors associated with suicide deaths. Population Trends 1993; 71: 34–42.

Clarke RV, Lester D. Toxicity of care exhausts and opportunity for suicide: comparison between Britain and United States. Journal of Epidemiology and Community Health 1987; 41: 114–120.

Cohen LJ, Test MA, Brown RL. Suicide and schizophrenia: data from a prospective community treatment study. American Journal of Psychiatry 1990; 147: 602–607.

Copas JB, Freeman-Browne DL, Robin AA. Danger periods for suicide in patients under treatment. Psychological Medicine 1971; 1: 400–404.

Cox JL, Murray D, Chapman G. A controlled study of the onset, duration and prevalence of postnatal depression. British Journal of Psychiatry 1993; 163: 27–31.

Crammer JL. The special characteristics of suicide in hospital in-patients. British Journal of Psychiatry 1984; 145: 460–463.

Davies DR. Malignant alienation. British Journal of Psychiatry 1994; 164: 697–698.

Dennehy JA, Appleby L, Thomas CS, Faragher BE. Case control study of suicide by discharged psychiatric patients. British Medical Journal 1996; 312: 1580.

Department of Health. The Health of the Nation. London: HMSO, 1992.

Department of Health. Saving Lives: Our Healthier Nation. London: HMSO, 1999.

Department of Health. The Prevention of Suicide. London: HMSO, 1994.

Diekstra R. Suicide and the attempted suicide: an international perspective. Acta Psychiatrica Scandinavica 1989; 80 (suppl. 354): 1–18.

Diekstra R. Towards a comprehensive strategy for prevention of suicidal behaviour. Acta Psychiatrica Scandinavica 1989; 80 (suppl. 354): 19–24.

Drake RE, Gates C, Whitaker A, Cotton PG. Suicide among schizophrenics: a review. Comprehensive Psychiatry 1985; 26: 90–100.

Durkheim, E. Suicide. A Study in Sociology, trans. Spalding JA, Simpson G. London: Routledge, 1952.

European Community Directive 91/441 L242, August 30, 1991. Statutory Instrument 1992, 2909.

Farberow NL, Ganzler S, Cutter F, Reynolds D. An eight year survey of hospital suicides. Life-Threatening Behaviour 1971; 1: 184–202.

Farmer RDT, Pinder RM. Why do fatal overdose rates vary between antidepressants? Acta Psychiatrica Scandinavica 1989; 80 (suppl. 354): 25–35.

Farmer RDT, Rohde J. Effect of availability and acceptability of lethal instruments on suicide mortality. Acta Psychiatrica Scandinavica 1980; 62: 436–446.

Flood RA, Seager CP. A retrospective examination of psychiatric case records of patients who subsequently committed suicide. British Journal of Psychiatry 1968; 144: 443–450.

Forster DP, Frost CEB. Medicinal self-poisoning and prescription frequency. Acta Psychatrica Scandinavica 1985; 71: 567–74.

Fradd SO. Selective serotonin reuptake inhibitors. British Medical Journal 1992; 305: 366.

Freemantle N, House A, Song F, Mason JM, Sheldon TA. Prescribing selective serotonin reuptake inhibitors as strategy for prevention of suicide. British Medical Journal 1994; 309: 249–253.

Garnier R, Bismuth C. Liver failure induced by paracetamol. British Medical Journal 1993; 306: 718.

Gissler M, Hemminki E, Lonnqvist J. Suicides after pregnancy in Finland, 1987–94: register linkage study. British Medical Journal 1996; 313: 1431–1434.

Glatt KM. Helpline: suicide prevention at a suicide site. Suicide and life-threatening behaviour 1987; 17: 299–309.

Goh SE, Salmons PH, Whittington RM. Hospital suicides: are there preventable factors? Profile of the psychiatric hospital suicide. British Journal of Psychiatry 1989; 154: 247–249.

Goldacre M, Seagroatt V, Hawton K. Suicide after discharge from psychiatric inpatient care. Lancet 1993; 342: 283–286.

Gunnel D, Frankel S. Prevention of suicide: aspirations and evidence. British Medical Journal 1994; 308: 1227–1233.

Guze SB, Robins E. Suicide and primary affective disorder. British Journal of Psychiatry 1970; 117: 437–438.

Harris EC, Barraclough B. Suicide as an outcome for mental disorders. British Journal of Psychiatry 1997; 170: 205–228.

Hawton K. Deliberate self-harm. Medicine International 1996; 24: 77–80.

Hawton K, Fagg J. Trends in deliberate self-poisoning and self-injury in Oxford 1976–90. British Medical Journal 1992; 304: 1409–1411.

Hawton K, Ware C, Mistry H, Hewitt J, Kingsbury S, Roberts D, Weitzel H. Paracetamol Self-poisoning – characteristics, prevention and harm reduction. British Journal of Psychiatry 1996; 168: 43–48.

Heikkinen ME, Isometsa ET, Marttunen MJ, Aro HM, Lonnqvist JK. Social factors in suicide. British Journal of Psychiatry 1995; 167: 747–753.

Isacsson G, Holmgren P, Wasserman D, Bergman U. Use of antidepressants among people committing suicide in Sweden. British Medical Journal 1994; 308: 506–509.

Isacsson G, Redfors I, Wasserman D, Bergman U. Choice of antidepressants: questionnaire survey of psychiatrists and general practitioners in two areas of Sweden. British Medical Journal 1994; 309: 1546–1549.

Kendell RE. Catalytic converters and prevention of suicide. Lancet 1998; 352: 1525.

Kendell RE, Chalmers JC, Platz C. Epidemiology of puerperal psychoses. British Journal of Psychiatry 1987; 150: 662–673.

Kendell RE, de Roumanie M, Ritson EB. Influence of an increase in excise duty on alcohol consumption and its adverse effects. British Medical Journal 1983a; 287: 809–811.

Kendell RE, de Roumanie M, Ritson, EB. Effect of economic changes on Scottish drinking habits 1978–82. British Journal of Addiction 1983b; 78: 365–379.

Kessel N. Self-poisoning – Part II. British Medical Journal 1965; 2: 1336–1340.

King E, Barraclough B. Violent death and mental illness. A study of a single catchment area over eight years. British Journal of Psychiatry 1990; 156: 714–720.

Kleiner GJ, Greston WM. Suicide in Pregnancy. Bristol: Wright, 1984.

Kraft DP, Babigian HM. Suicide by persons with and without psychiatric contacts. Archives of General Psychiatry 1976; 33: 209–215.

Kreitman N. The coal gas story. British Journal of Preventive Social Medicine 1976; 30: 86–93.

Kumar R, Robson KM. A prospective study of emotional disorders in childbearing women. British Journal of Psychiatry 1984; 144: 35–47.

Langley GE, Bayatti NN. Suicide in Exe Vale Hospital 1972–1981. British Journal of Psychiatry 1984; 145: 463–467.

Lester D. The availability of firearms and the use of firearms for suicide: a study of 20 countries. Acta Psychiatrica Scandinavica 1990; 81: 146–147.

Lewis G, Appleby L, Jarman B. Suicide and psychiatric services. Lancet 1994; 344: 822.

Linehan MM, Armstrong HE, Suarez A, Allmon D, Heard HL. Cognitive behavioural treatment of chronically parasuicidal borderline patients. Archives of General Psychiatry 1991; 48: 1060–1064.

Linehan MM, Goodstein JL, Nielson SL, Chiles JA. Reasons for staying alive when you are thinking of killing yourself: the Reason For Living inventory. Journal of Consulting and Clinical Psychology 1983; 51: 276–286.

Lloyd GG. Suicide in hospital: guidelines for prevention. Journal of the Royal Society of Medicine 1995; 88: 344–346.

Lonnqvist JK, Henriksson MM, Isometsa ET, Marttunen MJ, Heikkinen ME, Hillevi MA, Kuoppasalmi IK. Mental disorders and suicide prevention. Psychiatry and Clinical Neurosciences 1995; 49 (suppl. 1): S111–116.

Low AA, Farmer RDT, Jones DR, Rohde JR. Suicide in England and Wales: an analysis of 100 years, 1876–1975. Psychological Medicine 1981; 11: 359–368.

Martin RL, Cloninger R, Guze SB, Clayton PJ. Mortality in a follow-up of a 500 psychiatric outpatients. II. Cause-specific mortality. Archives of General Psychiatry 1985; 42: 58–66.

Meltzer ES, Kumar R. Puerperal mental illness, clinical features and classification: a study of 142 mother-and-baby admissions. British Journal of Psychiatry 1985; 147: 647–654.

Milne S, Alcorn A, Bell AJ. Selective serotonin reuptake inhibitors. British Medical Journal 1993; 306: 1126.

Monk M. Epidemiology of suicide. Epidemiologic Reviews 1987; 9: 51–69.

Morgan HG. Death Wishes: The Understanding and Management of Deliberate Self-Harm. Chichester: Wiley, 1979.

Morgan HG. How feasible is suicide prevention? Current Opinion in Psychiatry 1994; 7: 111–118.

Morgan HG. Suicide prevention and 'The Health of the Nation'. Psychiatric Bulletin 1993; 17: 135–136.

Morgan HG. Suicide prevention. Hazards on the fast lane to community care. British Journal of Psychiatry 1992; 160: 149–153.

Morgan HG, Priest P. Assessment of suicide risk in psychiatric in-patients. British Journal of Psychiatry 1984; 145: 467–469.

Moskowitz JM. The primary prevention of alcohol problems: a critical review of the research literature. Journal of Studies on Alcohol 1989; 50: 54–88.

NHS Health Advisory Service. Suicide Prevention: The Challenge Confronted. London: HMSO, 1994.

O'Donnell I, Farmer RDT. Suicidal acts on metro systems: an international perspective. Acta Psychiatrica Scandinavica 1992; 86: 60–63.

Office for National Statistics. Mortality Statistics: Cause, 1997. Series DH2 no. 24. London: HMSO, 1998.

Office for National Statistics. Mortality Statistics: Serial Tables 1841–1990. Series DH1 no. 25. London: HMSO, 1992.

Ohberg A, Vuori E, Ojanpera I, Lonnqvist J. Alcohol and drugs in suicides. British Journal of Psychiatry 1996; 169: 75–80.

Oliver RG, Hetzel BS. An analysis of recent trends in suicide rates in Australia. International Journal of Epidemiology 1973; 2: 91–101.

Paffenbarger RS. Epidemiological aspects of parapartum mental illness. British Journal of Preventive and Social Medicine 1964; 18: 189–195.

Paykel ES, Hart D, Priest RG. Changes in public attitudes to depression during the Defeat Depression Campaign. British Journal of Psychiatry 1998; 173: 519–522.

Pitt B. 'Atypical' depression following childbirth. British Journal of Psychiatry 1968; 114: 1325–1335.

Platt S. Suicide trends in 24 European Countries 1972–1984. In Moller MJ, Schnidike A, Welz R (eds), Current Issues in Suicidology. London: Springer, 1988, pp. 3–13.

Platz C, Kendell RE. A matched control study and family study of puerperal psychosis. British Journal of Psychiatry 1988; 153: 90–94.

Pokorny AD. A follow-up study of 618 suicidal patients. American Journal of Psychiatry 1966; 122: 1109–1116.

Pritchard C. New patterns of suicide by age and gender in the United Kingdom and the Western World 1974–1992; an indicator of social change? Social Psychiatry and Psychiatric Epidemiology 1996; 31: 227–234.

Proulx F, Lesage AD, Grunberg F. One hundred in-patient suicides. British Journal of Psychiatry 1997; 171: 247–250.

Pugh TF, Jerath BK, Schmidt WM, Reed RB. Rates of mental disease relating to child-bearing. New England Journal of Medicine 1963; 268: 1224–1228.

Rix S, Paykel ES, Lelliot P, Tylee A, Freeling P, Gask L, Hart D. Impact of a national campaign on GP education: an evaluation of the Defeat Depression Campaign. British Journal of General Practice 1999; 49: 99–102.

Roy A. Risk factors for suicide in psychiatric patients. Archives of General Psychiatry 1982; 39: 1089–1095.

Roy A. Suicide in chronic schizophrenia. British Journal of Psychiatry 1982; 141: 171–177.

Rutter M. Resilience: some conceptual considerations. Journal of Adolescent Health 1993; 14: 626–631.

Rutz W, von Knorring L, Walinder J. Long term effects of an educational program for general practitioners given by the Swedish Committee for the Prevention and Treatment of Depression. Acta Psychiatrica Scandinavica 1992; 85: 83–88.

Rutz W, Walinder J, von Knorring L, Rihmer Z, Pihlgren H. Prevention of depression and suicide by education and medication: impact on male suicidality. An update from the Gotland Study. International Journal of Psychiatry in Clinical Practice 1997; 1: 39–46.

Sainsbury P, Jenkins J, Levey A. The social correlates of suicide in Europe. In Farmer RDT, Hirsch SR (eds), The Suicide Syndrome. London: Croom-Helm, 1980, pp. 38–53.

Sainsbury P. Depression, suicide and suicide prevention. In Roy A (ed.), Suicide. Baltimore: Williams & Wilkins, 1986, pp. 73–88.

Sainsbury P. Suicide in London. Maudsley Monograph no. 1. London: Chapman & Hall, 1955.

Salmons PH. Suicide in high buildings. British Journal of Psychiatry 1984; 145: 469–472.

Sims A, O'Brien K. Autokabalesis: an account of mentally people who jump from buildings. Medicine, Science and the Law 1979; 19: 195–198.

Spooner JB, Harvey JG. Paracetamol overdosage – facts not misconceptions. Pharmaceutical Journal 1993; May: 706–707.

Steering Committee of the Confidential Inquiry into Homicides and Suicides by Mentally Ill People. Report of the Confidential Inquiry into Homicides and Suicides by Mentally Ill People. London: Royal College of Psychiatrists on behalf of the Steering Committee, 1996.

Surtees SJ. Suicide and accidental death at Beachy Head. British Medical Journal 1982; 284: 321–324.

Syverson CJ, Chavkin W, Atrash HK, Rochat RW, Sharp ES, King GE. Pregnancy-related mortality in New York City, 1980 to 1984. Causes of death and associated risk factors. American Journal of Obstetrics and Gynaecology 1991; 164: 603–608.

Temoche A, Pugh TF, McMahon B. Suicide rates among current and former mental institution patients. Journal of Nervous and Mental Disease 1964; 138: 124–131.

The North West Regional Health Authority Working Party on Suicide Prevention. A Health Service Suicide Prevention Strategy in the North West Region. Manchester: North West Regional Health Authority, 1996.

Vassilas CA, Morgan HG. General practitioners' contact with victims of suicide. British Medical Journal 1993; 307: 300–301.

Wagg AS, Aylwin SJB. Catalytic converter and suicide risk. Lancet 1993; 342: 1295.

Walk D. Suicide and community care. British Journal of Psychiatry 1967; 113: 1381–1391.

Watson JP, Elliott SA, Rugg AJ, Brough DI. Psychiatric disorder in pregnancy and the first postnatal year. British Journal of Psychiatry 1984; 144: 453–462.

Watts D, Morgan HG. Malignant Alienation: dangers for patients who are hard to like. British Journal of Psychiatry 1994; 164: 11–15.

Weir JG. Suicide during pregnancy in London: 1943–1962. In Kleiner GJ, Greston WM (eds), Suicide in Pregnancy. Bristol: Wright, 1984.

Wells N. Suicide and deliberate self-harm. London: Office of Health Economics, 1981.

World Health Organization. Changing Patterns in Suicide Behavior. Copenhagen: WHO, 1982.

World Health Organization. Health for all Targets. Summary of the Updated Edition. Copenhagen: WHO, 1992.

17

MENTALLY ILL PARENTS

Alain Gregoire

The impact of mental illness in the parents of dependent children goes beyond the suffering of the individual and the distress caused to those around. Parents caring for dependent children are undertaking the most important function in their lives, with far-reaching significance for them, their children and, collectively, for the species. Evidence is emerging of direct adverse effects of parental mental illness on children as well as a range of indirect effects. This is a time when partners have a greater need to function cooperatively but the demands on them at this time may make this all the more difficult. Mental illness can impair a parent's ability to function effectively and lead to relationship problems with profound effects on the other partner and on the children. This chapter will consider the impact of being a parent on the risk and nature of mental illness and the various effects of mental illness on parents, as well as the factors which affect these. Interventions to mitigate these effects will be explored.

MENTALLY ILL PARENTS: A CHALLENGE FOR SERVICES

The number of people who are parents of dependent children and suffer from mental illness is not known. Available data allow one to estimate proportions of mental health service users who are parents and the risk of mental illness among people who become parents.

Patients as parents

It seems likely from recent evidence that reproduction among people with severe mental illness differs little from the general population (Nimgaonkar et al. 1997, Lane et al. 1992) and people with bipolar disorders may have increased fertility. Older studies of schizophrenic populations found reduced reproductive rates, with evidence of a gradual increase from the 1930s to the 1950s (Ødegård 1960) and rates may now be increasing to match general population norms (Saugstad, 1989). It is not clear whether this is a change that reflects the move from institution to community-based care.

Sexuality and reproduction are important areas of functioning that receive little attention from services despite the increasing emphasis on normalization of functioning by clients and professionals. Women with schizophrenia have more sexual partners and more unwanted pregnancies than controls (Miller and Finnerty 1996). Clients want, but do not receive, attention to their sexuality (Pinderhughes et al. 1972) and contraceptive care for the mentally ill is largely neglected (Coverdale and Turbott 1997). This needs to be addressed, particularly as the advent of newer antipsychotic drugs, which do not cause hyperprolactinaemia and improve functioning, is leading to a spate of unplanned pregnancies (Pearson and Gregoire in press).

Varying figures have been presented for the proportion of mental health service users with dependent children. A case register study in Nottingham, UK, found that 25% of psychiatric referrals had children under 5 years of age (Oates 1988) and a study of children of adults with mental illnesses in south London had similar findings (Iddamalogoda and Naish 1993). A study of a case-managed population in the USA found that 9% had dependent children under 18 years of age (White 1995).

Does being a parent increase the risk of mental illness?

Brown and Harris (1978) demonstrated that having the care of three or more young children increased the risk of depression in women. Depression in women frequently dates back to a post-natal onset although this is often missed (Wisner et al. 1995). Several epidemiological studies of psychiatric disorder in the post-natal period have been conducted. These have demonstrated a 21-fold increase in the risk of psychosis post-natally (Kendell et al. 1987) and a 3-fold increase in the risk of developing depression (Cox et al. 1993) in the first 5 weeks post-partum, although the overall prevalence of non-psychotic depression appears not to be elevated in the 6 months post-partum. Women admitted to hospital with puerperal mental illnesses are more disturbed and have greater care needs than non-puerperal controls (Oates 1988). Those with post-natal psychotic disorders show more cognitive disorganization and homicidal thoughts than controls (Wisner et al. 1994). For women with a history of psychotic illness, pregnancy is also a time of risk for poor mental health, much of which goes unrecognized (McNeil et al. 1984a, b)

The risk of post-natal depression in fathers is not as high as in mothers, but the partners of women with post-natal mental illnesses have substantially increased rates of morbidity: 30% of partners of women with post-natal depression are depressed (Sharp et al. 1993) and 50% of partners of women admitted to a mother-

and-baby unit reach a level for definition of a psychiatric disorder (Lovestone and Kumar 1993). Fathers with a history of bipolar disorder have a 50% risk of relapse in the first post-partum year (Davenport and Adland 1982).

Are some parents more likely to have mental illness?

Little specific research exists identifying the risk factors for mental illness in parents. However, it is not unreasonable to generalize from studies of risk factors for mental illness generally as well as from the literature on puerperal disorders. Factors such as life events, social adversity, relationship conflicts and poor social support would seem as likely to apply to parents as to non-parents. Some caution must be applied to such generalization as several studies have indicated that in the case of puerperal relapse of psychotic illness, there was no association with social factors such as stresses or life events (McNeil 1988, Dowlatshahi and Paykel 1990, Marks et al. 1992). Kendell (1985) has described the factors associated with increased risk of puerperal psychosis. These include first pregnancy, previous psychosis, family psychiatric history and caesarean section. Correlates of non-psychotic post-natal depression include past psychiatric history, antenatal depression and anxiety, life events, social adversity and poor marital and social support (O'Hara 1997).

Also intriguing are findings of child characteristics that appear to be associated with parental mental illness. These include prematurity and neonatal illness (Stewart and Gangbar 1984) temperamental difficulties (Wolkind and DeSalis 1982, Field 1992, Murray et al. 1996), developmental delays (Sharp et al. 1995), behavioural problems (Zahn-Waxler et al. 1990) and emotional problems (Richman 1982). It is, therefore, not surprising that parents of children presenting at child mental health services have high rates of mental illness (Dover et al. 1994).

EFFECTS OF PARENTAL MENTAL ILLNESS

Most of the research on the effects of parental mental illness has focussed on mothers rather than fathers (Downey and Coyne 1990). This is probably because mothers remain the primary care givers in most societies, including countries like Sweden which has attempted, but largely failed, to engage fathers more in childcare through social and legislative changes. Fathers are also more elusive and difficult to engage in research, which creates practical obstacles to data collection and makes it more likely that samples who participate may be unrepresentative of the population. The literature reviewed below, therefore, refers to maternal mental illness unless otherwise stated.

Effects on the individual

Oates (1988) has shown that women admitted with severe mental illness post-natally have more severe symptoms and disability than a comparable non-postnatal group. This may be a feature of mental illness post-natally or of thresholds for admission at this time. There is nothing to suggest differences in the nature or expression of illnesses in parents at other times, and it can, therefore, be assumed that the suffering and disability caused to the individual are similar to that found in the general population.

Rates of suicide in severely mentally ill women are very high in the first post-natal year, when the risk is 70 times that at other times (Appleby et al. 1998). However, apart from this group, the overall rate of suicide in women post-natally is lower than the expected (Appleby 1991), suggesting a protective effect of the presence of dependent children on suicide in all except the most severely ill.

Effects on partners

About 50% of the partners of women admitted with severe post-partum mental illness suffer psychiatric illness themselves (Lovestone and Kumar 1993). Although not specific to parents, the literature on the impact of mental illness on partners and other carers documents their distress and the adverse effects on their social lives and work (Fadden et al. 1987).

Marital relationships often suffer following the birth of a child (Cowan and Cowan 1988). This effect is aggravated by parental mental illness, and the increased difficulties or breakdown in the relationship (Rutter and Quinton 1984) then perpetuate or worsen the illness and its effects. Mental illness appears to occur in both parents more often than expected (Rutter and Quinton 1984, Ballard et al. 1994). This could be due to the impact of illness in one parent on the other, the presence of shared risk factors such as social adversity or the effects of assortative mating. The latter has been demonstrated in a range of psychiatric disorders from schizophrenia (Parnas 1985) to somatization disorder (Zoccollilo and Cloninger 1985).

Effects on parenting behaviour

Some of the effects of severe mental illness on parenting behaviour are easily observable, but others are subtler and have only emerged from detailed studies of parental behaviour and, in particular, mother–infant interaction. Parents with schizophrenia or other severe and chronic psychotic illnesses show a range of disturbances of parenting including absent or limited intimacy and warmth, restricted cognitive and physical stimulation, exposure of the child to bizarre social behaviour or isolation and experiences of parental behaviour which can be confusing, frightening or, in extremes, terrorizing (Seeman 1996, Ragins et al. 1975, Sameroff et al. 1984). The following is a poignant example:

A schizophrenic mother of a five year old and eighteen month old boys was causing concern to family and neighbour because she was up with them at all hours, not dressing or feeding them properly and the elder son had not been taken to school for two weeks. Several times a day in the previous week they had been seen going to the end of the pier and looking out to sea, the children usually inadequately clothed. When I went to see her, her five year old son turned to me as she went out of the room and spoke of the father he did not know: 'Mummy says we should stand at the end of the pier and wait for him, because soon he will come back in his spaceship to fetch us'. He had tears in his eyes.

Rodnick and Goldstein (1974) found that poor pre-morbid functioning among mothers with an acute schizophrenic episode predicted greater severity and slower improvement or unresponsivity of parenting problems whereas good pre-morbid functioning was associated with significant improvements in parenting over 6 months. Among groups of severely mentally ill women admitted to mother-and-baby units in the post-natal period, parenting was most impaired in women with schizophrenia with lesser effects in bipolar disorder and unipolar depression, even when correcting for age, parity and marital status (Hipwell and Kumar 1996). In a series of women with schizophrenia admitted to a mother-and-baby unit, 50% were unable to care for their children long-term (Kumar et al. 1995). Mothers with depression are more likely to be negative, unsupportive and intrusive with their children (Zajicek and DeSalis 1979, Field et al. 1990). Some of the changes in reciprocal interaction between mother and infant as measured in laboratory situations are very subtle but are nevertheless of crucial importance to the development of the infant.

Less subtle effects are often readily observable in the clinical situation. This under-standing is no great feat of academic and clinical observation as parents themselves commonly describe these parenting difficulties, although in less technical terms such as 'I can't cope with the children'. The challenge to clinicians is to pay attention to this rather than merely accepting it as another inevitable result of the illness they are treating.

Effects on children

Over the past two decades evidence has been consistently accumulating of the effects of parental mental illness on almost every aspect of the development of the child. The evidence emerges from cross-sectional, and more recently from longitu-dinal studies as well as from observational studies of mother–child interactions and naturalistic studies of service outcomes. Effects on the child are demonstrable at the time of exposure to parental mental illness and later in childhood and adulthood, following parental recovery.

Emotional and behavioural problems

In their landmark study, Rutter and Quinton (1984) found double the rate of child psychiatric problems in children of mentally ill parents compared with controls.

One-third of these children had pervasive and persistent problems, in another one-third problems were transient and in the remainder no difficulties were found. The magnitude of this effect was not related to any particular diagnostic categories although findings from other studies suggest that maternal unipolar depression may have a particularly damaging effect (Hammen et al. 1987) and associations between a number of specified disorders in parents and psychological problems in their offspring emerge from several studies. Maternal chronic or recurrent depression appears to be associated with depression and eating disorder in teenage and adult daughters (Andrews et al. 1990). Offspring of mothers with somatization disorder have an increased risk of depression and suicide (Zoccolillo and Cloninger 1985, Livingstone 1993). The specific effects on children of psychotic symptoms in their parents can be both dramatic and damaging (Anthony 1970, Anthony 1986, Aldridge and Tagg 1998).

Attachment behaviour

Mother–infant interactions from 3 days and attachment behaviour at 1 year are adversely affected in women with a history of schizophrenia (Naslund et al. 1984. Persson-Blennow et al. 1984). In children of women with puerperal psychosis insecure avoidant attachment at 1 year is more likely in women who were manic (Hipwell et al. in press). Field et al. (1988) provide worrying evidence that the avoidant attachment seen in infants with post-natally depressed mothers generalizes to other non-depressed adult caregivers.

Effects on cognitive development

Several recent studies have examined the possible relationship between maternal depression and cognitive development of the infant. An association with reduced intellectual functioning emerges fairly consistently, with several studies suggesting an effect specific to maternal depression in the first post-natal year (Cogill et al. 1986, Hay and Kumar 1995, Sharp et al. 1995) which may be a particularly vulnerable period. Other possible vulnerability factors that emerge include male children, low socio-economic class and low birth weight. A large study by Murray (1992) suggested that depression did not have a direct effect on development but increased vulnerability to the adverse effects of lower social class and gender. The effects of depression on the infant may be mediated by the characteristic depressed interaction of mothers with their infants, particularly their patterns of speech (Murray et al. 1993). Studies published to date have demonstrated continued effects on prospective follow-up of children up to 5 years of age.

Abuse and neglect

Parents looking after infants and small children provide the emotional, physical and intellectual environment on which the child's quality of life, development and safety depend. Infants and young children are particularly vulnerable, as they are unable to anticipate or avoid harm. The earliest models for the aetiology of child abuse and neglect assumed that such parental behaviour stemmed from psychiatric disorder. There are a number of inherent dangers in this assumption. First, it leads to the false dichotomy between 'crazy abusers' – 'them' and 'sane non-abusers' – 'us'. Second, it suggests that people with mental illness are by definition 'potential abusers'. Finally, it sets up the unrealistic, impractical and, in some cases, falsely reassuring expectation that therapy or other treatment will be an effective treatment (Ross and Zigler 1983). The assumption is, therefore, potentially damaging to the process of identifying, preventing and dealing with abuse, to parents with mental illness who work hard to be good parents despite their illness; as well as to non-parents with mental illness who are affected by the negative public perceptions of mentally ill people as unpredictable and child abusing individuals.

Parental psychopathology is no longer accepted as the major aetiological factor in child maltreatment but its contribution as one of several factors in various forms of abuse is being clarified. Examining court records of seriously abused children, Taylor et al. (1991) found that there was evidence of mental illness (depression or schizophrenia) in 42% of mothers and 29% of parents had at some time received inpatient psychiatric treatment. Alcohol and drug abuse were common and associated with poor cooperation with services and criminality. Personality disorder was associated with a high likelihood of child removal. A study of parents with delinquent children showed a clear association with abuse and severe psychopathology, often psychotic in nature (Lewis and Balla 1976). Children of psychotic parents are more likely to suffer physical harm if they are involved in the content of the parental delusions or hallucinations (Rutter and Quinton 1984).

Death

A prospective study of offspring of women with schizophrenia and matched controls showed a doubled rate of foetal and neonatal death (8 versus 4%) (Reider et al. 1975). The risk of death by homicide also appears considerably increased in offspring of people with severe mental illness. A review of 100 cases of fatal child abuse in England and Wales found that parental psychiatric disorder was present in 35 cases, and in 25 the perpetrator parent was mentally ill (Falkov 1995). The UK Confidential Inquiry into Homicides and Suicides by Mentally Ill People found that one-third of the perpetrators were women and 85% of their victims were their young children (Department of Health 1996).

A study of all homicides in England showed 25% of victims to be children, mainly killed by their parents (Gibson 1975). In 90% of the maternal filicide cases, maternal psychiatric disorder was documented. However, d'Orban (1979) demonstrates that the majority of cases of neonaticides (child homicide in the first 24 hours post-partum) are not associated with maternal mental illness.

Psychiatric disorder appears to become a significant factor after this stage. Maternal psychiatric illness occurs in about one-third of infanticides occurring after 24 hours (Marks and Kumar 1993). Mentally ill mothers are more likely to kill more than one child and to then kill themselves (West 1965, d'Orban 1979, Marks and Kumar 1993). The presence of personality disorder appears to be a common risk factor in these studies, accounting for 43% of the women in d'Orban's study.

Mediating and modulating factors

Early research into associations between parental mental illness and child effects lacked the contextual perspective which permits a clearer understanding of processes involved and the other factors which modulate them. More recent studies have begun to document these often-complex interrelationships and point to the other factors involved, although the mediating processes remain poorly understood (Rutter 1997).

Factors relating to the parents, their psychopathology, the child and the wider environment have been identified. A full discussion of the influence of these factors is beyond the scope of this chapter but a brief overview gives a flavour of current understanding.

Parental factors

The quality of the marital relationship between parents has been repeatedly identified as important to various child outcomes in mentally ill and well parents (e.g. Rutter and Quinton 1984). Higher social class exerts a protective effect on cognitive development in children of women with post-natal depression (Hay and Kumar 1995, Sharp et al. 1995). Separation from, or early loss of, the mother's own parents increases the mother's difficulties caring for their newborn (Frommer and O'Shea 1973) and increases vulnerability to depression (Rodgers 1996a, b, Lloyd and Miller 1997). The presence of personality disorder has a compounding effect on most areas of outcome. Mentally ill women are more likely to smoke, have a poor diet and abuse alcohol or drugs in pregnancy, which all adversely affect child health.

In general, adverse effects on the child are more likely if the primary care giver is the parent with mental illness. In most societies the primary care giver is the mother but there is nevertheless evidence of effects of paternal mental illness in children which should not be ignored (Phares and Compas 1992).

Parental psychopathology

The importance of genetic transmission of predisposition varies according to the nature of the psychiatric disorder. The risk of developing schizophrenia or affective disorder in the children of affected parents is well established (Scourfield and McGuffin 1999) (Table 17.1).

Children of parents with bipolar disorder have an increased risk of bipolar and unipolar disorder whereas those of parents with unipolar depression have an increased risk of unipolar but not bipolar illness. Children of one parent with schizophrenia have an about 10-fold lifetime risk of developing the illness, but if both

Parental disorder	Risk to offspring (total population risk given in parentheses)
Schizophrenia (one parent) Schizophrenia (both parents)	13% risk of schizophrenia (1%) 45% risk of schizophrenia
Bipolar Affective Disorder	7.8% risk of bipolar disorder (1%) +11.4% risk of unipolar depression (3%)
Unipolar Depression	0.6% risk of bipolar disorder (1%) 9.1% risk of unipolar disorder (3%)

Table 17.1 – Risk of disorders in offspring of mentally ill parents (from Scourfield and McGuffin 1999).

parents are affected the risk is greatly increased to about 50%. Unfortunately the risk of both parents being affected by mental illness is increased by assortative mating as people with mental illness are more likely to develop relationships with mentally ill partners (Cantwell and Baker 1984, Parnas 1985) and indeed with criminal or personality disordered partners (Lewis and Balla 1976, Rutter and Quinton 1984).

The evidence from twin and adoption studies indicates a powerful genetic component to the transmission of risk in schizophrenia and to a lesser extent in bipolar disorder. The genetic component to the transmission of unipolar depression is less conclusive (McGuffin et al. 1994). The association between adverse childhood outcomes and parental mental illness appears to be less specific to the type of disorder (Rutter and Quinton 1984). Rather, it is the nature of parental symptoms and disability that are determining factors. For example, the adverse cognitive outcomes in offspring of women with post-natal depression appear related to maternal behaviour and speech patterns (Murray et al. 1993). Parental psychopathology that does not involve the child is less likely to lead to child psychiatric problems (Rutter 1996). Withdrawal, detachment, hostility and poor interpersonal competence appear to be particularly damaging parental characteristics across different parental diagnoses (Rodgers 1996, Rutter and Quinton 1984). Chronicity of symptoms and pre-morbid functioning are further important determinants of effect on parenting ability (Rodnick and Goldstein 1974, Andrews et al. 1990). Rutter and Quinton (1984) found that the presence of personality disorder in one parent increased the risk of psychiatric problems in the child, equivalent to cancelling out the protective effect of having one non-mentally ill parent. However, the adverse effect of personality disorder disappeared in the absence of parental hostility. In this study half of mentally ill fathers and one-quarter of mentally ill mothers had a personality disorder.

The wider context

A crucial influence on child outcomes is the child's wider environment, some aspects of which may result indirectly from the parental illness or may be correlates of the illness. Examples of effects of the illness include the higher rates of marital conflict, dysfunctional family situations and single parenthood among people with mental illness (Birtchnell and Kennard 1983, Rutter and Quinton 1984, Canino et al. 1990). The modulating effect of marital conflict is pronounced when considering the effects of maternal depression although less so in schizophrenia (Emery et al. 1982). Children of mentally ill parents are more likely to be taken into care which itself has demonstrable effects on parenting and child outcomes (Quinton and Rutter 1984, Wolkind and Kruk 1985, Coverdale and Turbott 1997).

Correlates of mental illness which have effects on child outcomes include greater social adversity, exposure to life events and poorer social supports (Bhugra and Leff 1993, Goodyear et al. 1993).

The child

Post-natal depression appears adversely to affect cognitive development in boys but not girls (Hay and Kumar 1994, Sharp et al. 1995). In addition, the effects appeared specific to exposure to maternal depression in the first rather than subsequent years. In Rutter and Quinton (1984), boys tended to show disturbance at an earlier stage than girls but over the 4-year follow-up the gender difference narrowed substantially. Bearsdslee et al. (1983) concluded in their review that infancy and adolescence might be particularly vulnerable periods for children of parents with affective disorders.

Temperamental differences in children emerge consistently as important factors governing parental behaviour towards children and children's response to various forms of adversity. Parental criticism and hostility is most likely to focus on a temperamentally 'difficult' child (Rutter and Quinton 1984) and features such as social responsiveness and activity appear to be protective (Garmezy 1984). Furthermore, some neonatal characteristics such as poor motor function and irritability appear to increase the risk of maternal depression (Murray et al. 1996).

HOW CAN SERVICES MEET THE CHALLENGE?

Parental mental illness presents a daunting challenge to services in its scale, the extent of its effects and the complexity of the solutions required to mitigate them. However, this challenge also offers an opportunity to engage in primary, secondary and tertiary prevention which is unique in the field of mental health and should be grasped (NHS Centre for Reviews 1997). Realising this opportunity requires services to work together at every level.

Prevention

Prevention is commonly divided into measures that prevent a disorder from occurring (primary prevention), those which prevent deterioration or relapse of a disorder (secondary prevention) and steps which can be taken to prevent or limit the consequences of a disorder such as disability and loss of employment (tertiary prevention). Such preventative measures can be applied in a general way to the whole population or can be targeted to individuals or groups known to be at high risk. Prevention of problems is usually more desirable than repair or cure. In the field of mental health realistic opportunities for prevention are still very limited because of our relative lack of knowledge about the disorders we are dealing with and their antecedents, our inability to control many of the factors which are known about and the cost implications of many of the generalized measures and some of the specific measures which could be applied (Lieh Mak 1994). Nevertheless, some evaluated examples of prevention in the field of severe mental illness do exist, for example pharmacological measures such as mood stabilizers to prevent relapse of bipolar affective disorders, continuation of antidepressants following recovery from depression to prevent relapse, family intervention to reduce expressed emotion and strategies to prevent suicide (see Chapters 2, 3 and 16). Most examples of targeted measures are forms of secondary or tertiary intervention and primary prevention strategies tend to be generalized and take the form of social policy.

Puerperal psychosis represents a unique opportunity to engage in specifically targeted primary prevention. Although only 1–2 per 1000 women develop puerperal psychosis following childbirth, the risk in those women who have a past history of affective psychosis is increased to about 50% (Dean et al. 1989, Marks et al. 1992a). Only very small trials of prophylaxis have been carried out using lithium with promising results (Stewart et al. 1991, Austin 1992) and antipsychotic prophylaxis also appears promising but has so far not been formally studied. Such women are readily identifiable antenatally but at present routine enquiry which might reveal such histories is rare in maternity care and services which can take preventative measures even rarer. Given the severity and impact of these disorders and the relative simplicity of possible preventative measures there seems little justification for this situation.

Attempts have been made to develop clinically useful screening instruments for the detection of women at high risk of post-natal depression but so far these instruments have lacked the specificity and sensitivity required for clinical use (Appleby et al. 1994, Cooper et al. 1996). General measures such as increasing education, fostering partner and other social support and improving early detection through education of professionals and screening must be relied upon. Nevertheless, women who have previously had a depressive illness are at a somewhat increased risk of post-natal depression and one study has demonstrated the effectiveness of antidepressant medication in reducing this risk (Wisner and Wheeler 1994).

Detection of mental illness among parents

Parents are often in contact with primary healthcare services and parents with social problems, who have a higher risk of psychiatric morbidity, are likely to be in contact with social services at some stage. Parents also tend to have contact with other parents and are targeted for child health literature. These various channels open up opportunities for educating parents about their own and their children's mental health, for offering them opportunities to present with mental health difficulties and for the early detection by others such as health visitors and general practitioners of mental health problems. If such early detection is followed by effective intervention, the impact on the individual and on others including the children is likely to be reduced as the duration and chronicity of mental illness is an important predictor of these effects.

Targeting those people with severe mental illness who are parents

It is obvious that a first step towards targeted intervention among people with severe mental illness is to identify which of these have dependent children. It is puzzling that even in services which have developed systematic methods of needs identification and case management such as the Care Programme Approach in the UK, no specific mention is made of clients needs as parents or of risks to children; despite the importance of these needs and risks. It seems likely that part of the reason for this neglect by services is that this is an area for which no single service has the knowledge, responsibility or skills.

In view of this lack of attention to the parenting function, it is not surprising that descriptions or evaluations of service models and interventions are rare, with the possible exception of services for women in the perinatal period (e.g. Oates 1988). Trail-blazing services such as the Schizophrenic Mothers Programme described by Waldo et al. (1987) receive little attention. It is of course difficult to develop services when there is so little literature on the outcomes of interventions and indeed on the specific predictors of outcome which might be used in the clinical setting (Appleby and Dickens 1993). This is no excuse for not attempting to develop services to meet such an important need but is of course a reason to ensure that any such service engages in evaluation of outcomes.

Working together

One of the principal challenges in reducing the impact of parental mental illness is the close collaboration required between various services which is notoriously difficult to achieve. Services such as those for child and adult mental health, primary care, and child and adult social services have different aims, philosophies and ways of working. Their effective collaboration often requires that one service, or indeed one individual, takes a lead. One such model is the development of specialist perinatal mental health services which bridge the divide between other agencies and have the knowledge and skills to help this group of clients and assist other services in doing so. Various elements of care which comprise such services including mother-and-baby inpatient units, day services and community based services have been described (Oates 1988, Cox et al. 1993b, Kumar et al. 1995).

In addition to interventions at an individual clinical level and at the level of services a greater emphasis on parental mental illness and its transgenerational effects is required at a policy level. Policy and strategic documents about adult mental illness rarely refer to the sorts of important issues described in this chapter. In the UK, for example, Health of the Nation documents on mental illness services, the Care Programme Approach, Supervision Registers and indeed the Mental Health Act make almost no mention of the particular problems and risks associated with mental illness among parents.

TREATMENT

Treatment of parental mental illness differs little from treatment of mental illness at any other time with two possible exceptions. First, consideration must be given to the dependent child or children and, second, special considerations apply to treatment given to women during pregnancy and post-natally.

Influence of dependent children on treatment

Admission to hospital of a parent can have a very disruptive effect on young children (Hawes and Cottrell 1999) which needs to be balanced against the exposure of children to severe disturbance in a parent's mental state or any potential risk to the child's safety. In the case of children up to the age of 12–18 months and where facilities are available, admissions of mothers with their infants to a specialist mother-and-baby inpatient unit can be advantageous. Such units have the facilities and skills needed to treat the maternal mental illness whilst assessing and supporting the mother's care for the child and the mother–child relationship.

Where admission of the parents of older children is necessary consideration should be given to appropriate contact. There will be times on all inpatient units when it could be inappropriate or harmful for a child to visit a parent and on some units, for example psychiatric intensive care units, it may be inappropriate all the time. Provision must, therefore, be made for contact to take place in more appropriate surroundings. The mental state of the parent and any potential risk to the child must be regularly reviewed. Specific considerations apply to psychotherapeutic interventions with mentally ill parents. First, the evidence that duration of parental illness is a determinant of the extent of the effects on the child means that interventions most likely to deliver the most rapid benefits in the circumstances should be selected. Second, as there is evidence that parent/child relations can remain disturbed after recovery of the illness, therapy should focus on the client's parenting function as well as the mental illness. Examples of interventions for severe mental illness with a particular focus on parenting have been described with beneficial effects on both the mental illness and parenting (Waldo et al. 1987, Cox et al. 1993b, Cooper and Murray 1997).

Treatment of perinatal disorders

It is reasonable to assume that treatments for mental illnesses are equally effective in pregnancy and post-natally as they are at any other time. Thus, studies examining response to treatment post-natally confirm the effectiveness of counselling and various forms of brief therapy for post-natal depression (Holden et al. 1989, Cooper and Murray 1997) and of treatment with fluoxetine (Appleby et al. 1997). Antipsychotics are also effective but there is some suggestion that women post-natally may be more sensitive to extrapyramidal side-effects. A number of special considerations also apply to treatments at this time.

First, consideration needs to be given to the possible effects on the child of psychotropic drugs taken during pregnancy and breastfeeding. With almost all drugs formal advice given by drug companies and official bodies recommends caution in prescribing during pregnancy and breastfeeding, unless evidence of harm to the child exists when more stringent restrictions are advised. The advice of caution is not particularly helpful to the clinician who is trying to advise the patient on the most appropriate treatment and is trying to balance uncertain risks against the need to treat the disorder. Evaluation of adverse effects on the child from use in pregnancy and breastfeeding in humans usually comes only from cumulative clinical experience coupled with voluntary reporting to regulatory bodies, pharmaceutical companies or in the literature. Controlled trials of drugs which include women who are pregnant or breastfeeding are extremely rare because funding bodies, pharmaceutical companies and ethics committees judge the risks involved to be unacceptable. It is paradoxical that the evidence base on drug-adverse effects is particularly weak in circumstances which cause particularly strong concerns among patients and clinicians. It follows that more information tends to be available on older drugs.

A full discussion of the available data is outside the scope of this chapter, but the principal clinical conclusions can be summarized as follows.

Antidepressants

Only one controlled trial of antidepressant treatment for depression occurring specifically in the post-natal period has been carried out (Appleby et al. 1997). This showed that treatment with fluoxetine was more effective than placebo in the treatment of non-psychotic post-natal depression and, interestingly, that it was as effective as six sessions of cognitive behaviourally orientated counselling, although the combination of the two was no more effective than either on their own. These findings confirm what one might expect from the literature on non-psychotic depression generally and it is at present reasonable to assume that antidepressants are as effective post-natally as they are at other times. However, women are generally more reluctant to take any prescribed drugs during pregnancy and when breastfeeding. They are also more likely to be put off by side-effects, particularly sedation which is not only troublesome during the day but, unlike patients who are not caring for young children, nocturnal sedation can also be a problem when caring for an infant.

Tricyclic antidepressants appear to be safe in pregnancy. Altshuler et al. (1996) have collected data from a variety of sources on 300 000 live births in women who took tricyclic antidepressants in pregnancy. There was no evidence from this data of any increase in malformations. For most tricyclic antidepressants low levels are found in breast milk and no significant adverse effects on the baby. Follow-up on breastfed infants has been carried out for as long as 2 years in the case of imipramine and between 3 and 5 years in the case of dothiepin (Wisner et al. 1996). The evidence for SSRI antidepressants is less extensive. Eli Lilly, the makers of fluoxetine, has information on over 1000 women who have taken fluoxetine during pregnancy with no evidence of significant dangers to the child. Fluoxetine does pass into breast milk, with an infant receiving about 10% equivalence of the maternal dose but with no observable adverse effect. Sertraline was undetectable in breast milk with no effects observed. Overall, however, the data available on SSRI antidepressants in pregnancy and breast feeding is far from complete and continued caution and vigilance should be observed.

Antipsychotics

There is no evidence of teratogenicity arising from the use of the older antipsychotics (e.g. chlorpromazine, haloperidol) in pregnancy (McElhatton 1992). Cases of *in utero* exposure to phenothiazines near term leading to tremor, hypertonia and hyper reflexia, which can persist in the neonate for several weeks, have been described. In general, minimal levels of the older antipsychotics appear in breast milk but sedative effects on the infant, which are dose-related, have been reported. Very little or no experience is available on the effects of the newer atypical antipsychotics in pregnancy and breastfeeding and considerable caution and vigilance must, therefore, be applied.

Mood stabilizers

Lithium exposure in the first trimester is associated with an increased risk of Ebsteins Abnormality. The exact level of risk has been difficult to ascertain as this is a rare disorder, occurring in the general population at a rate of 1:20 000 and the research methodology used will affect the likely accuracy of the result. The most recent evidence suggests that the risk of Ebsteins Abnormality in women taking lithium in the first trimester is not higher than 1:700 (Zalzstein et al. 1990). Exposure in the second and third trimester can lead to abnormalities in neonatal thyroid and renal function tests but no other abnormalities in infants have been found in follow-up over 5 years (Schou 1976). If lithium is prescribed during pregnancy monitoring of levels must be carried out more frequently and dosage adjustments made due to changes in lithium excretion and fluid volumes during pregnancy. There appears to be a significant risk of toxicity in the infant in breastfeeding women and, therefore, either lithium or breastfeeding should be avoided.

The risk of neural tube defect is increased in infants of women taking carbamazepine and sodium valproate in pregnancy (Koch et al. 1992). These should, therefore, be avoided in pregnancy or doses minimized and divided throughout the day. Folate supplementation may confer protection in such cases. Early antenatal screening for neural tube defects is also appropriate. Carbamazepine and valproate appear to be safe in breastfeeding as low levels appear in milk and no evidence has emerged of serious effects on the infant although some cases of drowsiness have been reported.

Benzodiazepines

Current evidence suggests that exposure to benzodiazepines in the first trimester may be associated with an increased risk of oral cleft (Dolovich et al. 1998). Benzodiazepines should, therefore, be avoided if possible and antenatal screening for oral cleft is appropriate. Benzodiazepines during breastfeeding can cause drowsiness and poor feeding in the infant.

Hormones

There is an increased rate of hypothyroidism post-natally and there is a clear association between abnormalities of thyroid function and post-natal affective disorder (Harris 1993).

Progesterone has been widely and popularly advocated as a treatment and prophylaxis for puerperal mental health problems, and is still commonly prescribed for this purpose by general practitioners, obstetricians and even psychiatrists despite the complete absence of any sensible evidence for effectiveness. The first double-blind, randomized placebo-controlled trial of progesterone administration post-natally was published by Lawrie et al. (1998) and demonstrated an **increased** risk of developing postnatal depression in the group treated with progesterone.

One double-blind, randomized, placebo controlled trial of oestradiol treatment for severe non-psychotic post-natal depression has been carried out which showed an improvement in the oestradiol treated group at 1 month which persisted for the 6 months of treatment and the effects were maintained at follow-up (Gregoire et al. 1996).

High-risk families: when children can't wait for effective treatment

Jones (1987) provides a useful review of some of the features of families that present a high risk of continuing harm to children (Table 17.2). He describes families with many of these factors as 'untreatable'. Although this is debatable in theory, in practice

- Evidence of past neglect/abuse/serious injury/sadistic treatment/premeditated torture

- Child involved in psychopathology

- Parental conflict involving the child

- Lack of empathic feelings towards the child or parental hostility towards child/children

- Lack of understanding of difficulty/motivation to overcome it

- Denial of problems/treatment refusal

- Learning disability/severe personality disorder/substance abuse co-morbidity

- Munchausen by Proxy

- Failure to thrive

Table 17.2 – Factors associated with a high risk of continuing abuse to children.

children suffering harm or at high risk of harm cannot wait indefinitely for things to change. Although much of the literature on such risk factors does not relate specifically to parents who have a mental illness it is nevertheless helpful to consider them as they are probably equally valid in this context and indeed there is a considerable degree of overlap with those risk factors described elsewhere in this chapter.

SUMMARY

From the moment a child is born the risk of mental illness is greater in parents than non-parents, although most of the research available to date has been carried out on mothers rather than fathers. Reproduction among people with severe mental illnesses appears to be little different to the general population. Parents with severe mental illnesses experience not only the suffering and disability but also an impairment of parenting and a deterioration of relationships; their partners have increased rates of mental illness and a negative impact on most areas of development of their children as well as increases in accidents and abuse have been demonstrated. Mental Health and Social Services have a unique opportunity to engage in primary and secondary intervention of illness and disability but, despite this, parental mental illness receives relatively little attention from services.

References

Aldridge S, Tagg G. Spurious childhood psychosis induced by schizophrenia in the parent. Advances in Psychiatric Treatment 1998; 4: 39–43.

Altshuler LL, Cohen L, Szuba MP et al. Pharmacologic management of psychiatric illness during pregnancy: dilemmas and guidelines. American Journal of Psychiatry 1996; 153: 592–605.

Andres B, Brown GW, Creasey L. Intergenerational links between psychiatric disorders in mothers and daughters: the role of parenting experiences. Journal of Child Psychology and Psychiatry 1990; 31: 1115–1129.

Anthony EJ. The influence of maternal psychosis on children – folie … deux. In Anthony EJ, Benedeck T (eds), Parenthood. Boston: Little Brown, 1970.

Anthony EJ. Terrorizing attacks on children by psychotic parents. Journal of the American Academy of Child Psychiatry 1986; 25: 326–335.

Appleby L. Suicide during pregnancy and in the first postnatal year. British Medical Journal 1991; 302: 137–140.

Appleby L, Dickens C. Mothering skills of women with mental illness. British Medical Journal 1993; 306: 348–349.

Appleby L, Gregoire A, Platz C et al. Screening women for high risk of postnatal depression. Journal of Psychosomatic Research 1994; 38: 539–545.

Appleby L, Mortenson PB, Faragher EB. Suicide and other causes of mortality after post-partum psychiatric admission. British Journal of Psychiatry 1998; 173: 209–211.

Appleby L, Warner R, Whitton A et al. A controlled study of fluoxetine and cognitive–behavioural counselling in the treatment of postnatal depression. British Medical Journal 1997; 314: 932–936.

Austin M-PV. Puerperal affective psychosis: is there a case for lithium prophylaxis? British Journal of Psychiatry 1992; 161: 692–694.

Ballard CG, Davis R, Cullen PC et al. Prevalence of postnatal psychiatric morbidity in mothers and fathers. British Journal of Psychiatry 1994; 164: 782–788.

Beardslee WR, Bemporad J, Keller MB et al. Children of parents with major affective disorder: a review. American Journal of Psychiatry 1983; 140: 825–832.

Belsky J, Vondra J. Lessons from child abuse: the determinants of parenting. In Cicchetti D, Carlson V (eds), Child Maltreatment – Theory and Research on the Causes and Consequences of Child Abuse and Neglect. Cambridge: Cambridge University Press, 1989.

Birtchnell J, Kennard J. Marriage and mental illness. British Journal of Psychiatry 1983; 142: 193–198.

Bools C, Neale B, Meadow R. Munchausen syndrome by proxy: a study of psychopathology. Child Abuse and Neglect 1994; 18: 773–788.

Briscoe M. Identification of emotional problems in postpartum women by health visitors. British Medical Journal 1986; 292: 1245–1248.

Brown GW, Harris T. Social Origins of Depression. London: Tavistock, 1978.

Brughra TS. Support and Personal Relationships. In Bennett D, Freeman H (eds), Community Psychiatry: The Principles. London: Churchill Livingstone, 1991a.

Canino GJ, Bird HR, Rubio-Stipec M et al. Children of parents with psychiatric disorder in the community. Journal of the American Academy of Child and Adolescent Psychiatry 1990; 29: 398–406.

Cantwell D, Baker L. Parental illness and psychiatric disorders in at risk children. Journal of Clinical Psychiatry 1984; 45: 503–507.

Cogill SR, Caplan HL, Alexandra H et al. Impact of maternal postnatal depression on cognitive development of young children. British Medical Journal 1986; 292: 1165–1167.

Cooper PJ, Murray L. The impact of psychological treatments of postpartum depression on maternal mood and infant development. In Murray L, Cooper PJ (eds), Postpartum Depression and Child Development. New York: Guildford, 1997.

Cooper PJ, Murray L, Hooper R et al. The development and validation of a predictive index for postpartum depression. Psychological Medicine 1996; 26: 627–634.

Coverdale JH, Turbott SH. Family planning outcomes of male chronically ill psychiatric outpatients. Psychiatric Services 1997; 48: 1199–1200.

Cowan PA, Cowan CP. Changes in marriage during the transition to parenthood. In Michaels, Goldberg (eds), The Transition to Parenthood – Current Theory and Research. Cambridge: Cambridge University Press, 1988.

Cox JL, Garrard J, Cookson D et al. Development and audit of Charles Street Parent and Baby Day Unit, Stoke-on-Trent. Psychiatric Bulletin 1993b; 17: 711–713.

Cox JL, Murray D, Chapman G. A controlled study of the onset, duration and prevalence of postnatal depression. British Journal of Psychiatry 1993a; 163: 27–31.

Cummings EM, Davies PT. Maternal depression and child development. Journal of Child Psychology and Psychiatry 1994; 35: 73–112.

D'Orban PT. Women who kill their children. British Journal of Psychiatry 1979; 134: 560–571.

Davenport YB, Adland MS. Postpartum psychosis in female and male bipolar manic depressive patients. American Journal of Orthopsychiatry 1982; 52: 288–297.

Dean C, Kendell RE. The symptomatology of puerperal illness. British Journal of Psychiatry 1981; 139: 128–133.

Dean C, Williams JR, Brockington IF. Is puerperal psychosis the same as bipolar manic depressive disorder? A family study. Psychological Medicine 1989; 19: 637–647.

Department of Health. Report of the Confidential Inquiry into Homicides and Suicides by Mentally Ill People. London: HMSO, 1996.

Dolovich LR, Addis A, Regis Vaillancourt JM et al. Benzodiazepine use in pregnancy and major malformations or oral cleft: meta-analysis of cohort and case-control studies. British Medical Journal 1998; 317: 839–843.

Dover SJ, Leahy A, Foreman DM. Parental psychiatric disorder: clinical prevalence and effects on default from treatment. Child Care Health and Development 1994; 20: 137–143.

Dowlatshahi D, Paykel ES. Life events and social stress in puerperal psychoses: absence of effect. Psychological Medicine 1990; 20: 655–662.

Downey F, Coyne JC. Children of depressed parents: an integrative review. Psychological Bulletin 1990; 108: 50–76.

El-Guebaly N, Offord DR. The competent offspring of psychiatrically ill parents. Canadian Journal of Psychiatry 1980; 25: 457–467.

Emery R, Weintraub S, Neale J. Effects of marital discord on the school behaviour of children of schizophrenic, affective disordered, and normal parents. Journal of Abnormal Psychology 1982; 16: 215–225.

Fadden G, Bebbington P, Kuipers L. The burden of care: the impact of functional psychiatric illness on the patient's family. British Journal of Psychiatry 1987; 150: 285–292.

Falkov A. Study of Working Together 'Part 8' Reports – Fatal child Abuse and Parental Psychiatric Disorder: An Analysis of 100 Area Child Protection Committee Case Reviews Conducted Under the Terms of Part 8 of Working Together under the Children Act 1989. London: Department of Health, 1995.

Field T. Infants of depressed mothers. Development and Psychopathology 1992; 4: 49–66.

Field T, Healy B, Goldstein S et al. Infants of depressed mothers show 'depressed' behaviour even with non-depressed adults. Child Development 1988; 59: 1569–1597.

Field T, Healy B, Goldstein S et al. Behaviour-state matching and synchrony in mother–infant interactions of non depressed versus depressed dyads. Developmental Psychology 1990; 26: 7–14.

Frommer EA, O'Shea G. Antenatal identification of women liable to have problems managing their infants. British Journal of Psychology 1973; 123: 149–156.

Garmezy N. Stress resistant children: the search for protective factors. In Stevenson J (ed.), Recent Research into Developmental Psychopathology. Monograph supplement no. 4 to the Journal of child Psychiatry and Psychology. Oxford: Pergamon, 1984.

Gibson E. Homicide in England and Wales 1967–1971. Home Office research study no. 31. London: HMSO, 1975.

Goodyear IM, Cooper PJ, Vize CM et al. Depression in 11–16 year old girls: the role of past parental psychopathology and exposure to recent life events. Journal of Child Psychology and Psychiatry 1993; 34: 1103–1115.

Gregoire AJP, Kumar R, Everitt B et al. Transdermal oestrogen for treatment of severe post-natal depression. Lancet 1996; 347: 930–933.

Hammen C, Gordon D, Burge D et al. Maternal affective disorders, illness, and stress: risk for children's psychopathology. American Journal of Psychiatry 1987; 144: 736–741.

Harris B. A hormonal component to postnatal depression. British Journal of Psychiatry 1993; 163: 403–405.

Hawes V, Cottrell D. Disruption of children's lives by maternal psychiatric admission. Psychiatric Bulletin 1999; 23: 153–156.

Hawton K, Roberts J, Goodwin G. The risk of child abuse among mothers who attempt suicide. British Journal of Psychiatry 1985; 146: 486–489.

Hay DF, Kumar R. Interpreting the effects of mothers' postnatal depression on children's intelligence: a critique and re-analysis. Child Psychiatry and Human Development 1995; 25: 165–181.

Hipwell AE, Goossens FA, Melhuish EC et al. Severe maternal psychopathology, 'joint' hospitalisation and infant–mother attachment. Development and Psychopathology (in press).

Hipwell AE, Kumar R. Maternal psychopathology and prediction of outcome based on mother–infant interaction ratings (BMIS). British Journal of Psychiatry 1996; 169: 655–661.

Holden JM, Sagovsky R, Cox JL. Counselling in a general practice setting: controlled study of health visitor intervention for postnatal depression. British Medical Journal 1989; 298: 223–226.

Iddamalagoda K, Naish J. 'Nobody Cared About Me'. Unmet Need Among Children in West Lambeth Whose Parents are Mentally Ill. London: West Lambeth Community Health Trust, 1993.

Jones DPH. The untreatable family. Child Abuse and Neglect 1987; 11: 409–420.

Kauffman C, Grunebaum H, Cohler B, Gamer E. Superkids: competent children of psychotic mothers. American Journal of Psychiatry 1979; 136: 1398–1402.

Kendell RE. Emotional and physical factors in the genesis of puerperal mental disorders. Journal of Psychosomatic Research 1985; 29: 3–11.

Kendell RE, Chambers JC, Platz C. Epidemiology of puerperal psychoses. British Journal of Psychiatry 1987; 150: 662–673.

Kendell RE, Rennie D, Clarke JA et al. The social and obstetric correlates of psychiatric admission in the puerperium. Psychological Medicine 1981; 11: 341–350.

Koch S et al. Major and minor birth malformations and anti-epileptic drugs. Neurology 1992; 42: 83–88.

Kumar R, Marks M, Platz C et al. Clinical survey of a psychiatric mother-and-baby unit: characteristics of 100 consecutive admissions. Journal of Affective Disorders 1995; 33: 11–22.

Lane A, Mulvany M, Kinsella A et al. Evidence for increased fertility in married male schizophrenics. Schizophrenia Research 1992; 6: 94.

Lawrie TA, Hofmeyr GJ, De Jager M et al. A double-blind randomised placebo controlled trial of postnatal norethisterone enanthate: the effect on postnatal depression and serum hormones. British Journal of Obstetrics and Gynaecology 1998; 105: 1082–1090.

Lewis DO, Balla DA. The Parents: Clinical and Epidemiological Findings in their Delinquency and Psychopathology. New York: Grune & Stratton, 1976.

Lieh Mak F. Psychosocial aspects of preventive psychiatry. In Christodoulou GN, Kontaxakis VP (eds), Topics in Preventive Psychiatry. Basel: Karger, 1994.

Livingstone R. Children of people with somatization disorder. Journal of the American Academy of Child and Adolescent Psychiatry 1993; 32: 536–544.

Lloyd C, Miller PMCC. The relationship of parental style to depression and self-esteem in adulthood. Journal of Nervous and Mental Disease 1997; 185: 655–663.

Lovestone S, Kumar R. Postnatal psychiatric illness: the impact on partners. British Journal of Psychiatry 1993; 163: 210–216.

Margision FE. Infants of mentally ill mothers: the risk of injury and its control. Journal of Reproductive and Infant Psychology 1990; 8: 137–146.

Marks M, Kumar R. Infanticide in England and Wales. Medicine Science and the Law 1993; 33: 329–339.

Marks MN, Wieck A, Checkley SA et al. Contribution of psychological and social factors to psychotic and non-psychotic relapse after childbirth in women with previous histories of affective disorder. Journal of Affective Disorders 1992a; 29: 253–264.

Marks MN, Weick A, Seymour A et al. Women whose mental illnesses recur after childbirth and partners' levels of expressed emotion during late pregnancy. British Journal of Psychiatry 1992b; 161: 211–216.

McElhatton PR. The use of phenothiazines during pregnancy and lactation. Reproductive Toxicology 1992; 6: 475–490.

McGuffin P, Owen MJ, O'Donovan MC et al. Seminars in Psychiatric Genetics. London: Royal College of Psychiatrists, 1994.

McNeill TF. Women with nonorganic psychosis: psychiatric and demographic characteristics of cases with versus without postpartum psychotic episodes. Acta Psychiatrica Scandinavica 1988; 78: 603–609.

McNeil TF, Kaij L, Malmquist-Larsson A. Women with nonorganic psychosis: mental disturbance during pregnancy. Acta Psychiatrica Scandinavica 1984a; 70: 127–139.

McNeil TF, Kaij L, Malmquist-Larsson A. Women with nonorganic psychosis: pregnancy's effect on mental health during pregnancy. Acta Psychiatrica Scandinavica 1984b; 70: 140–148.

Miller L, Kramer R, Warner V et al. Intergenerational transmission of parental bonding among women. Journal of the American Academy of Child and Adolescent Psychiatry 1997; 36: 1134–1139.

Miller LJ, Flinnerty M. Sexuality, pregnancy and child bearing among women with schizophrenia-spectrum disorders. Psychiatric Services 1996; 47: 502–506.

Miller WH, Resnick MP, Williams MH, Bloom JD. The pregnant psychiatric inpatient – a missed opportunity. General Hospital Psychiatry 1980; 12: 373–378.

Murray L. The impact of postnatal depression on infant development. Journal of Child Psychology and Psychiatry 1992; 33: 543–561.

Murray L, Kempton C, Woolgar M et al. Depressed mothers' speech to their infants and its relation to infant gender and cognitive development. Journal of Child Psychology and Psychiatry 1993; 34: 1083–1101.

Murray L, Stanley C, Hooper R et al. The role of infant factors in postnatal depression and mother–infant interactions. Developmental Medicine and Child Neurology 1996; 38: 109–119.

Naslund B, Persson-Blennow I, McNeill T et al. Offspring of women with nonorganic psychosis: infant attachment to the mother at 1 year of age. Acta Psychiatrica Scandinavica 1984; 69: 231–241.

NHS Centre for Reviews and Dissemination, University of York. Mental health promotion in high risk groups. Effective Health Care 1997; 3: 1–12.

Nimgaonkar VL, Ward SE, Agarde H, Weston N, Gangnli R. Fertility in schizophrenia: results from a contemporary US cohort. Acta Psychiatrica Scandinavica 1997; 95: 364–369.

Oates M. The development of an integrated community orientated service for severe postnatal mental illness. In Kumar R, Brockington I (eds), Motherhood and Mental Illness, vol. 2. London: Wright, 1988.

O'Hara MW. The nature of postpartum depressive disorders. In Murray L, Cooper PJ (eds), Postpartum Depression and Child Development. New York: Guildford, 1997.

Ødegård Ø. Marriage rate and fertility in psychotic patients before admissions and after discharge. International Journal of Social Psychiatry 1960; 6: 25–33.

Parnas J. Mates of schizophrenic mothers – a study of assortative mating from the American–Danish high risk project. British Journal of Psychiatry 1985; 146: 490–497.

Persson-Blennow I, Naslund B, McNeill T et al. Offspring of women with nonorganic psychosis: mother–infant interaction at three days of age. Acta Psychiatrica Scandinavica 1984; 70: 149–159.

Phares VE, Compas BE. The role of fathers in child and adolescent psychopathology. Psychological Bulletin 1992; 111: 387–412.

Pinderhughes CA, Barrabee Grace E, Reyna LJ. Psychiatric disorders and sexual functioning. American Journal of Psychiatry 1972; 128: 96–102.

Quinton D, Rutter M. Parents with children in care – 1. Current circumstances and parenting. Journal of Child Psychology and Psychiatry 1984; 25: 211–229.

Radke-Yarrow M, Nottlemann E, Martinez P et al. Young children of affectively ill parents: a longitudinal study of psychosocial development. Journal of the American Academy of Child and Adolescent Psychiatry 1992; 31: 68–77.

Ragins N, Schachter J, Elmer E et al. Infants and children at risk for schizophrenia. Journal of Child Psychiatry 1975; 14: 150–177.

Richards JR. Postnatal depression and infant development. British Medical Journal 1991; 302: 1336.

Rieder RO, Rosenthal D, Wender P et al. The offspring of schizophrenics: foetal and neonatal deaths. Archives of General Psychiatry 1975; 32: 200–211.

Richman N, Stevenson J, Graham PA. Pre-school to School: A Behavioural Study. London: Academic Press, 1982.

Rodgers B. Reported parental behaviour and adult affective symptoms: 1. Associations and moderating factors. Psychological Medicine 1996a; 26: 51–61.

Rodgers B. Reported parental behaviour and adult affective symptoms: 2. Mediating factors. Psychological Medicine 1996b; 16: 63–77.

Rodnick EH, Goldstein MJ. Premorbid adjustment and the recovery of mothering function in acute schizophrenic women. Journal of Abnormal Psychology 1974; 83: 623–628.

Ross C, Zigler E. Editorial. Treatment issues in child abuse. Journal of the American Academy of Child and Adolescent Psychiatry 1983; 22: 305–308.

Rutter M. Maternal depression and infant development: cause and consequence; sensitivity and specificity. In Murray L, Cooper P (eds), Postpartum Depression and Child Development. New York: Guildford, 1987.

Rutter M, Quinton D. Parental psychiatric disorder: effects on children. Psychological Medicine 1984; 14: 853–880.

Sameroff AJ, Barocas R, Seifer R. The early development of children born to mentally ill women. In Watt NF, Anthony EJ, Wynne LC, Rolf J (eds), Children at Risk for Schizophrenia: A Longitudinal Perspective. New York: Cambridge University Press, 1984.

Scourfield J, McGuffin P. Familial risks and genetic counselling for common psychiatric disorders. Advances in Psychiatric Treatment 1999; 5: 39–45.

Schou M. What happened to the lithium babies? A follow-up study of children born without malformations. Acta Psychiatrica Scandinavica 1976; 54: 193–197.

Seeman MV. Neuroleptic prescription for men and women. Social Pharmacology 1989; 3: 219–236.

Seeman MV. The mother with schizophrenia. In Gopfert M, Webster J, Seeman MV (eds), Parental Psychiatric Disorder. Cambridge: Cambridge University Press, 1996.

Sharp D, Hay DF, Pawlby S et al. The impact of postnatal depression on boys' intellectual development. Journal of Child Psychology and Psychiatry 1995; 36: 1315–1336.

Silverman MM. Children of psychiatrically ill parents: a prevention perspective. Hospital and Community Psychiatry 1989; 40: 1257–1265.

Stewart D, Gangbar R. Psychiatric assessment of competency to care for a new-born. Canadian Journal of Psychiatry 1984; 29: 583–569.

Stewart DE, Klompenhouwer JE, Kendell RE et al. Prophylactic lithium in puerperal psychosis: the experience of three centres. British Journal of Psychiatry 1991; 158: 393–397.

Taylor CG, Norman J, Murphy M et al. Diagnosed intellectual and emotional impairment among parents who seriously mistreat their children: prevalence, type and outcome in a court sample. Child Abuse and Neglect 1991; 15: 389–401.

Thiels C, Kumar R. Severe puerperal mental illness and disturbances of maternal behaviour. Journal of Psychosomatic Obstetrics and Gynaecology 1987; 7: 27–38.

Waldo MC, Roath M, Levine W et al. A model programme to teach parenting skills to schizophrenic mothers. Hospital and Community Psychiatry 1987; 38: 1110–1111.

West DJ. Murder Followed by Suicide. London: Heinemann, 1965.

White CL, Nicholson J, Fisher WH et al. Mothers with severe mental illness caring for children. Journal of Nervous and Mental Disease 1995; 183: 398–403.

Wisner KL, Peindl KS, Hanusa BH. Psychiatric episodes in women with young children. Journal of Affective Disorders 1995; 34: 1–11.

Wisner KL, Peindl KS, Hanusa BH. Symptomatology of affective and psychotic illnesses related to childbearing. Journal of Affective Disorders 1994; 30: 77–87.

Wisner KL, Perel JM, Findling RL. Antidepressant treatment during breast-feeding. American Journal of Psychiatry 1996; 153: 1132–1137.

Wisner KL, Wheeler SB. Prevention of recurrent postpartum major depression. Hospital and Community Psychiatry 1994; 45: 1191–1196.

Wolkind SN, DeSalis W. Infant temperament, maternal mental state, and child behaviour problems. In Porter R, Collins GM (eds), Temperamental Differences in Infants and Young Children. London, Publ?, 1982.

Wolkind SN, Kruk S. From child to parent: early separation and adaptation to motherhood. In Nicol AR (ed.), Longitudinal Studies in Child Psychology and Psychiatry: Practical Lessons from Research Experience. Chichester: Wiley, 1985.

Zahn-Waxler C, Ianotti RJ, Cummings EM et al. Antecedents of problem behaviours in children of depressed mothers. Development and Psychopathology 1990; 26: 51–59.

Zajicek E, DeSalis W. Depression in mothers of young children. Child Abuse and Neglect 1979; 3: 833–835.

Zalzstein E, Koren F, Einarson T et al. A case-control study on the association between first trimester exposure to lithium and Ebstein's anomaly. American Journal of Cardiology 1990; 65: 817–818.

Zoccolillo M, Cloninger CR. Parental breakdown associated with somatisation disorder (hysteria). British Journal of Psychiatry 1985; 147: 443–446.

MONITORING EFFECTIVENESS AND INCREASING KNOWLEDGE: EDUCATION, AUDIT AND RESEARCH

Jed Boardman

INTRODUCTION

Previous chapters have highlighted the breadth and heterogeneous nature of the concept of severe mental illness. What is not in dispute is the need to identify and provide effective services for those with severe mental illness and their carers and families. Education, research and audit have important contributions to make in this area. This chapter is not intended as a comprehensive review of this field but will use as a means of illustration some of the work examining the reduction in size of the asylum population in the UK and the relocation of services in the community. It will also examine the contribution of audit to this area and gives some examples of audit projects and tools. The need for both public education and staff education will be highlighted in relation to the evidence from existing research.

THE DEMISE OF THE ASYLUM – DE-INSTITUTIONALIZATION

> There they stand, isolated, majestic, imperious, brooded over by the gigantic water tower and chimney combined, rising unmistakable and daunting out of the countryside. … It is out of duty to err on the side of ruthlessness. For the great majority of these establishments there is no appropriate use. (Enoch Powell 1961)

Many will recognize this quote. It was supported by a statistical prediction of a reduction of the numbers of residents of such institutions and their eventual emptying by 1970 (Tooth and Brooke 1961). These predictions prompted several early local studies, many of which may now be considered to be audit projects, describing the asylum population.

Gore and Jones (1961) surveyed the patients in Menston Hospital, Yorkshire, in June 1959, which at that time had 2351 residents. The majority was under 65 years of age, many had no contact with the outside world, and few had been used to occupations that would have suited them for outside employment. Two-thirds had schizophrenia. This extensive, but simple, survey led the authors to the insightful conclusion that 'The evidence suggests that in this hospital at least, the Ministry's assumption that 'none will remain in sixteen years or a little more' is likely to be fulfilled' (Gore and Jones 1961). One had to wait until the 1980s before the first asylum closed (BMJ 1993, Groves 1993).

Other such studies followed in Friern, North London (Christie Brown et al. 1977), Tooting Bec, Southeast London (Bewley et al. 1975, 1981, Fottrell et al. 1975) and Glenside Hospital, Bristol (Cooper and Early 1961). The Glenside study evolved into a series of quinquennial surveys that provided a continuing story of the evolution of a large mental hospital in the post-war years (Early and Magnus 1966, Early and Nicholas 1977, 1981, Ford et al. 1987). These studies all made similar findings and highlighted similar concerns. The institutions had declining numbers of residents but generally the core population was increasing in age, they were handicapped by their psychiatric conditions, often had coexisting physical illnesses, were socially isolated and had rarely been out of hospital. Importantly, the studies pointed to the need for extensive re-provision of services if the institutions were to close. The evidence they presented was in conflict with the earlier predictions of the government and reinforced the conclusions of Gore and Jones (1961).

As the numbers of residents of asylums fell in the 1960s and 1970s, the inevitable question arose concerning those patients who would have been admitted had there been sufficient beds. The answer to this was found within two concepts: the **revolving door** patient and the **new long-stay** (NLS) patient. As the number of residents fell the number of patients who were re-admitted to hospital rose, possibly reflecting the inadequacy of alternative psychiatric provision. In addition, there was a growing number of younger patients who had been admitted after the drive to empty the asylums but who had protracted stays in hospital. These NLS patients became subject to increasing attention as they were perceived as presenting a particular challenge for the re-provision of residential services (Magnus 1967, Wing 1971, Eason and Grimes 1976, Mann and Cree 1976). They were of concern in several other countries whose asylum populations were dwindling (Hafner and Klug 1982, Rud and Noreik 1982, Taube et al. 1983, Craig et al. 1984, Kastrup 1987).

It is important to be clear about what is meant by the NLS if their number is to be counted. A recent national survey of this group defined them as those individuals, aged 18–64 years on admission to a psychiatric unit, whose stay had been between

6 months and 3 years (Lelliott et al. 1994). Returns from 59 UK mental health services in 1992 revealed 905 NLS patients, a mean prevalence of 6.1 per 100 000 population with a rate of accumulation of 1.3 per 100 000 per year (Lelliott and Wing 1994, Lelliott et al. 1994). These patients were characterized by two subgroups: one of predominantly younger men aged 18–34 years who had a history of violence and dangerous behaviour and were often formally detained; and another of older (55–67 years) married or previously married women with affective disorders or dementia who were at risk of non-deliberate self-harm. This survey population represented a shift in the characteristics of this group since a previous survey in 1972 (Mann and Cree 1976) revealing a higher proportion of men, single people, those with schizophrenia, those with formal admissions and multiple admissions. As English hospitals, by 1992, had reduced their long-stay bed provision, almost one-third of the NLS in England were on acute psychiatric wards (Lelliott and Wing 1994). The patients' state, both their level of disturbance or handicap, and the lack of suitable alternative accommodation conspired to keep this group in hospital. In 1992 the opinion of the psychiatric staff caring for the patients was that 61% would be better placed in a non-hospital setting. Almost half were thought to require a community-based residential setting, but unfortunately over half of this group remained in hospital because no suitable community placement was available (Lelliott and Wing 1994).

As we journeyed into the 1980s, Health Districts were instructed to close their asylums. A further series of studies examining the suitability for placement of long-stay hospital residents emerged. By the late 1980s almost all health districts still had a long-stay hospital with a dwindling and residual population. Several studies indicated that the populations were mainly elderly and suffered from schizophrenia; they were often severely disabled with multiple problems in the areas of symptoms, behaviour, personal functioning, social skills and physical health (Mann and Cree 1976, Levene et al. 1985, Ford et al. 1987, Curson et al. 1988, Carson et al. 1989, Chong and Abbott 1990, Clifford et al. 1991, Pryce et al. 1991, O'Driscoll et al. 1993, Smyth et al. 1997). As detailed in the earlier studies, these patients remained isolated in the hospital and were thought of as being difficult to place outside the hospital unless some supervised accommodation could be found. For example, Clifford et al. (1991) surveyed long-stay populations in five hospitals and found that only 3% were thought able to live independently, 26% required low dependency accommodation and 71% required high dependency accommodation.

In keeping with the earlier studies these later studies were essentially simple to carry out (although labour-intensive) but yielded important results for planning purposes. They often used more detailed instruments to measure the patients' state than the previous studies that utilized simple descriptive protocols and head counts.

Follow up of patients discharged from mental hospitals

In retrospect, the 'post-hospital adjustment of chronic mental patients' (Brown et al. 1958) provided the basis for one of the major areas of study in social psychiatry: the impact of the family environment on relapse in schizophrenia. Two hundred and twenty-nine patients aged 20–65 years who had been in hospital for more than 2 years and subsequently discharged from seven mental hospitals between 1949 and 1956 were shown to have mixed success in adjusting to life outside the asylum (Brown et al. 1958). Over two-thirds remained out of hospital for more than 1 year and two-thirds of these showed full or partial social adjustment. Those who were healthier at discharge, who gained employment and who were not returned to their family environment generally did better. Given the importance of post-hospital adjustment there are too few studies in this area. Those that are available show mixed results. Johnstone et al.'s (1984) follow-up of individuals with schizophrenia discharged from Shenley Hospital showed that many had enduring psychotic symptoms and handicaps and almost one-third had lost contact with psychiatric services. Twenty years later, the situation may have changed little, with continuing high levels of disability being the norm along with shortcomings in the area of social care provision (O'Brien 1992, Jones et al. 1997). The TAPS study (see below), however, suggests that if community provision of residential care is well organized then desirable outcomes for the majority of those with severe mental illness can be obtained. It is important to note that the availability of residential care for these patients is highly variable between health districts and one of the consequences of diversification has been a reduction in the proportion of such facilities being available to those with severe disability (Lelliott et al. 1996).

The Team for the Assessment of Psychiatric Services (TAPS) study

In 1993 the Northeast Thames Regional Health Authority (NETRHA) announced its intention to close the two large institutions at Friern and Claybury. An independent research programme was funded to follow up the progress of all long-stay patients in their community placements for the duration of the closure programme. This TAPS study (Leff 1993, 1997) has provide some of the finest data on the outcome of patients who were relocated from the large institutions. The principal design of the study was to describe all existing patients in the two hospitals and to compare successive cohorts of 'leavers' with those 'stayers' who remained in the hospitals. The research team used a battery of schedules to provide baseline measures and outcomes. The main findings for the long-stay non-demented patients are shown in Table 18.1.

Twelve-month outcome for cohorts 1–8 ($n = 671$ successfully followed up)

- Seven of 671 patients lost to follow-up
- No increase in deaths or suicide
- Two imprisoned
- 15% re-admitted to hospital
- No change in positive symptoms (hallucinations/delusions)
- Reduction in negative symptoms (7% lost entirely)
- Small reduction in social behavioural problems
- No deterioration in physical health, but an increase in immobility and incontinence in the older patient
- Domestic and community skills improved
- Increase in freedom — appreciated by patients
- More than 80% want to stay in community homes
- Increased perceived helpfulness of medication — fewer problems with compliance
- Increase in size of social networks — patients made more friends, gained acquaintances and service contacts

Five-year outcome follow-up of cohorts 1–4 ($n = 359$ successfully followed up)

- 54 deaths over 5 years
- Five suicides — no increase in suicide rate
- No patient imprisoned during years 1–5
- Low levels of assaults and other criminal behaviour (more likely to be victim than perpetrator of crime)
- No patients lost of follow-up
- No change in positive symptoms
- Negative symptoms reduced
- More freedom — 80% wish to stay
- Continuing small increase in community skills
- Increase in domestic skills in first year, then declines to above baseline levels
- Increase perceived helpfulness of medication
- Improvement in physical health. But an increase in immobility and incontinence with a resultant increase in needs for physical nursing care
- Decrease contact with relatives
- Patients gain acquaintances and friends and made more contacts

Table 18.1 – The TAPS study — outcome for the long-stay non-demented population.

RESEARCH AND AUDIT OPPORTUNITIES

Four projects

While the TAPS study was a well-funded and ambitious project, the description of in-patient populations is not beyond the resources of many departments of psychiatry and audit departments. There are many examples of good audit projects (Smith 1992) and below are four that relate to the severely mentally ill.

Study 1

A description of a long-stay hospital population; a survey of long-stay and rehabilitation wards at one mental hospital (Boardman 1992 unpublished data)

This survey was carried out at St Edwards Hospital near Leek, North Staffordshire. The hospital, built in 1897, was planned for closure before 2000. The survey was carried out to assist in this planning process. All patients identified on one census day were included and the staff completed the FACE profile (Clifford 1993). This profile had also been used in the national survey on the NLS (Lelliott et al. 1994). One hundred and fifty-one patients (30 per 100 000 population), of whom 35 were NLS, were surveyed. Their overall characteristics were similar to those found in the surveys quoted above: 60% male, 37% aged over 65 years, 64% never married, 58% had been in hospital for more than 3 years and one-third for more than 20 years. Almost 60% had schizophrenia, 70% had some existing psychotic symptoms and one-third had moderate or severe physical problems.

Of particular interest were those factors that would make it difficult to move these patients to other accommodation and what type of care would be suitable for them. Five variables were pertinent to examining the chances of discharge:

- Risk of a violent or dangerous incident
- Deliberate risk to self
- Non-deliberate risk to self
- Socially unacceptable behaviour
- Problems with personal functioning

The main results for these are shown in table 2. Only 17 of the patients were not rated on any of the five variables and all of these had been admitted within the previous year. Of these 55% were rated on at least three of the variables. Sixteen patients were rated on all five variables and many were rated as severe. When asked to rate the patients' current ability to lead a normal life, for 40% of the patients their ability was severely, very severely or overwhelmingly curtailed, with 30 patients being largely or entirely dependent on others.

	n	%
Risk of violence (or other dangerous incident) if discharged		
Non/minimal	81	54.0
Low	24	16.0
Medium	21	14.0
High	24	16.0
Deliberate risk to self if discharged		
Non/minimal	109	74.1
Low	16	10.9
Medium	14	9.5
High	8	5.4
Non-deliberate risk to self if discharged		
Non/minimal	46	31.1
Low	37	25.0
Medium	36	24.3
High	29	19.6
Socially unacceptable behaviour		
Non/minimal	67	44.4
Low	30	19.9
Medium	30	19.9
High	24	15.9
Overall personal functioning		
Little/no problem	34	22.5
Mild problem	58	38.4
Moderate problem	47	31.1
Severe problem	12	7.9

Table 18.2 – Survey of long-stay and rehabilitation wards at one mental hospital.

What was gained from carrying out this survey?

- The survey identified three broad groups of patients: the first group of around 40 patients who were severely handicapped and needed continuing care, a further group of around 40 who were less handicapped and for whom non-hospital placement was probably achievable. Finally, the remainder (almost half the patients) who could be placed in less dependent settings and for whom there might be a need to create suitable community placements.

- Patients had received an individual needs assessment that could be used to plan their rehabilitation programme and could form a baseline against which progress could be measured.

- The basis for planning the district's resettlement programme. The survey suggested that attention should be given to three areas: the provision of appropriate aftercare facilities, continuing rehabilitative efforts and the provision of continuing care facilities.

Study 2

Follow-up of long-stay hospital population; a follow-up survey of patients in one mental hospital (Boardman 1995 unpublished data).

To assist further in the closure plans a second survey was carried out 18 months after the original. The general outcome of the original cohort was examined in addition to examining the group of patients who were resident on the wards 18 months later. Twenty new patients who were resident on the census day were included. Of the original cohort, 97 remained in hospital; 43 had been discharged and 11 had died. There were now 117 patients on the long-stay and rehabilitation wards and when they were compared overall with the original cohort of 151 they were more handicapped, more difficult to place and less likely to live independently.

The information obtained from the follow-up study could be used in a variety of ways, but it is useful to consider two matters: what are the differences between those patients who remained in hospital and those who were discharged or died? How stable are the conditions of those who remained in hospital?

Comparison of those who remained in hospital with those who were discharged revealed:

- The discharged group was younger and contained more women.

- The discharged group had spent less time in hospital.

- Those with functional psychoses were more likely to remain in hospital than the other patients.

- Patients who were discharged were more likely to have an extended or moderate social network before admission.

- Those who remained in hospital were more likely to be rated at high risk of incurring a violent or otherwise dangerous incident if discharged from hospital, more likely to be at high risk of non-deliberate self-harm and to have severe problems with socially unacceptable behaviour.

- Those who remained in hospital were more likely to have high levels of poor personal functioning.

The staff were generally accurate in their prediction of overall placement for those who were discharged: 90% of those who were discharged were thought able to live outside hospital at the time of the first survey.

There were 97 patients who were in hospital at the time of the first survey and remained there. Their condition tended to remain stable and the overall condition of 70% had not altered or had changed only mildly. Some patients had improved, but there was a tendency for these to be replaced by an equal number who had deteriorated.

What was learned from this second study?

- There had been no overall accumulation of patients and the loss of patients from the hospital population had not been matched by admissions giving a fall in the total in-patient population by 22%.

- There had been a tendency for the easier-to-place, less handicapped patients to be discharged first. The ward staff accurately predicted these discharges.

- Two factors appeared to prevent placement outside of hospital: the extent of the patients' handicaps and the availability of suitable placements.

- Those remaining in hospital had enduring, and sometimes deteriorating, handicaps. Many of these require placement in a high-staffed setting.

Study 3

Follow-up of a discharged cohort out of hospital: aftercare for people with schizophrenia (Jones et al. 1997)

This study examined the aftercare given to a group of patients with schizophrenia following their discharge from acute psychiatric units in North Durham. The main features of the study were:

- Data were collected from routine sources (case notes and Care Programme Approach [CPA] data) and from a semi-structured interview with patients and carers.

- The Health of the Nation (HoNOS) scales were used to assess the clinical state of the patients (Wing et al. 1998).

- Of the cohort of 77 patients, 66 were followed up over a 2–3-year period.

The main findings of the study were:

- High use of in-patient facilities. Over half of the patients had a least one in-patient readmission.

- The majority remained in contact with services, but this was mainly in the form of routine outpatient appointments.

- 31% remained on a CPN caseload; 19% on a social workers caseload.

- None committed offences.

- 40% of those who were not employed used daycare facilities.

- HoNOS revealed high levels of continuing disability. For example, half had major problems with activities of daily living.

- Most users and carers were satisfied with the services received, but carers were more critical than the patients were.

This study should be compared with an audit of community care provision conducted in Lambeth, South London (Melzer et al. 1991), which revealed poor outcome and a substantial risk that patients would fall through the net of care.

Study 4

Description of the users of components of a service; monitoring of new patient contacts at two Community Mental Health Centres (Boardman and Bouras 1988, Boardman 1997)

Routine monitoring of contacts with a service can be helpful; not only in revealing trends, but also in examining whether the components of a service are attracting their targeted patient groups. One of the early Community Mental Health Centres in the UK, the Mental Health Advice Centre (MHAC) in Lewisham, South-east London (Boardman and Bouras 1988), had routinely recorded all new contacts with the three main components of the service: the multi-professional walk-in service (MPT), the crisis intervention team (CIT) and the routine out-patient clinic (OPC). Trends in contact showed a steady increase in walk-in service referrals, a fall in new outpatient contact and changing number of crisis team contacts (figure 1). The walk-in facility attracted mainly those individuals with adjustment and other non-psychotic disorders, whereas the crisis team referrals consisted of 40% of individuals with psychotic disorders. These patterns of contact lead to criticisms that the MHAC may not be adequately targeting those patients with Severe Mental Illness (Sayce et al. 1991), especially as there was no team that addressed the continuing needs of this group of users. These findings eventually led to the establishing of a continuing care team (Beer et al. 1995).

When a new Community Mental Health Centre (CMHC) was set up in 1992 (Boardman 1997), the service components were again routinely monitored

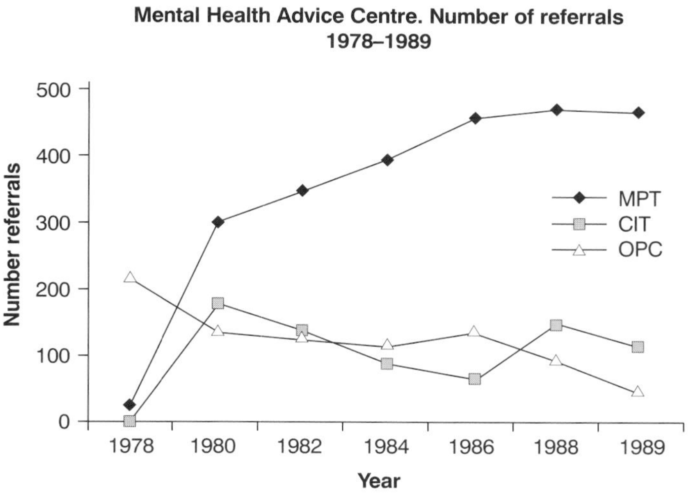

**Mental Health Advice Centre. Number of referrals
1978–1989**

Figure 18.1 – Percentage referrals with functional psychoses: MPT, 9%; CIT, 40%; OPC, 12%

(Table 18.3). In this case there was a walk-in facility but no crisis team. However, there was a community in-patient unit attached to the CMHC that focussed on those with severe mental illness, a multi-professional team which prioritized those with SMI and a group of CPNs who worked directly with general practitioners. The figures suggested that the service components were successful in serving those groups that they targeted and almost all discharges from the in-patient unit had a key worker in the team. It was notable that the general practice attached CPN were seeing a large number of patients who were rising in number, a phenomenon similar to that seen in the Lewisham walk-in service.

The studies outlined above are all relatively simple to carry out and can be readily undertaken with minimal resources and may be considered as routine parts of the audit or monitoring process for a service. They may be facilitated by the use of routine databases, case registers and an effective audit department. They do not represent studies conducted by research teams with specific grants of which there are many fine examples (e.g. Tyrer and Creed 1995). Many of them dealt with the collection of readily available data and not all of them involved collecting data directly from patients. However, the use of baseline data collection and the measuring of individual patient outcomes are important in the assessment of services, and such measures will form part of the minimum data set to be introduced in the UK (Glover et al. 1997).

Measuring tools

What instruments are available to measure individual patient outcomes? Those

	1992	1993	1994	1995	1996	% OF REFERRALS WITH FUNCTIONAL PSYCHOSES
Duty Professional referrals	34*	226	257	272	244	15%
Team referrals	76**	80	88	106	79	14%
Outpatient referrals	235	190	139	155	143	12%
Community inpatient admissions	5+	57	74	74	63	67%
Community Psychiatric Nurse direct referrals	111	115	304	520	725	0%

* October — December only

** August — December only

+ December only

Table 18.3 – Referrals to Lyme Brook Mental Health Centre (1992–96).

outlined in Table 18.4 do not comprise a comprehensive list, but includes those which may be useful in assessing individuals with severe mental illness. When choosing a suitable instrument the following should be taken into consideration:

- Is the instrument appropriate for its intended use? Is it right for the population? Does it measure the dimensions that you want it to? (e.g. symptoms as opposed to satisfaction?).

- Is the instrument too broad or too narrow for the intended use?

- Does the instrument have a theoretical underpinning that is not appropriate for the intended use?

- Is the instrument feasible to administer? For example, is it too long? Can it be self-administered or does it require an interview? Can the data be routinely obtained?

- Can the instrument be easily scored? How can it be analysed? What are the appropriate statistical methods? Does it give an overall score or subscores?

- Has the instrument been used in other studies? Can these form comparisons to the present use?

- Can the instrument readily detect change?

- Is the there published evidence of good reliability and validity?

For further information of the above, see the larger texts on the subject (e.g. McDowell and Newell 1987, Parry and Watts 1989, Freeman and Tyrer 1992, Oppenheim 1992).

Present State Examination (PSE) (Wing *et al.* 1974)
Schedules for Clinical Assessment in Neuropsychiatry (SCAN) (Wing *et al.* 1989)
Structured Clinical Interview (SCID) (Spitzer *et al.* (1985)
Brief Psychiatric Rating Scale (BPRS) (Overall and Gorman 1962)
Global Assessment of Functioning (GAF) (Jones *et al.* 1995)
Health of the Nation Outcome Scales (Wing *et al.* 1998)
Manchester Scale (Krawiecka *et al.* 1977)
Social Behavioural Schedule (SBS) (Wykes and Sturt 1986)
Social Behavioural Assessment Schedule (SBAS) (Platt *et al.* 1980)
Camberwell Assessment of Need (CAN) (Slade *et al.* 1996)
Lancashire Quality of Life Scales (LQL) (Oliver *et al.* 1997)
Involvement Evaluation Questionnaire (IEQ) (Shene and Van Wijngaarden 1993)
REHAB Scale (Baker and Hall 1998)
FACE Schedules (Clifford 1993)
The Community Placement Questionnaire (Clifford *et al.* 1991)
The Verona Service Satisfaction Schedule (VSSS) (Ruggeri *et al.* 1994)

Table 18.4 – Measurement tools useful in audit/research for those with severe mental illness.

In many studies a range of instruments may be required to measure more than one dimension of the outcomes. Areas that may be considered are:

- Administrative data – include personal, demographic and clinical data that may be readily accessible from routine sources
- Symptom data
- Social functioning
- Quality of life
- Satisfaction
- Carer burden
- Needs

The value of research to patients with severe mental illness

This chapter has avoided mention of 'what research needs to be done' for fear of creating a shopping list of areas that many would contest and would be in need of almost immediate revision. There is, however, room to comment on the value of research. Here one needs to look at the recipients of research; first, the practitioners but ultimately the patients and a wider society.

Mental health professionals draw on a range of strategies that are supposed to have known beneficial effects on the natural histories of mental illness, but these interventions all have the capacity to cause harm as well as benefit, and professionals, with the best of intentions, can inadvertently harm as well as help. The absence of an adequate knowledge base for much of the care provided has been highlighted (Cochrane 1971) and it is the purpose of research to update this and to contribute to the creation of professionals who do more good than harm. The introduction of such elements into the daily working lives of UK health workers such as clinical audit, the National R&D strategy, regional and local R&D committees, promotion of Evidence-based Medicine and the Cochrane database have significant contributions to make in this area. While it is recognized that many practitioners will be research consumers rather than research producers, there is a need to produce up-to-date and stimulated professionals who operate in an enquiring ethos within their services and research can contribute to this.

The service user is not merely a recipient of research, but may have a more reciprocal role to play in the creation of questions for enquiry and change of focus for research to better inform decisions about healthcare. This involvement of users represents a move towards the democratization of the research process in which professionals, users, carers and a broader society all have a stake. The aim of research should be to provide a rational and systematic basis for the provision of mental health services; whether this bears fruit will only be seen in the future.

EDUCATION

Public attitudes towards mental illness

Patients with severe mental illnesses are a marginalized group who are little understood by the public at large and who are perceived in terms of media images of madness and danger. It is generally true that the public's view of mental illness has been characterized by negative and rejecting attitudes (Cumming and Cumming 1957, Nunally 1961, MacLean 1969, D'Arcy and Brockman 1976). However, these views are not inevitable and some surveys have found more accepting and tolerant attitudes (Lemkau and Crocetti 1962, Meyer 1964, Ring and Schein 1970). These contradictory findings may reflect methods used in the studies (McPherson and Cocks 1983) but certainly highlight the complex and often contradictory views that we hold towards many issues, not least towards mental illness and the mentally ill. Over time attitudes may have become more liberal (Bentz and Edgerton 1971, Kirk 1974) but are just as likely to have remained static (Olmstead and Durham 1976, Green et al. 1987, Angermeyer and Matschinger 1997). A recent study carried out in the Midlands of England (Brockington et al. 1993) showed some evidence of increasingly positive attitudes towards mental illness, but many respondents continue to give negative and stigmatizing responses. Attitudes vary according to social groups with older, less educated and lower socio-economic groups showing less favourable attitudes (Sellick and Goodyear 1985). Those with personal experiences if mental illness or the mentally ill tend to show more favourable responses (Angermeyer and Matschinger 1997).

Studies on attitudes, and the associated concept of stigma, had their heyday in the 1950s and 1960s, but with the increased interest in community psychiatry and the closure of large asylums there has been a resurgence of interest in these areas (Hayward and Bright 1997). Stigma refers to the negative effects of a label placed on a group, in this case the mentally ill. There appears to be several factors underlying these negative effects (Hayward and Bright 1997):

- Dangerousness – the perception of this in physical terms or as a threat to personal mental stability
- Responsibility – the attribution of this in terms of 'self-inflicted' illness or 'weakness' and the ideas of 'choice' and 'responsibility'
- Prognosis – the belief that mental disorders have a bleak outlook
- Social interaction – seen as difficult with those with mental illness, perhaps reflecting a discomfort at being able to understand their acts or to be able to identify with them

Given the complexity of our attitudes and the associated stigma, what may be their effects?

- User perceptions and experiences – many people with a mental illness face widespread discrimination across several areas of life. The title of a MIND survey, 'Not just sticks and stones', reflects that this discrimination is not just at the level of perceptions but represents material injustices. Almost half of those interviewed reported being abused or harassed in public and 14% had been physically attacked. One-quarter had been forced to move house because of harassment. One-third had been dismissed from their jobs or forced to resign, and half reported that health professionals had unfairly treated them because of their psychiatric history or current diagnosis.
- Employment – the prospects of employment may be grim for many of those with severe mental illness and this may be a reflection of the severity of their handicaps and the lack of sheltered workplace schemes. However, if they can work on the open market, they face the discriminatory practices from public companies that are reluctant to employ and believe those with a history of mental illness (Manning and White 1995). More enlightened attitudes from employers are required and the Employers Forum on Disability, an employers organization funded and managed

by employers to recruit, retain and develop disabled people may be important in this area (Scott-Parker 1997). Those with mental illness require a range of employment opportunities from supported to open employment. Changes towards increasing service and computer-based work may be an advantage for those with mental illness, provided they are not caught among the marginalized in the growing Network Society and discounted (Castals 1996). Legal redress may be available to those with mental illness in the form of the Disability Discrimination Act, but there may be ambivalence towards regarding service users as disabled by practitioners and user organizations (Scott-Parker 1997). In addition, the UK Governments emphasis on helping the long-term unemployed move from dependence to self-sufficiency may be encouraging.

- Help seeking and engagement – several studies of the public's knowledge of mental illness have highlighted the gap between this and that of mental health professionals. While this may reflect a need for public education campaigns it is also necessary for professionals to develop a better understanding of the publics 'common sense' views of mental illness. The narrowing of such knowledge gaps may assist in promoting insight and willingness to take part in therapy especially for those groups who are difficult to engage (Johnson and Orrell 1995, Sainsbury Centre for Mental Health 1998).

- Resistance to de-institutionalization – the phenomenon of 'Not in my backyard' (NIMBY) has media credibility and may conspire to block the development of local housing schemes for the ex-residents of institutions. Public attitudes on this matter are often contradictory as highlighted by two recent studies (Reda 1995a, 1996, Woolf et al. 1996a). In both studies the majority of people was against the closure of the psychiatric hospitals but nevertheless welcomed the opening of smaller community-based units. Interestingly, many members of the public saw the closure of hospitals as a political cost-saving exercise. The contradictory public opinions are presumably fuelled by a political agenda that is often inconsistent and the paradoxical media portrayal of institutional scandal and community neglect.

- Success of community services – public acceptance of mentally ill people in the community may be central to the success of community services and may depend on their perception of disasters in this area (Ritchie et al. 1994) and on the type of behaviours that can be tolerated (Furnham and Rees 1988). Therapeutic effects of patients' rehabilitation and their social integration may be counteracted by public rejection (Dear and Taylor 1988). Frequent relapses of the mentally ill may lead to sense of failure and public mistrust in the services.

Public education – two studies

Two recent studies have thrown some light on what may be done to assist in liaison with the public at a local level.

Study 1: 'Attitudes towards community mental healthcare for residents in North London' (Reda 1995a)

This study was associated with the TAPS project and examined public opinion in the neighbourhoods of the residencies into which those relocated from Friern and Claybury were placed. The opinions of near neighbours were compared with those of more distant neighbours. The main findings were:

- No differences between the attitudes of the two groups of neighbours

- Most people did not distinguish between mental illness and mental handicap

- Mental illness was associated with violence, physical assault, difficult communication and bizarre behaviour

- Almost half were against the decision to close mental hospitals, but nevertheless often welcomed the opening of community facilities

- Almost all chose treatment in psychiatric hospitals for their relatives but preferred treatment in the community for themselves

- Opinions were divided about whether former psychiatric patients could live in the community with appropriate support

- Two-thirds thought it was important to prepare residents before the opening of mental health facilities and 80% would like to be told of this beforehand

Study 2: 'Public education for Community Care' (Woolf et al. 1996a–d)

This study evaluated a local public education campaign centred on the opening of supported housing in south London for ex-residents of Tooting Bec Hospital. The study compared two areas, one without and one with the campaign. The main findings were:

- The public attitudes expressed were similar to those seen in the Reda (1996a) study.

- Those exposed to the education campaign showed only a small increase in knowledge, but a significant lessening of fearful and rejecting attitudes.

- Those exposed to the education campaign made more social contact with patients and staff of the supported housing.

- The social contact appeared to be directly associated with the improved attitudes rather than directly with the education.

Current campaigns

Changing public attitudes to mental illness and combating stigma are now high on the agenda of the UK government. Several national and international organizations have instituted or are planning campaigns in these areas:

- UK Royal College of Psychiatrists – 'Every family in the land'; launched in 1998 is a 5-year campaign to increase public and professional understanding of mental disorders and related mental health problems, thereby to reduce the stigmatization and discrimination against people suffering from them and to close the gap between the differing beliefs of healthcare professionals and the public about useful mental health interventions.

- UK Department of Health – a number of initiatives are being developed with user and carer organizations to tackle the issue of stigma. In addition, they are working in collaboration with Focus on Mental Health (a consortium of voluntary and statuary mental health organizations), mounting conferences on stigma and social exclusion in ethnic minorities.

- MIND – this UK mental health charity has recently launched a national campaign, RESPECT, aimed at creating a fair deal for people with mental health problems not only in the public eye, but also in working life and as citizens. In addition, MIND is launching a project aimed at schools, 'Bird and a Word', and there is a joint initiative between MIND and the Health Education Authority aimed at children and young people.

- World Health Organization – the WHO is developing a new educational programme on schizophrenia that is targeted not only at the general public, but also at patients and their families, mental health workers and general practitioners.

- World Psychiatric Association – it is planning a worldwide anti-stigma campaign.

What do we need to do?

Negative public attitudes towards those with mental illness reflect a prejudice and discrimination that has common links to other areas of life such as racism and sexism. To alter such practices will take time and will need action at many social and political levels. At the governmental level, there needs to be consistency with all policies that affect mental health services and those with mental health problems both within and between departments. In addition, a notion of citizenship needs to be developed within a framework of constitutional reform that can take us beyond the restrictive concepts of being subjects and consumers. National campaigns are welcome especially those created between agencies and user groups. However, these may need to work closely with the media and challenge their contradictory approach to the mentally ill. The importance of popular culture should not be forgotten, for example the portrayal of mental illness in current television soap operas. The evidence presented above suggests that local educational campaigns can be effective and the lessons learned from these seem to be that the attitudes of specific sections of the population need to be targeted.

The image of mental health services needs to be improved; in terms of the standards of treatments offered, the quality of the staff and their training, and the quality of the buildings associated with the services. This poor public image needs to be deflected away from the alienating and crumbling buildings of the past where there appeared to be no hope of recovery to a more positive service which can attract both public trust and a cadre of high quality recruits who can contribute to the future success of services. These matters are of central importance if public respect for community care is to be gained and the stigma associated with mental illness reduced.

Staff education and training

Health workers in general

Health workers are members of the public and share public attitudes towards those with mental illness. Their attitudes are also amenable to change and this may be borne in mind when considering their training. Health workers at all levels and all disciplines require education regarding those with mental illness that they see. However, given the frequency of contact that primary care services have with those with severe mental illness (Kendrick et al. 1994) they must be considered of particular priority (Bindman et al. 1997).

Mental health workers

A recent review of training for mental health staff (Sainsbury Centre for Mental Health 1997) concluded that improvements in training can be achieved within the framework of the existing professions, but that there is a need to establish both the core competencies of staff and the distinctive competencies required by each profession. These sentiments will probably find favour among many professionals but it remains to define the core and distinctive competencies.

Other matters to consider are:

- Preparation for emptying the asylums – staff need to be well prepared for such moves and require training in the skills to manage the ex-residents in the community settings (Reda 1995b, Ardagh-Walter et al. 1997).

- Avoidance of burnout – working in community settings may be satisfying but may result in professional casualties (Prosser et al. 1996). Adequate resources, staff support and supervision, and appropriate acquiring of skills are important factors.

- Equipping professional with the ability to deliver treatments for which there is evidence of effectiveness – the diffusion of innovations may be slow but there is now growing evidence for effective treatments for those with severe mental illness. Psychosocial interventions for those with schizophrenia are an example of this and it is recognized that too few professional are equipped with the skills necessary to deliver such effective interventions (Gournay 1995).

- Multidisciplinary and multi-agency working – the importance of multidisciplinary teams is well recognized as is the importance of the working together of the large number of agencies who have a role to play in helping those with mental illness (Hancock et al. 1997). With the move towards a range of locally based services, staff now have to be prepared to work in multi-professional teams, in a variety of settings, across agencies and with a variety of purchasing and service delivery models. There may be a mismatch between current training arrangements and future service needs, and barriers to multidisciplinary and multi-agency training exist within the configurations of current professional boundaries (Sainsbury Centre for Mental Health 1997).

- Development of the skills of non-professional workers who work with the mentally ill – the development of the tier of healthcare support workers and their equivalent in social services and housing agencies has been an important addition to users with whom they may form a different but important therapeutic relationship. These personnel may be particularly important in the care of those who are difficult to engage with services (Sainsbury Centre for Mental Health 1997, 1998).

SUMMARY

Research

Statistical predictions in the early 1960s suggested the emptying of the UK asylums by the 1970s. Early descriptive research on asylum populations pointed to clear barriers to the emptying of the large institutions. Follow-up of patients discharged from these psychiatric hospitals reveals poor outcomes, but more desirable outcomes can be achieved through well-organized provision of residential care. Good-quality studies in this area can be undertaken with minimal resources and can be carried out as part of routine audit and monitoring. The value of research should be at least to reduce harm, at best to provide a rational basis for the provision of mental health services that can contribute to a broader social world.

Education

The public's view of mental illness is complex and contradictory and, while it may have changed over time, remains generally negative and rejecting. Such attitudes and stigma affect those with mental illness in many ways including: users' perspectives and experiences, employment, help seeking and engagement, resistance to de-institutionalization and the success of community services. Local public education, which can be tackled at a series of levels, can be effective in lessening fearful and rejecting attitudes and increase social contact with patients. Health staff in areas other than mental health share public attitudes towards mental illness. Efforts must be made to provide them with appropriate education and training.

Mental health professionals must be trained to deliver treatments for which there is evidence for effectiveness. Multidisciplinary training is appropriate to modern practice and should include the development of skills for non-professionals who work with those with mental illness.

References

Angermeyer MC, Matschinger H. Social distance towards the mentally ill: results of representative surveys in the Federal Republic of Germany. Psychological Medicine 1997; 27: 131–141.

Ardagh-Walter N, Naik P, Tombs D. Staff attitudes to a psychiatric hospital closure. Psychiatric Bulletin 1997; 21: 139–141.

Baker R, Hall J. REHAB: a new assessment instrument for chronic psychiatric patients. Schizophrenia Bulletin 1988; 14: 97–111.

Bentz WK, Edgerton JW. The consequences of labelling a person as mentally ill. Social Psychiatry 1971; 6: 29–33.

Beer D, Cope S, Smith J, Smith R. The crisis team as part of comprehensive local services. Psychiatric Bulletin 1995; 19: 616–619.

Bewley T, Bland JM, Ilo M et al. Census of mental hospital patients and life expectancy of those unlikely to be discharged. British Medical Journal 1957; 4: 671–675.

Bewley T, Bland M, Mewchen D, Walch E. 'New Chronic' patients. British Medical Journal 1981; 283: 1161–1164.

Bindman J, Johnson S, Wright S et al. Integration between primary and secondary services in the care of the severely mentally ill: patients and practitioners' views. British Journal of Psychiatry 1997: 171; 169–174.

BMJ. Government lacks data on mental hospital closures. British Medical Journal 1993; 306: 475–476.

Boardman AP. Lyme Brook Mental Health Centre Annual Report for 1996. University of Keele, Academic Unit of Social and Community Psychiatry, Keele, 1997.

Boardman AP, Bouras N. The Mental Health Advice Centre in Lewisham. Health Trends 1998; 20: 59–63.

Brockington IF, Hall P, Levings J, Murphy C. The Community's tolerance of the mentally ill. British Journal of Psychiatry 1993; 162: 93–99.

Brown GW, Carstairs GM, Topping G. Post-hospital adjustment of chronic mental patients. Lancet 1958; ii: 685–689.

Carson J, Shaw L, Wills W. Which patients first: a study from the closure of a large mental hospital. Health Trends 1989; 21: 117–120.

Castells M. The Information Age: Economy, Society and Culture, vol. I: The Rise of the Network Society. Oxford: Blackwell, 1996.

Chong S, Abbott P. Which patients first?: a study from the closure of a large psychiatric hospital. Health Trends 1990; 22: cov. iii.

Christie Brown JRW, Ebringer L, Freedman LS. A Survey of a long-stay psychiatric population: implications for community services. Psychological Medicine 1977; 7: 113–126.

Clifford P. FACE Profile. London: Research Unit, Royal College of Psychiatrists, 1993.

Clifford P, Charman A, Webb Y, Best S. Planning for community care long-stay populations of hospitals scheduled for rundown or closure. British Journal of Psychiatry 1991; 158: 190–196.

Cochrane AL. Effectiveness and Efficiency: Random Reflections On Health Services. London: Nuffield Provincial Hospitals Trust, 1972.

Cooper AB, Early DF. Evolution in the mental hospital. British Medical Journal 1961; 1: 1600–2603.

Craig TJ, Goodman AB, Seegal C et al. The dynamics of hospitalization in a defined population during deinstitutionalization. American Journal of Psychiatry 1984; 141: 782–785.

Cumming E, Cumming J. Closed Ranks: An Experiment in Mental Health Education. Cambridge, MA: Harvard University Press, MA, 1957.

Curson DA, Patel M, Liddle PF, Barnes TRE. Psychiatric morbidity of a long stay hospital population with chronic schizophrenia and implications for future community care. British Medical Journal 1988; 297: 819–822.

D'Arcy C, Brockman J. Changing public recognition of psychiatric symptoms? Journal of Health and Social Behaviour 1976; 17: 302–310.

Dear M, Taylor S. Not On Our Street: Community Attitudes to Mental Health Care. London: Pion, 1988.

Early DF, Magnus RV. Population trends in a mental hospital. British Journal of Psychiatry 1966; 112: 595–597.

Early DF, Nicholas M. 'Dissolution of the Mental Hospital': fifteen years on. British Journal of Psychiatry 1977; 130: 117–122.

Early DF, Nicholas M. Two decades of change: Glenside Hospital population surveys 1960–80. British Medical Journal 1981; 282: 1446–1449.

Eason RJ, Grimes JA. In-patient care of the mentally ill: a statistical study of future provision. Health Trends 1976; 8: 13–19.

Ford M, Goddard C, Lansdall-Welfare R. The Dismantling of the Mental Hospital? British Journal of Psychiatry 1987; 152: 479–485.

Fottrell E, Peermohamed F, Kothari R. Identification and definition of a long-stay mental hospital population. British Medical Journal 1975; 4: 675–677.

Freeman C, Tyrer P (eds). Research Methods in Psychiatry, 2nd edn. London: Gaskell, 1992.

Furnham A, Rees. Lay theories of schizophrenia. International Journal of Social Psychiatry 1988; 34: 212–221.

Glover G, Knight S, Melzer D, Pearce L. The development of a new minimum data set for specialist mental healthcare. Health Trends 1997; 29: 48–51.

Gore CP, Jones K. Survey of a long-stay mental hospital population. Lancet 1961; ii: 544–546.

Gournay K. Mental Health Nurses working purposefully with people with severe and enduring mental illness – an international perspective. International Journal of Nursing Studies 1995; 32: 341–351.

Green DE, McCormick IA, Walkey FH, Taylor AJW. Community attitudes to mental illness in New Zealand twenty-two years on. Social Science and Medicine 1987; 24: 417–422.

Groves T. Closing mental hospitals. British Medical Journal 1993; 306: 471–472.

Hafner H, Klug J. The impact of an expanding community mental health service on patterns of bed usage: evaluation of a four year pattern of implementation. Psychological Medicine 1982; 12: 177–190.

Hancock M, Villeneau L, Hill R. Together We Stand – Effective Partnerships. London: Sainsbury Centre for Mental Health, 1997.

Hayward P, Bright JA. Stigma and Mental Illness: a critique and review. Journal of Mental Health 1997; 6: 345–354.

Johnson S, Orrell M. Insight and psychoses: a social perspective. Psychological Medicine 1995; 25: 515–520.

Johnstone EC, Owens DGC, Gold A, Crow TJ, Macmillan JF. Schizophrenic patients discharged from hospital – a follow-up study. British Journal of Psychiatry 1984; 145: 586–590.

Jones E, Alexander J, Howarth P. Out of hospital: after-care for people with schizophrenia. Health Trends 1997; 28: 128–131.

Jones SH, Thornicroft G, Coffey M, Dunn G. A brief mental health outcome scale: reliability and validity of the Global Assessment of Functioning (GAF). British Journal of Psychiatry 1995; 166: 654–659.

Kastrup M. Prediction and profile of the long-stay population. Acta Psychiatrica Scandinavica 1987; 76: 71–79.

Kendrick T, Burns T, Freeling P, Sibbald B. Provision of care to general practice patients with disabling long-term mental illness: a survey in 16 practice. British Journal of General Practice 1994; 44: 301–305.

Kirk SA. The impact of labelling on rejection of the mentally ill: an experimental study. Journal of Health and Social Behaviour 1974; 15: 108–117.

Krawiecka M, Goldberg D, Vaughan M. A standardized psychiatric assessment scale for rating chronic patients. Acta Psychiatrica Scandinavica 1977; 59: 70–79.

Leff J. The TAPS Project: evaluating community placement of long-stay psychiatric patients. British Journal of Psychiatry 1993; 162 (suppl. 19).

Leff, J (ed.). Care in the Community Illusion or Reality? Chichester: Wiley, 1997.

Lelliott P, Audini B, Knapp M, Chisholm D. The Mental Health Residential Care Study: Classification of facilities and description of residents. British Journal of Psychiatry 1996; 169: 139–147.

Lelliott P, Wing J, Clifford P. A national audit of new long-stay psychiatric patients I: Method and description of the cohort. British Journal of Psychiatry 1994; 165: 160–169.

Lelliott P, Wing J. A national audit of new long-stay psychiatric patients II: Impact on services. British Journal of Psychiatry 1994; 165: 160–169.

Lemkau PO, Crocetti GM. An urban populations opinion and knowledge about mental illness. American Journal of Psychiatry 1962; 118: 692–700.

Levene LS, Donaldson LJ, Brandon S. How likely is it that a District Health Authority can close its large mental hospitals? British Journal of Psychiatry 1985; 147: 150–155.

MacLean U. Community attitudes to mental illness in Edinburgh. British Journal of Preventive and Social Medicine 1969; 23: 45–52.

Magnus RV. 'The New Chronics'. British Journal of Psychiatry 1967; 113: 555–556.

Mann SA, Cree W. 'New' long-stay psychiatric patients: a national sample survey of fifteen mental hospitals in England and Wales 1972/73. Psychological Medicine 1976; 6: 603–606.

Manning C, White PD. Attitudes of employers to the mentally ill. Psychiatric Bulletin 1995; 19: 541–543.

McDowell I, Newell C. Measuring Health: A Guide to Rating Scales and Questionnaires. Oxford: Oxford University Press, 1987.

McPherson IG, Cocks FJ. Attitudes towards mental illness: influence of data collection procedures. Social Psychiatry 1983; 18: 57–60.

Melzer D, Hale AS, Malik SJ, Hogman GA, Wood S. Community care for patients with schizophrenia one year after hospital discharge. British Medical Journal 1991; 303: 1023–1026.

Meyer JK. Attitudes towards mental illness in a Maryland community. Public Health Reports 1964; 79: 769–772.

Nunally JC. Popular Conceptions of Mental Health: Their Development and Change. New York: Holt, Rinehart, Winston, 1961.

O'Brien J. Closing the asylum: where do all the former long-stay patients go? Health Trends 1992; 24: 88–90.

O'Driscoll C, Wills W, Leff J, Margolis M. The TAPS project 10: the long-stay populations of Friern and Claybury hospitals. British Journal of Psychiatry 1993; 162 (suppl. 19): 30–35.

Oliver JPJ, Huxley S, Priebe WK. Measuring the quality of life of severely mentally ill people using the Lancashire Quality of Life Profile. Social Psychiatry and Psychiatric Epidemiology 1997; 32: 76–83.

Olmstead DW, Durham K. Stability of mental health attitudes: a semantic differential study. Journal of Health and Social Behaviour 1976; 17: 35–41.

Oppenheim AN. Questionnaire Design, Intervening and Attitude Measurement, 2nd edn. London: Pinter, 1992.

Overall JE, Gorman DR. The brief Psychiatric Rating Scale. Psychological Reports 1962; 10: 799–812.

Parry G, Watts FN (eds). Behavioural and Mental Health Research: A Handbook of Skills and Methods. London: Lawrence Erlbaum Associates, 1989.

Platt S, Weymann A, Hirsch S et al. The Social Behaviours Assessment Schedule (SBAS). Rationale, contents, scoring and reliability of a new interview schedule. Social Psychiatry 1980; 15: 43–55.

Prosser D, Johnson S, Kiupers E et al. Mental Health 'Burn-out' and job satisfaction among hospital and community-based mental health staff. British Journal of Psychiatry 1996; 169: 334–337.

Proulx F, Lesage AD, Grunberg F. One hundred In-patient suicides. British Journal of Psychiatry 1997; 171: 247–250.

Pryce IG, Griffiths RD, Gentry RM et al. The nature and severity of disabilities in long-stay psychiatric in-patients in South Glamorgan. British Journal of Psychiatry 1991; 158: 817–821.

Reda S. Attitudes towards community mental healthcare of residents in North London. Psychiatric Bulletin 1995a; 19: 731–733.

Reda S. Staff perception of their roles during the transition of psychiatric are into the community. Journal of Psychiatric and Mental Health Nursing 1995b; 2: 13–22.

Reda S. Public opinions about preparation required before closing psychiatric hospitals. Journal of Mental Health 1996; 5: 407–420.

Ring S, Schein L. Attitudes towards mental illness and the use of caretakers in the black community. American Journal of Orthopsychiatry 1970; 40: 710–716.

Ritchie JH, Dick D, Lingham R. The Report of the Inquiry into the Care and Treatment of Christopher Clunis. London: HMSO, 1994.

Rud J, Noreik K. Who became long-stay patients in a psychiatric hospital. Acta Psychiatrica Scandinavica 1982; 65: 1–14.

Ruggeri M, Dall'Agnola R, Agostini C, Bisoffi G. Acceptability, sensitivity and content validity of the VECS and VSSS in measuring expectations and satisfaction in psychiatric patients and their relatives. Social Psychiatry and Psychiatric Epidemiology 1994; 29: 265–276.

Sainsbury Centre for Mental Health. Pulling Together: The Future Order and Training of Mental Health Staff. London: Sainsbury Centre for Mental Health, 1997.

Sainsbury Centre for Mental Health. Keys to Engagement. London: Sainsbury Centre for Mental Health, 1998.

Sayce E, Craig TKJ, Boardman AP. Community Mental Health Centres in the United Kingdom. Social Psychiatry and Psychiatric Epidemiology 1991; 26: 14–20.

Schene AH, van Wijngaarden B. Involvement Evaluation Questionnaire (IEQ). Amsterdam: University of Amsterdam, 1993.

Scott-Parker S. Mental Health Policy and Employment. Mental Health Review 1997; 2: 26–28.

Sellick K, Goodyear J. Community attitudes towards mental illness: the influence of contact and demographic variables. Australia and New Zealand Journal of Psychiatry 1985; 19: 293–298.

Slade M, Phelan M, Thornicroft G, Parkman S. The Camberwell Assessment of Need (CAN): comparison of assessments by staff and patients of the needs of the severely mentally ill. Social Psychiatry and Psychiatric Epidemiology 1996; 31: 109–113.

Smith R. Audit in Action. London: BMJ Publ., 1992.

Smyth C, Mohan A, Buckley C, Clarke A. Where to? A survey of the residual population of a district mental hospital and their predicted placement needs. Irish Journal of Psychological Medicine 1997; 14: 105–108.

Spitzer RL, Williams JBW, Gibbon M. Instruction Manual for the Structured Clinical Interview for DSM-III-R (SCID). New York: Biometrics Research Department, New York State Psychiatric Institute, 1985.

Taube CA, Thompson JW, Rosenstein MJ et al. The 'chronic' mental hospital patient. Hospital and Community Psychiatry 1983; 34: 611–615.

Tooth GC, Brooke EM. Trends in the mental hospital population and their effect on future planning. Lancet 1961; i: 710–713.

Tyrer P, Creed F (eds). Community Psychiatry in Action: Analysis and Prospects. Cambridge: Cambridge University Press, 1995.

Wing JK. How many psychiatric beds? Psychological Medicine 1971; 1: 188–190.

Wing JK, Bahor T, Brugha T et al. SCAN: Schedules for Clinical Assessment in Neuropsychiatry. Archives of General Psychiatry 1989; 47: 589–593.

Wing JK, Beevor AS, Curtis RH et al. Health of the Nation Outcome Scales (HoNOS). British Journal of Psychiatry 1998; 172: 11–18.

Wing JK, Cooper JE, Sartorius N. The Description and Classification of Psychiatric Symptoms: An Instruction Manual for the PSE and CATEGO System. Cambridge: Cambridge University Press, 1974.

Wolff G, Pathare S, Craig T, Leff J. Who's in the lion's den? Psychiatric Bulletin 1996a; 20: 68–71.

Wolff G, Pathare S, Craig T, Leff J. Community attitudes to mental illness. British Journal of Psychiatry 1996b; 168: 183–190.

Wolff G, Pathare S, Craig T, Leff J. Community knowledge of mental illness and reaction to mentally ill people. British Journal of Psychiatry 1996c; 168: 191–198.

Wolff G, Pathare S, Craig T, Leff J. Public education for community care. British Journal of Psychiatry 1996d; 168: 441–447.

Wykes T, Sturt E. The measurement of social behaviour in psychiatric patients: an assessment of the reliability and validity of the SBS schedule. British Journal of Psychiatry 1986; 148: 1–11.

INDEX

A

ABC model, schizophrenia therapy, 307–10, 316
accident and emergency departments, suicide
    risk detection, 330
accommodation
    housing, 218–20
    specialist provision, 219–20
    supported, 25
    women, 203
acetylcholine *see* anticholinesterases
activities of daily living, schizophrenia, 26
acute stress disorder, 72–73
acute *vs* chronic mental illness, community
    mental health teams, 215
admission rates, 187
    anorexia nervosa, 87
    district level prediction, 193
adolescence, anorexia nervosa outcome, 89
adoption studies, schizophrenia, 13
advocacy
    old age mental care, 247
    see also MIND
affect
    flattening, 17
    inappropriate, 17
affective disorders, 33–52
    with anorexia nervosa, 95
    with body dysmorphic disorder, 112
    prevalence, 185 (Table)
    with somatoform pain disorder, 116
    see also named affective disorders
affiliation (interpersonal theory), 159–60
African-Caribbeans, schizophrenia, 11–12, 195
age groups
    depression, 39
    risk of violence, 265
agitation, depression and dementia, 146
agnosia, 139
agoraphobia, 57, 61, 62–63
akathisia, 22
alcohol
    antisocial personality disorder, 169
    anxiety disorders, 74, 75
    elderly people, 137–38
    social phobia, 63
    suicide, 323
algorithms, schizophrenia drug treatment, 23
alienation
    community care and, 211
    malignant, 330–31
All Saints Hospital, Birmingham, family
    interventions for schizophrenia, 300

α2-adrenergic agonists, post-traumatic stress
    disorder, 71
alprazolam, panic disorders, 60
Alzheimer's disease, 140–43
    anticholinesterases, 145, 248
    vs depression, 140
    schizophrenia, 137
amitriptyline, elderly people, 130
amyloid precursor protein, gene, 142
Andrews, J.D.W, feedback loops and personality,
    167
anger
    family interventions for schizophrenia, 299
    personality disorders, 159
anorexia nervosa, 85–97, 101
anticholinesterases, 145, 248
anticonvulsant drugs
    for mania, 46
    pregnancy and post-natal period, 358
antidepressants, 44
    anxiety disorders, 74, 75, 77
        generalized anxiety disorder, 74, 75
    bulimia nervosa, 100
    dementia, 146
    dysthymia, 46
    elderly people, 129–31
    long-term, 47–48
    perinatal, 356–57
    puerperal depression prevention, 353
    suicide, 326
    see also named types
antipsychotic drugs, 20
    early intervention strategies, 306
    generalized anxiety disorder, 74–75
    Lewy body dementia, 144
    mania, 45, 132
    paraphrenia, 136
    pregnancy, 357
    on schizophrenic prodromes, 303
    unplanned pregnancies, 344
    see also 'atypical' antipsychotics
antisocial personality disorder, 162
    DSM-IV, 158
    outcome, 170–71
anxiety
    co-morbidity with depression, 39–41
    with conversion disorder, 111
    elderly people, 134
    prevalence, 185 (Table)
anxiety disorders, 53–84
    with anorexia nervosa, 95
    elderly people, 134
    hypochondriasis, 113

anxiety disorders (continued)
    mixed anxiety and depressive disorder, 37
'anxiety management', 78
aphasia, 139
apolipoprotein E, 142
appointees, Social Security benefit collection,
    147
apraxia, 139
Aricept (donepezil hydrochloride), 145
Asians
    needs assessment and, 195
    women, suicide, 186
assaults, on mental patients, 203
assertive community treatment services, 209
assortative mating, 351
asylums see mental hospitals
attachment behaviour, mother–child, 348
'atypical' antipsychotics, 21, 24
    community care, 209
    first-episode schizophrenia, 20
    maximum security care, 263
    old age, 137
audit
    mental hospitals, 367–80
    public education, 383
    somatoform disorders, 289
Audit Commission
    on community care, 202
    'Finding a Place', 2–3
auditory hallucinations see voices
Australia, sedative drugs and suicide, 325–26
Autoneed, 182
avoidant attachment, 348
avoidant personality disorder, 158
    vs social phobia, 64
Axis I and Axis II personality disorders, 168–69

B

bail hostels, 274
barbiturates, 135
    suicide, 325
behaviour therapy see cognitive behaviour
    therapy
behaviours, vs traits, 158
beliefs
    in ABC model, 307–8
    anorexia nervosa vs schizophrenia, 87
    delusions as, 312–14
    on psychotherapy of psychosis, 311, 312
benevolence, voices, 310
benzodiazepines
    acute stress disorder, 72
    anxiety disorders, 55 (Table)
        generalized anxiety disorder, 73–74, 75
    elderly people, 135
    obsessive-compulsive disorder and, 68

panic disorders, 59–60, 77
post-traumatic stress disorder, 70
pregnancy and puerperium, 358
schizophrenia, 20
social phobia, 65
bereavement, mania, 43
β-adrenergic blockers
    generalized anxiety disorder, 74
    panic disorders, 60
    social phobia, 65
Bethlem Royal Hospital, Gresham Ward, 247
biofeedback, constipation, 291
biological depressive symptoms, 35
biopsychosocial model, personality disorders,
    165–68
bipolar affective disorder, 37–38
    aetiology, 43
    fertility, 343
    parents, 350, 351 (Table)
    post-natal relapse in fathers, 345
    prevalence, 39
    as severe mental illness, 7
    treatment, 45–46, 47–48
Birmingham, All Saints Hospital, family
    interventions for schizophrenia, 300
birth weight, anorexia nervosa, 94
Black Caribbeans, schizophrenia, 11–12, 195
Blackburn, R., on personality disorder and
    criminality, 163–64
Bleuler, E., 11
blood flow see cerebral blood flow
body dysmorphic disorder, 112–13
    ICD-10, 109
body mass index, anorexia nervosa, 89
borderline personality disorders
    depression, 168–69
    outcome, 170
    self-injury, 328
brain
    Alzheimer's disease, 142–43
    anorexia nervosa, 96
    paraphrenia, 136
    personality disorders, 166
    schizophrenia, 15
    see also cerebral blood flow
breast milk
    psychotropic drugs, 356, 357
    vs schizophrenia, 14
brief depression see recurrent brief depression
Briquet's syndrome see somatization disorder
British Medical Association, GMSC on care
    programme approach, 3–4
bromocriptine, on mania, 43
'Building Bridges' (Department of Health), 4–5,
    234–35
bulimia nervosa, 85, 86, 97–101
burden of disease, 5

conversion disorder, 111–12
schizophrenia on families, 294, 296
buspirone
anxiety disorders, 54, 55 (Table)
generalized, 74, 75
post-traumatic stress disorder, 71
Butler Committee (Report), 258, 259 (Table),
273

C

Camberwell Assessment of Need, 179–80
Camberwell Dementia Case Register, 248
Camberwell Family Interview, 297
Canada, forensic psychiatry, 257
car exhaust fumes, suicide, 324–25
carbamazepine
mania, 46, 133
post-traumatic stress disorder, 71
pregnancy and post-natal period, 358
carbon monoxide poisoning, suicide, 324
Cardinal Needs Schedule, 181–82
care management (DoH), 207, 240
NHS and Community Care Act 1990, 233
care plans, individual, 234
Care Programme Approach, 207, 222, 233–36
BMA GMSC on, 3–4
key workers, 240
carers
dementia, 146
stress criterion (Cardinal Needs Schedule), 181
Caribbeans, schizophrenia, 11–12, 195
Carr-Hill et al., resource requirement prediction,
193
Carson, D., risk management systems, 271
case loads see work loads
case management, community care, 206–7,
222–23
casualty departments, suicide risk detection, 330
catalytic converters, suicide prevention, 325
categorical definitions, 157–59
centralization, health care prioritization, 2–3
cerebral blood flow
phobias, 135
schizophrenia, 15
Certificates of Incapacity, 147
Challenge Funds, 208
change agents, 214
Chichester, old age suicide rates fall, 328
child abuse, 348–49
personality disorders from, 167
risk factors, 358–59
childbirth, women, suicide, 327–28
childhood of patients
conduct disorder, criminality and violence,
171, 265

personality disorders, 166–67
children
depression, 39
education on mental illness, 384
feeding, eating disorders in mothers, 95, 98–99
of mentally ill parents, 345, 347–51, 352
treatment of parents and, 355–56
Chiswick, D., future forensic psychiatry services,
276
cholinergic neurotransmission, dementia, 145
chronic fatigue syndrome see neurasthenia
citalopram, panic disorders, 59
class see socio-economic class
classification
anxiety disorders, 56
personality disorders, 157–59
cleft, oral, benzodiazepines, 358
clinic rooms, somatoform disorders, 289
clinical psychologists, schizophrenia and, 26
clomipramine
obsessive-compulsive disorder, 68
panic disorders, 58–59
clonazepam, panic disorders, 77
clonidine, post-traumatic stress disorder, 71
clozapine, 15, 24, 263
Clunis Inquiry, 4, 203
Clusters, personality disorders (DSM-IV),
157–58
coal gas, suicide, 324
cognitive behaviour therapy
anxiety disorders, 54–56, 77–78, 79
generalized anxiety disorder, 75
body dysmorphic disorder, 113
bulimia nervosa, 99, 100–101
elderly people, 135
hypochondriasis, 114
inpatient care, 221
post-natal depression, 356
psychoses, 307–15, 316
resource requirements, 287–88
cognitive impairment
depression, 129
parental depression, 348, 351, 352
commissioning vs purchasing, forensic psychiatry
services, 261
communal living, 220
community care, 201–6
elderly people, 252–54
Lambeth, audit, 376
public education studies, 383
suicide and, 328–29
community care plans, 232–33
community management, schizophrenia, 25–27
Community Mental Health Centres, 376–77
community mental health teams, 26, 211–18
panic disorder, 79–80
work loads, 202

community psychiatric nurses
  case load distribution, 202
  court diversion schemes, 275
  prioritization and, 3
co-morbidity
  anorexia nervosa, 95, 96
  anxiety disorders, 53
  generalized anxiety disorder, 73
  anxiety with depression, 39–41
  body dysmorphic disorder, 112
  bulimia nervosa, 99
  conversion disorder, 111
  in elderly people, 251
  forensic psychiatry services, 262
  hypochondriasis, 113
  obsessive-compulsive disorder, 66–67
  panic disorder, 57
  personality disorders and other Axis I
    disorders, 168–69
  post-traumatic stress disorder, 71–72
  social phobia, 63
complementary medicine, unipolar depression,
  45
complementary reactions (interpersonal theory),
  160–61
compliance
  antidepressants, anxiety disorders, 77
  schizophrenia treatment, 21, 27
  see also non-cooperation
compulsions, 67
computer programs
  MINI, 193–94
  self-treatment of anxiety disorders, 78
conditional discharge
  Mental Health Act Restriction Orders, 272
  repeat offences, 273
conduct disorder (childhood), criminality and
    violence, 171, 265
Confidential Inquiry into Homicides and
    Suicides by Mentally Ill People, 332–33
  fatal child abuse, 349
confidentiality, risk assessment and, 268
confusional states see delirium
constipation, biofeedback, 291
consultant physicians, somatoform disorders,
  286
consulting rooms, somatoform disorders, 289
containment, somatoform disorder patients,
  283–84
contextual factors, risk assessment, 265–66
continuing care, old age mental care, 251–52
contraceptive requirements, schizophrenia, 344
conversion disorder, 111–12
  ICD-10, 109
cooperation criterion (Cardinal Needs
    Schedule), 181
coordination problems, community mental

health teams, 214–15
coping strategies, relatives of schizophrenics,
  294–95
Coping Strategy Enhancement, 314–15
coroners, anorexia nervosa, 92
cortisol, depression, 42
cost-effectiveness
  definition of needs, 177
  family interventions for schizophrenia, 299
  treatment of somatoform disorders, 289–91
costs
  anorexia nervosa inpatient care, 87
  depression, 34
  drug treatment of Alzheimer's disease, 248
  elderly people, 244
  schizophrenia, 11
counselling, interpersonal, anxiety disorders,
  78–79
court diversion schemes, 203, 273–75
Court of Protection, 147
CPA see Care Programme Approach
crime, mental patients as victims, 203
criminality
  age, 170–71
  personality disorders, 162–65
criminology, risk management, 271–72
crisis management, anxiety disorders, 78–79
criticism, by relatives of schizophrenics, 294
cumulative risk, suicide, 332
cyproheptadine, post-traumatic stress disorder,
  71

D

Damasio, A.R., somatic marker hypothesis, 166
dangerousness
  perception, 381
  vs risk, 264
day care, 218
  elderly people, 253
day centres
  provision rates, 187
  statutory, 218
  waiting lists, 220
death see mortality
Defeat Depression Campaign, 323–24
definitions
  of needs, 177–78
  personality disorder, 155, 156–57
  severe mental illness, 1–9
de-institutionalization, 136, 201, 252, 367–71
delirium, 133–34
  mania-like features, 132
delusions, 16, 17
  ABC model, 308–9
  body dysmorphic disorder and, 112
  dementia, 139

mania, 132
paraphrenia, 135
psychotherapy, 312–14, 316
violence, 266
and voices, 310, 315
demand, definition, 178
dementia, 138–46
care deficits, 246, 247–48
depression, 129, 139, 140, 146
frontal lobe type, 144
mania, 132
schizophrenia, 137
denial, family interventions for schizophrenia, 299
dental problems, bulimia nervosa, 99
Department of Health
'Building Bridges', 4–5, 234–35
guidelines on risk assessment, 267–69
Prevention of suicide, 334
public education, 384
'Spectrum of Care', 2, 238
suicide prevention targets, 321–22, 330
see also Health of the Nation; National Health
Service
dependence, interpersonal, 40
depression, 33–48
with anorexia nervosa, 95
borderline personality disorders, 168–69
with conversion disorder, 111
Defeat Depression Campaign, 323–24
dementia, 129, 139, 140, 146
elderly people, 127–31, 246, 248–49
general practitioner training, 329
parenting impairment, 347
in parents, 344–45, 348, 352
personality of relatives, 166
post-natal, 327, 345
prevalence, 38–39, 185 (Table)
somatoform disorders and, 286
see also named types
deprivation-weighted population approach,
needs assessment, 190–96
diagnosis
panic disorder, 58
personality disorders, 159–61
schizophrenia, 17–19
somatoform disorders, 283
see also misdiagnosis
Diagnostic and Statistical Manual of Mental
Disorders *see DSM-III; DSM-IV*
'dimensional' approach
affective disorders, 40
personality, 157, 166
Diogenes syndrome, 138
disability, discrimination, 382
Disability Adjusted Life Years, 5
disasters in care

homicides and risk assessment, 269
long-term care for elderly, 252
discharged patients
from mental hospitals, 370–71, 374, 375–76
schizophrenia, 202, 375–76
DISH (dispersed intensively supported housing),
219–20
disorganization, schizophrenia, 17
dispersed intensively supported housing, 219–20
dispositional factors, risk assessment, 264–65
District General Hospitals
acute inpatient units, 250–51
targets for bed numbers, 188
district level, needs assessment, 193
diversion schemes *see* court diversion schemes
divorce, suicide and, 328
docosahexanoic acid, 14
doctors, attitudes to depression, 38
domestic gas, suicide, 324
domiciliary visits, elderly people, 253
dominance (interpersonal theory), 159–60
domuses, 252
donepezil hydrochloride, 145
dopamine hypothesis, 15
dopaminergic neurotransmission
depression, 42
mania, 43
parkinsonian side-effects of antipsychotics,
21–22, 132
dothiepin, breast-feeding, 357
double depression, 46
Down's syndrome, Alzheimer's disease, 141–42
Driver and Vehicle Licensing Authority, 148
driving, dementia, 148
drug abuse *see* substance abuse
drug resistance, schizophrenia, 24
DSM-III, somatization disorder, 115
DSM-IV
affective disorders, 35
anxiety disorders, 56
dysthymia, 36
obsessive-compulsive disorder, 67
paraphrenia, 136
personality disorders, 157–59
schizophrenia, 17–18
somatoform disorders, 109–10
dual diagnoses, community mental health teams,
216
duration
anorexia nervosa, 86
antidepressant treatment, 47–48, 131
for definition of severe mental illness, 7
family interventions for schizophrenia, 299
illness in parents, 355
treatment of generalized anxiety disorder, 75
dysdiadochokinesis, anorexia nervosa, 96
dyskinesia, tardive, 24

dysmorphophobia, 67
dysphoria, schizophrenia relapse prodrome, 301–3, 304
dysthymia, 36, 46
   elderly people, 135

E

early intervention strategies, schizophrenia, 301–17
Early Sign Questionnaire, Herz, M.I., 302, 303
Early Signs Scale, 306
eating disorders, 85–108
Ebstein's anomaly, lithium, 357
economics
   anorexia nervosa, 87
   anxiety disorders, 79
   definition of needs, 177
   elderly people, 244
   somatoform disorders, errors, 286
economies of scale, 224
education, 380–86
   bulimia nervosa, 100
   psychosocial, on schizophrenia, 26–27
   of public opinion, 380–85, 386
   of staff, 385
elation, 37
elderly people *see* old age
electroconvulsive therapy
   depression, 131
   schizophrenia, 21
Emery Report, 258
emission controls (car exhaust), suicide prevention, 325
emotional environment, schizophrenia, 14–15
empathy, engagement in psychotherapy, 311
empathy disorders, anorexia nervosa, 95–96
Employers Forum on Disability, 381–82
employment
   of mentally ill people, 381–82
   see also unemployment
Enduring Power of Attorney, 147–48
engagement
   cognitive therapy, psychoses, 310–12
   family interventions for schizophrenia, 299
   public education and, 382
England and Wales, forensic psychiatry, 257–82
enquiries *see* inquiries
environmental factors, schizophrenia, 13–15
Epidemiologic Catchment Area survey
   neurotic disorders in elderly people, 134–35
   obsessive-compulsive disorder, 66
   somatization disorder, 115
   violence risk, 267
epidemiology
   Alzheimer's disease, 140–41

anxiety disorders, 76
bulimia nervosa, 86, 97–98
delirium, 133
depression, 38–39, 127–28
eating disorders, 86, 97–98
elderly people, 127–28, 134–35
mania, 131
needs assessment, 184–86
panic disorder, 80
ESQ (Early Sign Questionnaire), 302, 303
ethnic groups
   community care, 211
   needs assessment and, 194
   see also Asians; Caribbeans
European Community, old age care, 245–46
evaluation beliefs, in ABC model, 308, 313
'Every Family in the Land' (Royal College of Psychiatrists), 384
Exelon (rivastigmine), 145
exhaust fumes, suicide, 324–25
exposure therapy, 62, 63
   obsessive-compulsive disorder, 69
expressed emotion, relatives of schizophrenics, 294–97
extrapyramidal side-effects, antipsychotics, 21–22, 132
Eysenck, H.J., on personality, 156–57

F

FACE profile, 372
Falloon, I., definition of severe mental illness, 4
families
   discharged patients and, 370
   high-risk, 358–59
family interventions, schizophrenia, 27, 293–300, 315–16
family members, violence to, 265–66
famine, Holland, 95
fathers, post-natal mental illness, 344–45, 346
feedback loops, personality (Andrews), 167
feeding of offspring
   eating disorders in mothers, 95, 98–99
   see also breast milk
fertility, 343–44
   anorexia nervosa, 94
fibromyalgia, 116
'Finding a Place' (Audit Commission), 2–3
first-episode schizophrenia, 20
Five Factor Model, personality, 157, 158 5-HT
   see selective serotonin re-uptake inhibitors; serotonin
flattening of affect, 17
fluoxetine
   breast-feeding, 357
   obsessive-compulsive disorder, 68

panic disorders, 59
post-natal depression, 356
fluvoxamine, panic disorders, 59, 61
flying phobia, 63
Focus on Mental Health, public education, 384
forensic psychiatry services, 257–82
fractures (trauma), anorexia nervosa, 96
free care, *vs* means-tested care, 252
frontal lobe lesions, mania, 132
frontal lobe type dementia, 144
functional illness, old age inpatient units, 250
funding, BMA on, 3–4

G

galanthamine, 145
gas, suicide, 324
gatekeeping, general practitioners, 3, 253
General Medical Services Committee (BMA), on
care programme approach, 3–4
general practitioners, 3, 210
anxiety disorders, 76
community mental health teams, liaison with,
214, 217
depression, training on, 329
old patients, 125–26, 253
psychosis, early recognition, 306
somatoform disorders, 284, 286
suicide and, 329–30
generalized anxiety disorder, 73–76
elderly people, 135
genetics
Alzheimer's disease, 141–42
depression, 42
inheritance of mental illness, 350, 351
personality, 166
schizophrenia, 12–13
geography, service needs, 196–97
geriatrics, and old age mental care, 250–51
Gillberg, C et al., on anorexia nervosa, 89
Gilles de la Tourette's syndrome, obsessive-
compulsive disorder and, 67
Glancy Report, 258, 259 (Table)
Glenside Hospital, studies, 368
Global Burden of Disease study, 5
Goldberg, D., Huxley, P., needs assessment, 186
Goodmayes Hospital, old age mental care, 247
Gore, C.P, Jones, K., Menston Hospital study,
368
Gotland, services on suicide, 329
Government documents
elderly people, 127
see also Department of Health; inquiries
'graduates', 136–37
Great Ormond Street hospital, anorexia nervosa,
89
Grendon prison, 262

Gresham Ward, Bethlem Royal Hospital, 247
Grounds, A.T., future forensic psychiatry
services, 276
group living, 220
Guardianship Orders, 273
Gunn, J., risk management, 269–70
'Guys model', old age mental care, 254
Gwynne Report, prison medical service, 258

H

Hachinski score, vascular dementia, 143
halfway houses, anorexia nervosa, 97
hallucinations, 16, 17
dementia, 139–40
paraphrenia, 135
see also voices
haloperidol
delirium, 134
mania, 132
schizophrenia, 20
Handcock, M., Villaneu, L., joint strategies, local
authorities, 224
hanging, suicide, 324
harassment, of mentally ill people, 381
Hare Psychopathy Checklist, 162–63
head trauma, protection against post-traumatic
stress disorder, 70
Health Advisory Service (NHS), *Suicide
prevention: the challenge confronted*, 334
health care staff
education and training, 385
management of somatoform disorder patients,
288
vs patients, needs assessment, 180
research and, 380
Health of the Nation (Department of Health)
scales, 375–76
on suicide, 321, 322, 330
Health Service Indicators, 182
suicide rates, 185
health service policy
anxiety disorders, 76, 79–80
elderly people, 127
parents, 354–55
Herz, M.I, Early Sign Questionnaire, 302, 303
high intensity care *see* inpatient care
High Security Psychiatric Services
Commissioning Board, 261, 276
historical aspects, forensic psychiatry, 258–62
historical factors, risk assessment, 265
Holland, famine, 95
home environment, schizophrenia, 14–15
Home Office, on remand to prison, 274
homelessness, 204
needs assessment and, 195–96
schizophrenia, 25, 204

homicides
  of children, 349–50
  Zito Trust Report, 236
  see also Confidential Inquiry into Homicides
hospital admission rates *see* admission rates
Hospital Orders, Mental Health Acts, 257
hostels, anorexia nervosa, 97
House, A., inpatient liaison service for
    somatoform disorders, 286
House of Commons, Social Services Committee,
    on inpatient bed requirements, 188
housing, 218–20
  see also accommodation
5-HT *see* selective serotonin re-uptake
    inhibitors; serotonin
'Hybrid Orders', prison and hospital, 263
hypoalert delirium, 134
hypochondriasis, 113–14
hysteria *see* somatization disorder

I

ICD-10
  affective disorders, 35
  anxiety disorders, 56
  obsessive-compulsive disorder, 67
  paraphrenia, 135–36
  personality disorders, 157, 158–59
  schizophrenia, 17, 19 (Table)
  somatoform disorders, 109–10
image beliefs, in ABC model, 307
imipramine
  breast-feeding, 357
  panic disorder, 58–59, 77
Impact Message Inventory (Kiesler), 160
independent services, effect on NHS long-stay
    care, 251
individuals, needs assessment, 178–82, 234
infanticides, 349–50
inference beliefs, in ABC model, 307–8
influenza virus, schizophrenia, 14
informants, personality disorders, 161–62
inner-city districts, needs assessment, 194
innovation problems, Madison, Wisconsin,
    213–14
inpatient care
  anorexia nervosa, 85, 87, 96
  attached to Community Mental Health
    Centre, 377
  bed numbers reduction, 201
  community mental health teams, liaison, 214
  community role, 214, 220–21
  delirium incidence, 133
  depression in elderly people, 128
  eating disorders, 86–87
  elderly people, units for, 250–51
  parents and children, 355

schizophrenia, 19–20
somatoform disorders, 286
suicide and, 41, 326, 330–31
targeting, 3
women, 203
see also admission rates; mental hospitals
inquiries, 240–41 (Table), 261–62
  Clunis Inquiry, 4, 203
  see also Confidential Inquiry into Homicides
    and Suicides by Mentally Ill People
insight, anorexia nervosa, 87
institutionalization, 201
institutions
  old people in, 125, 128
  see also mental hospitals; residential care
integration, services, 210, 221–25, 277
integrative therapies, bulimia nervosa, 101
interim secure units, 260
International Classification of Diseases *see* ICD-
    10
interpersonal counselling, anxiety disorders,
    78–79
interpersonal dependence, 40
interpersonal diagnosis, personality disorders,
    159–61
interviews
  for delusional content of voices, 315
  personality disorders, 161
intramuscular antipsychotics
  first episode, 20
  long-term, 22, 24
intrauterine growth retardation, anorexia
    nervosa, 94–95
intrusive thoughts, 69
investment, treatment of anxiety disorders, 79
ischaemic score, vascular dementia, 143
isolation
  for delirium, 134
  in strip cell, 275

J

Jarman, B. et al., resource requirement
    prediction, 193
Jarman scores, 190
Joint Planning Teams, 233
joint strategies (Handcock and Villaneu), 224
junior physicians, somatoform disorder patients,
    283–84

K

key workers, 210, 234
  care management (DoH), 207, 222, 240
    (Table)
kidneys, anorexia nervosa, 96
Kiesler, D.J., Impact Message Inventory, 160

Kings Fund London Commission Mental Health Report, 231

L

Lambeth, community care, audit, 376
late paraphrenia, 135–36
L-dopa, on mania, 43
'Learning the Lessons' (Zito Trust Report), 236
lectures, bulimia nervosa, 100
Leeds, somatoform disorder case, 290
lethal means, reduction, 324–26
Lewisham, Mental Health Advice Centre, 376
Lewy body dementia, 144
liaison psychiatry services, somatoform disorder patients and, 284–91
life events
    depression, 42–43
    schizophrenia, 14
life expectancy, 126
limbic system, personality disorder, 166
link workers, CMHT and primary health care teams, 217–18
Lipowski, Z.J., inpatient service for somatoform disorders, 286
lithium, 45–46
    elderly people, 132–33
    pregnancy, 357–58
    puerperal psychosis, 353
local authorities
    community mental health care, 222–23
    housing and, 219
    social services departments, care management, 207
Local Authority Profile of Social Services, 187, 188 (Table)
local operational definitions, 5–6
local service provision, 182–84
localities, integration, 224–25
locums, psychogeriatric posts, 249
lofepramine, 130
London Borough of Westminster, Riverside NHS Trust and, 222–23
loneliness, 205
long-stay patients, 367–77
    see also continuing care; new long-stay patients
long-term management
    affective disorder, 47–48
    intramuscular antipsychotics, 22, 24
low-dose antipsychotic treatment, 22
Lyme Brook Mental Health Centre, 376–77, 378 (Table)

M

Macarthur Risk Assessment study, 265
MADD (mixed anxiety and depressive disorder), 37
Madison, Wisconsin, innovation problems, 213–14
magnetic stimulation, depression, 44
maintenance therapy, schizophrenia, 22, 24
malevolence, voices, 310
malignant alienation, suicide and, 330–31
managers, community mental health teams, 215
Manchester
    liaison service for somatoform disorders, 290
    suicide and general practice consultations, 329–30
    University, Confidential Inquiry into Homicides and Suicides by Mentally Ill People, 332–33
mania, 37–38, 43, 45–46
    elderly people, 131–33
manic stupor, 133
manuals, self-treatment
    anxiety disorders, 78
    bulimia nervosa, 100
marital relationships
    on children, 350, 352
    risk of violence, 265
market model, National Health Service reforms, 2
Marks' exposure with response prevention, 69
mating, assortative, 351
means-tested care, vs free care, 252
measuring tools, outcome studies, 377–79
media, the, 384
medico-legal issues, old age psychiatry, 147–48
medium secure units, 259–60, 276
memory, depression vs dementia, 140
Menston Hospital, 368
Mental Health Act
    risk management and, 272–73
    Section 117, 235
Mental Health Act 1959, 258
Mental Health Act 1983, Section 38, 263
Mental Health (Scotland) Act 1984, 257
Mental Health (Patients in the Community) Act 1995, Supervised Discharge Orders, 237–38, 273
Mental Health Act Commission, ward visits, 221
Mental Health Advice Centre, Lewisham, 376
mental health care staff see health care staff
mental health services see specialist mental health services
mental hospitals
    closure, 136, 201, 252, 367–71
    inadequate care of elderly, 246
Mental Illness Needs Index, 192–94
Mental Illness Specific Grants, 208
mianserin, 130
MIND
    'Not Just Sticks and Stones', 381

MIND *(continued)*
  public education, 384
  'Treatment, Care and Security', 261
Minghella, E., Ford, R., on community mental
  health teams, 216
MINI (Mental Illness Needs Index), 192–94
misdiagnosis, conversion disorder, 111
misinterpretations, panic disorders, 61
mixed anxiety and depressive disorder, 37
moclobemide, social phobia, 65
Modernising Mental Health Services (DoH 1998),
  208
monitoring
  for schizophrenia relapse, 306–7
  see also audit
monoamine oxidase inhibitors
  anxiety disorders, 55 (Table)
  obsessive-compulsive disorder, 68
  panic disorders, 59
  post-traumatic stress disorder, 71
  social phobia, 65
mood stabilizers, post-traumatic stress disorder,
  71
Morgan, H.G and Russell, G.F.M., anorexia
  nervosa, 88, 89
mortality
  anorexia nervosa, 92, 94
  bulimia nervosa, 98
  children of mentally ill parents, 349–50
  mania, 132
  personality disorders, 171
mothering
  anorexia nervosa, 95
  bulimia nervosa, 98–99
  see also parenting; parents
motivational enhancement therapy, anorexia
  nervosa, 97
MRC Needs for Care Schedule, 180–81
Mullen, P.E., risk management, 270
multidisciplinary working, 386
  community mental health teams, 211–12
multi-infarct dementia, 141, 143
multi-somatoform disorder, 117
murders *see* homicides

N

nail-biting, 67
narcissistic personality disorder, outcome, 172
National Assistance Act 1948, removal to place of
  safety, 148
National Health Service
  continuing care, 252
  Executive report 1996, 24-hour nursed care,
    238, 239 (Table)
  forensic psychiatry, future policy, 277

Health Advisory Service, *Suicide prevention: the
  challenge confronted*, 334
  and local care integration, 224–25
  reforms, 2–3, 192–93
  see also Department of Health
National Health Service and Community Care
  Act 1990, 232–33
  on housing, 219
National Service Framework, 235, 238–39
national strategies, suicide prevention, 333–34
natural history *see* outcome studies
nature, nurture and, 167
needs assessment, 177–200, 233–34
  NHS and Community Care Act 1990, 233
  somatoform disorders, 287–89
Needs for Care Schedule, MRC, 180–81
needs for services, *vs* needs for care, 181
negative symptoms, 17, 20–21
neglect (child), 348–49
neonatal death, 349
Netherlands, famine, 95
Network Society, 382
neural tube defects, risk of anticonvulsants, 358
neurasthenia, 117–18
  ICD-10, 109
neuroleptics, obsessive-compulsive disorder and,
  68
neurosis
  anxiety disorder as, 54
  elderly people, 134–35
neurosurgery, depression, 44
neurotransmitters
  depression, 42
  mania, 43
  panic disorders, 59
  personality, 166
  schizophrenia, 15
  see also anticholinesterases; parkinsonian side-
    effects
new long-stay patients, 368–69
night consultations, 214
nightmares, post-traumatic stress disorder,
  cyproheptadine, 71
NIMBY ('Not in my backyard'), 382
non-cooperation, family interventions for
  schizophrenia, 299
non-steroidal anti-inflammatory drugs,
  Alzheimer's disease, 142, 146
noradrenergic neurotransmission
  depression, 42
  panic disorders, 59
North-West Regional Health Authority, suicide
  prevention strategy, 334–35
'Not in my backyard' (NIMBY), 382
'Not Just Sticks and Stones' (MIND), 381
nurture, nature and, 167

O

obsessions, 67
  as intrusive thoughts, 69
obsessive-compulsive disorder, 66–69
  with body dysmorphic disorder, 112
  elderly people, 135
obstetric complications, schizophrenia, 14
occupational activities, schizophrenia, 25–26
oestrogens
  Alzheimer's disease, 142, 145–46
  post-natal depression, 358
Office of Population Censuses and Surveys
    (OPCS), 182
old age
  mental health care models, 243–56
  psychiatric illnesses persisting to, 136–37
  severe mental illness, 123–54
  suicide rates, 328
onychophagia, 67
operational definitions, local, 5–6
oral cleft, benzodiazepines, 358
organic illness, old age inpatient units, 250
osteoporosis
  anorexia nervosa, 96
  bulimia nervosa, 99
outcome studies
  anorexia nervosa, 89–92, 93
  bulimia nervosa, 98
  measuring tools, 377–79
  personality disorders, 169–72
  schizophrenia, 304
    family intervention, 297–98
outpatient assessment, elderly people, 253
outpatient care, somatoform disorders, 286
'Oxford' model, cognitive behaviour therapy,
    panic disorders, 60–61, 80

P

pain see somatoform pain disorder
panic attacks, 57
panic control treatment, 60–61
panic disorder, 56
  antidepressants, 77
  elderly people, 135
  health service policy, 79–80
  with hypochondriasis, 113
paracetamol, suicide, 324, 325
paraphrenia, 135–36
parenting, mental illness, 346–47
  see also child abuse; mothering
parents, 343–66
  with anorexia nervosa, 95
  schizophrenics living with, 25
  separation from, 350

with somatization disorder, 115, 348
  suicide and, 327–28
parkinsonian side-effects, antipsychotics, 21–22,
    132
paroxetine
  obsessive-compulsive disorder, 68
  panic disorders, 59, 77
passivity phenomena, 16
pathoplastic effect, 168
patient admission rates see admission rates
PELiCAN, 180
perfectionism, anorexia nervosa, 96
perinatal disorders see post-natal mental illness;
    pregnancy
perinatal mortality, anorexia nervosa, 94
persecutory delusions, 135, 136
person evaluations, 308
personality
  anorexia nervosa, 95–96
  depression and, 40–41
  normal, 156–57
Personality Diagnostic Questionnaire – Revised,
    161
personality disorders, 155–76
  with body dysmorphic disorder, 112
  depression and, 40–41
  forensic psychiatry services, 262–63
  future policy, 276–77
  hypochondriasis, 113
  infanticide, 350
  in parents, 351
  somatization disorder, 115
  somatoform disorders, 109
  statutory supervision on, 272–73
  see also avoidant personality disorder
personality traits, 157
phenelzine
  panic disorders, 59
  social phobia, 65
phenothiazines see antipsychotic drugs
phobias
  elderly people, 135
  specific, 61–66
physicians, consultant, somatoform disorders,
    286
physostigmine, 145
Pick's disease, 144
pilot practices, panic disorder, 80
place of safety, removal to (National Assistance
    Act 1948), 148
point prevalence
  anxiety disorders, 76
  depression, children, 39
  recurrent brief depression, 39
  schizophrenia, 12
policy
  de-institutionalization, 206–8

policy *(continued)*
  United Kingdom developments, 231–42
  see also health service policy
populations
  needs assessment, 182–97
  suicide prevention, 322–26
  see also epidemiology; public opinion
positive symptoms, 16–17, 20–21
positron emission tomography, schizophrenia,
  15, 17
Post, Felix, old age mental care, 247
postgraduate training, somatoform disorders,
  288–89
post-natal mental illness, 344–46
  on children, 352
  personality disorder, 169
  prevention, 353
  suicide, 327
  thyroid function, 358
  treatment, 356–58
post-traumatic stress disorder, 69–72
poverty (financial), 204–5
poverty of thought, 17
Powell, Enoch, on mental hospitals, 367
Powell, R. and Slade, M., on definitions of severe
  mental illness, 6
Power of Attorney, 147–48
predictors, prognosis in personality disorders,
  172
pregnancy
  anorexia nervosa, 94–95
  bulimia nervosa, 98–99
  mental illness, 344
   treatment, 356–58
  suicide rates, 327
  unplanned, antipsychotic drugs, 344
presbyophrenia, 132
pressure of speech, 37
prevalence, 184–85
  affective disorders, 185 (Table)
  anorexia nervosa, 86
  anxiety, 185 (Table)
  bulimia nervosa, 98
  depression, 38–39, 185 (Table)
  mania, 131
  mental disorder, 1
  panic disorder, 80
  schizophrenia, 11–12, 185 (Table)
prevention, 352–53
  parental mental illness and, 352–53
  schizophrenia relapses, 301–17
  suicide, 321–41
Prevention of suicide, Department of Health, 334
primary care, 210
  anxiety disorders, 76
  community mental health teams and, 217
  vs specialist care, prioritization, 2–3

primary prevention, 352
primary sociopaths, 163
prioritization, 1–4
prison medical service, Gwynne Report, 258
prisons
  mental illness, 203
  personality disorders, 262–63
  psychiatry in, 275
  remand to, 274
  transfer of inmates to hospitals, 261, 263
probation hostels, 274
probation services, risk management, 272, 274
'problem families', 300
prodromes, schizophrenia relapse, 301–4
progesterone, 358
prognosis *see* outcome studies
propentofylline, 145
protective factors, suicide, 326–29
  mental health service provision, 331–32
provision, definition, 178
pseudodementia, 129
psychiatrists
  court diversion schemes, 274
  and mental health care targeting, 214
  for old age care, 247, 249
  risk assessment, 263–64
  somatoform disorder services, 284–85
psychodynamic therapy, anxiety disorders, 78–79
psycho-educational treatment, bulimia nervosa,
  100
psychological treatment
  acute stress disorder, 73
  anorexia nervosa, 96–97
  anxiety disorders, 54–56, 77–79
   generalized anxiety disorder, 75–76
  bipolar affective disorder, 46
  depression, 131
   unipolar, 45
  dysthymia, 46
  obsessive-compulsive disorder, 69
  panic disorders, 60–61
  post-traumatic stress disorder, 71–72
  psychotic illness, 293–320
  social phobia, 65–66
  specific phobias, 62–63
psychologists, schizophrenia and, 26
psychomotor poverty, 17
psychopathy, 162–65
  forensic psychiatry services, 262
  social integration *vs* reoffending, 171
psychosexual function
  anorexia nervosa, 94–95
  bulimia nervosa, 98–99
  schizophrenia, 344
'psychosomatic' wards, 112
psychotherapy, community mental health teams
  and, 211–12

psychotic illness
  anorexia nervosa as, 87
  child maltreatment, 349
  post-natal, 327, 344
  psychological treatment, 293–320
  as severe mental illness, 7
  see also schizophrenia
psychotic symptoms, depression, 35
public health issues, 34 (Table)
public opinion
  on depression, 38
  education of, 380–85, 386
public transport, 196
Public Trust Office, 147
puerperal mental illness *see* post-natal mental
  illness; pregnancy
purchasing authorities (NHS), 192–93

Q

quality of life, needs, 204–5
questionnaire data
  anxiety disorders, 76
Personality Diagnostic Questionnaire – Revised,
  161
quiet delirium, 134

R

reactance, psychological, 313
reactions, complementary (interpersonal theory),
  160–61
reality distortion, schizophrenia, 17
rebound psychosis, clozapine, 263
receivers, 147
recurrent brief depression, 36, 46–47
  age groups, 39
recurrent unipolar depression, 35
  duration of treatment, 47
Reda study, 383
Reed Report, 261, 262, 263, 273–74
  A.T. Grounds on, 276
  on terminology, 163
referrals, restricted acceptance, 288
refugees, needs assessment and, 195
regional secure units, 260
  criticisms, 259 (Table)
Regional Specialised Commissioning Groups,
  261
rehousing, paraphrenia, 136
relapses
  post-natal, 344–45
  schizophrenia, 22, 27
    family intervention, 297–98
  prevention, 301–17
remand to prison, 274

reports, risk assessment, 270
research
  mental hospitals, 367–80
  somatoform disorders, 289
residential care
  housing, 218–20
  inadequate homes, 205
  provision rates, 187
  requirements (J.K. Wing), 189
  see also institutions; mental hospitals
'resistant' depression, 47
resource allocation, community mental health
  teams, 215, 216
RESPECT (MIND), public education, 384
Restriction Orders, Mental Health Act, 272
retirement, 125
reversible inhibitors of monoamine oxidase
  (RIMA)
  anxiety disorders, 55 (Table)
  panic disorders, 59
  social phobia, 65
review meetings, 234
revolving door patients, 368
risk assessment
  Department of Health guidelines, 267–69
  forensic psychiatry services, 263–69
  Gunn on, 270
risk factors, suicide, 322–24
  see also protective factors
risk management, 269–73
risk-reducing behaviour
  panic disorders, 61
  social phobia, 65–66
risperidone, 15
rituals
  compulsions, 67
  panic disorders, 61
rivastigmine, 145
Riverside NHS Trust, London Borough of
  Westminster and, 222–23
Royal College of Psychiatrists
  'Every Family in the Land', 384
  inpatient bed requirements, 188
  old age care, 249
  risk assessment, 268
  secure beds requirement, 277

S

safety
  mental health services, 203
  see also security; Supervision Register
Sainsbury Mental Health Initiative, 212–13, 215
St Edwards Hospital, Leek, audit, 372–74
Salford, 188
Saving lives: our healthier nation (DoH), suicide
  prevention targets, 321, 322

scale, economies of, 224
scandals *see* disasters in care
schema maintenance (Young), 168
schizophrenia, 11–31
    anorexia nervosa *vs*, beliefs, 87
    child maltreatment, 349
    discharged patients, 202, 375–76
    early intervention strategies, 301–17
    family interventions, 27, 293–300, 315–16
    fertility, 343–44
    first episode, 20
    forensic psychiatry services, 262, 263
    inheritance, 350–51
    late onset, 136
    loss of social contact, 205
    outcome, *vs* borderline personality disorders,
        170
    parents with, 346–47
    persisting to old age, 136–37
    prevalence, 11–12, 185 (Table)
    public education (WHO), 384
    violence, 266, 267
    see also relapses
schizotypal personality disorder, outcome, 172
SCL-90, 301–2
Scotland, Mental Health Act 1984, 257
screaming, trazodone, 146
'seamless service', forensic psychiatry, 277
season of birth, schizophrenia, 13
seasonal affective disorder, 39, 44
secondary prevention, 352–53
secondary sociopaths, 163
Section 38, Mental Health Act 1983, 263
Section 117, Mental Health Act, 235
sectorization, 196, 197, 210
security
    bed requirements, 277
    risk management, 269–70
    see also safety
Security in NHS Psychiatric Hospitals, Working
        Party on, 258
sedative drugs
    schizophrenia, 20
    suicide, 325–26
selective serotonin re-uptake inhibitors, 44
    anxiety disorders, 54, 55 (Table)
    generalized anxiety disorder, 74, 75
    body dysmorphic disorder, 113
    breast-feeding, 357
    elderly people, 130
    obsessive-compulsive disorder, 68
    panic disorders, 59
    post-traumatic stress disorder, 71
    social phobia, 65
    suicide and, 326
selegiline, 145
self-help groups, anxiety disorders, 78

self-help treatments, bulimia nervosa, 100
self-injury
    postnatal, 327
    in prisons, 275
    recurrent, 158
    risk, 204
self-neglect, 138
self-poisoning, drugs, 324, 325–26
self-reporting, personality disorders, 161
semi-manualized psychological treatment,
        unipolar depression, 45
sequential care model, bulimia nervosa, 100
serotonin
    antagonists, 55 (Table), 60, *see also* buspirone
        generalized anxiety disorder, 74, 75
    depression, 42
    obsessive-compulsive disorder, 68
    panic disorders, 59
sertraline
    breast-feeding, 357
    panic disorders, 59
service provision
    vs deprivation-weighted needs assessment,
        191–92
    local, 182–84
    targets, 188–90
seven ages of man (Shakespeare), 124
severe mental illness, definition, 1–9
severity criterion (Cardinal Needs Schedule),
        181
sexual abuse, personality disorders, 167
sexual function *see* psychosexual function
Shakespeare, W., seven ages of man, 124
Shenley Hospital, discharged patients study, 370
situational phobias, 62–63
Skodol, A.E., on personality disorder, 156
Slater, E., on hysteria, 114
Snowden, P.R., 270
soap operas, 384
social contact, loss, 205
social deprivation, 190–94
social effects, severe mental illness, 5
social factors, 193
    depression, 42–43
    personality disorders, 166–67, 171
social functioning
    anorexia nervosa, 94 (Table), 96
    bulimia nervosa, 99
social phobia, 63–66
    with body dysmorphic disorder, 112
Social Security benefits, appointees, 147
social services
    dementia, 146
    elderly people, 127
    parents, 353–54
Social Services Committee, House of Commons,
        on inpatient bed requirements, 188

socio-economic class
  anorexia nervosa, 96
  parents and children, 350
  risk of violence, 265
  schizophrenia, 14
somatic depressive symptoms, 35
somatic marker hypothesis (Damasio), 166
somatization, 110
  depression, 128
  schizophrenia relapse, 304
somatization disorder, 114–16
  elderly people, 135
  general practice, 284
  parents with, 115, 348
somatoform autonomic dysfunction, ICD-10, 109
somatoform disorders, 109–21
  services for, 283–92
somatoform pain disorder, 116
  cost-effectiveness of treatment, 289–90
Special Health Authorities, 261
Special Hospitals
  Emery Report, 258
  future policy, 276–77
  personality disorders, 262
Special Hospitals Service Authority, 260
Special Hospitals Treatment Resistant
    Schizophrenia Research Group, on
    clozapine, 263
specialism, and community mental health teams,
    212–16
specialist mental health services
  anxiety disorders, 76
  eating disorders, 86–87
  education and training, 385
  parents, 354–55
  on suicide rates, 328–29, 331
  targeting resources, 2–3
specific phobias, 61–66
'Spectrum of Care' (Department of Health), 2,
    238
St Edwards Hospital, Leek, audit, 372–74
standardized mortality rates
  anorexia nervosa, 92, 94
  suicide and pregnancy, 327
statutory supervision, 272–73
stealing, bulimia nervosa, 99
'step-down' units, 221
stigma, 18, 205–6, 236, 381
Strathdee, G., Thornicroft, G., service provision
    targets, 188–89, 194
stress
  acute stress disorder, 72–73
  post-traumatic stress disorder, 69–72
strip cells, 275
stroke
  anxiety, 135

dementia, 143
  mania, 132
substance abuse
  antisocial personality disorder, 169
  forensic psychiatry services, 262
somatoform pain disorder, 116
  violence, 267
suicide, 41
  anorexia nervosa, 94
  antisocial personality disorder, 171
  body dysmorphic disorder, 112
  loneliness, 205
  mortality rates, 34, 41
  narcissistic personality disorder, 172
  needs assessment, 185–86
  personality disorders, 170
  post-natal, 346
  prevention, 321–41
  in prisons, 275
Suicide prevention: the challenge confronted, NHS
    Health Advisory Service, 334
Supervised Discharge Orders, Mental Health
    (Patients in the Community) Act 1995,
    237–38, 273
supervision
  risk management, 270
statutory, 272–73
Supervision Register, 235–36
supported accommodation, 25
surgery
  and body dysmorphic disorder, 112–13
  brain, depression, 44
systems, services as, 210

T

tacrine, 145
TAPS study (Team for the Assessment of
    Psychiatric Services study), 370–71
tardive dyskinesia, 24
targeting resources
  community mental health teams, 213–14
  specialist mental health services, 2–3
targets
  service provision, 188–90
  suicide prevention, 321–22, 330
Team for the Assessment of Psychiatric Services
    study, 370–71
teeth, bulimia nervosa, 99
television, 384
temperament, 166
  of children, 352
ten-point plan (1993), 207–8
tertiary prevention, 353
'third age', 125
Thornicroft, G.
  district level admission rates, 193

Thornicroft, G. *(continued)*
    see also Strathdee, G., Thornicroft, G.
thought broadcasting, 16
thought chaining, 308
thought disorder, 16–17
thought insertion, 16
thought withdrawal, 16
'threat/control override' symptoms, 266–67
thyroid function, post-natal mental illness, 358
tiers, Care Programme Approach, 222, 234–35
time *see* duration
time-scale, and risk management (Carson), 271
tolerance, benzodiazepines, 74
Tourette syndrome, obsessive-compulsive
        disorder and, 67
training, 385
    for family interventions for schizophrenia, 300
    somatoform disorders, 288–89
traits, 157
transcranial magnetic stimulation, 44
trauma (physical)
    anorexia nervosa, 96
    see also child abuse
trauma (psychological)
    acute stress disorder, 72–73
    post-traumatic stress disorder, 69–72
trazodone, 130
    screaming, 146
treatability, personality disorder and criminality,
        164–65
'Treatment, Care and Security' (MIND), 261
trial leave, 273
trichotillomania, 67
tricyclic antidepressants, 44
    anxiety disorders, 55 (Table)
        generalized anxiety disorder, 74, 75
    elderly people, 130
    obsessive-compulsive disorder, 68
    panic disorder, 58–59
    post-traumatic stress disorder, 70
    pregnancy, 357
    social phobia and, 65
    suicide, 326
Tulip Outreach Service, 211 24-hour cover,
        community mental health teams, 214 24-
        hour nursed care, NHS Executive report
        1996, 238, 239 (Table)
twin studies
    bipolar affective disorder, 43
    schizophrenia, 12–13

U

undifferentiated somatoform disorder, 117
unemployment, 204–5
    needs assessment and, 196

schizophrenia, 25–26
    suicide, 323
unidisciplinary working, 211–12
unipolar depression
    burden of disease, 5
    in parents, 348, 350, 351 (Table)
    recurrent, 35, 47
    treatment, 43–45
United Kingdom
    old age care, 243–56
    policy developments, 231–42
    see also National Health Service
urban environment
    bipolar affective disorder, 39
    schizophrenia, 14
USA
    forensic psychiatry, 257
    prisons, mental illness, 203
    see also Epidemiologic Catchment Area survey
utilization, definition, 178

V

vacancy, psychogeriatric posts, 249
valproic acid
    for mania, 46, 133
    pregnancy and post-natal period, 358
vascular dementia, 141, 143
victims of crime, mental patients as, 203
violence
    suicide, 326
    see also risk assessment
violence inhibitory mechanism, 166
vision-based community care, 208–9
vitamin E, 145
voices (auditory hallucinations)
    ABC model, 309–10
    psychotherapy, 314–15, 316
voluntary services *see* independent services

W

Walker, N., on risk management, 271–72
walk-in service, Lewisham MHAC, 376
Waltham Forest, care integration, 222–23
Westminster, Riverside NHS Trust and, 222–23
Wing, J.K., needs assessment, 186–87, 189–90,
        191, 194
Wing, J.K., Morris, B., on de-institutionalization,
        206
winter birth, schizophrenia, 13–14
women
    childbirth, suicide, 327–28
    depression, 38–39
    mental patients, safety problem, 203, 221
    risk of violence, 264–65

Woolf study, 'Public Education for Community
    Care', 383
work
    disability, somatization disorder, 115
    schizophrenia, 25–26
work loads
    community mental health teams, 202
    community psychiatric nurses, 202
    key workers, 222
work schemes, 218
Working Party on Security in NHS Psychiatric
    Hospitals, 258
World Health Organization, public education on
    schizophrenia, 384

worry, 75, 76

Y

Young, J.E., schema maintenance, 168

Z

zimelidine, panic disorders, 59
Zito Trust Report, 236
zuclopenthixol, 20
Zurich criteria, recurrent brief depression, 36